TCRN Study Guide

Trauma Certified Registered Nurse Exam Prep with 650+ Practice Questions and Clinical Scenarios

Nedrial TestPrep

TCRN Study Guide: Trauma Certified Registered Nurse Exam Prep with 650+ Practice Questions and Clinical Scenarios

Disclaimer: This study guide is designed to help you prepare for the Trauma Certified Registered Nurse (TCRN) examination. While we have made every effort to ensure the accuracy and completeness of the information presented, this guide is not affiliated with or endorsed by the Board of Certification for Emergency Nursing (BCEN). The content is based on publicly available information about the TCRN exam and current evidence-based trauma nursing practices. Always refer to the official BCEN resources for the most current exam content outline and requirements.

The information in this book is not intended to replace clinical judgment or serve as medical advice. Always follow your institution's policies and protocols and consult with appropriate healthcare professionals when making clinical decisions.

Published by: Nedrial TestPrep

First Edition: 2025

Printed in the United States of America

TABLE OF CONTENTS

About This Guide

Welcome to your comprehensive TCRN exam preparation resource. If you're reading this, you've already taken an important step toward advancing your career in trauma nursing. The Trauma Certified Registered Nurse certification demonstrates your specialized knowledge and commitment to excellence in trauma care, and this guide is designed to help you achieve that goal.

Why This Guide is Different

Most study guides give you content to memorize. This one teaches you how to think like a trauma nurse. You'll find detailed explanations that go beyond simple facts, helping you understand not just what happens in trauma situations, but why it happens and how to respond effectively. Every concept is explained with real-world context because understanding the "why" behind trauma care makes the "what" easier to remember.

What You'll Find Inside

This guide contains everything you need to prepare for the TCRN exam:

Comprehensive Content Review: Each chapter breaks down complex trauma concepts into understandable sections. You won't find vague overviews here. Instead, you'll get detailed explanations that prepare you for both the exam and real-world practice.

650+ Practice Questions: These aren't just random questions. Each one is carefully designed to mirror the style and difficulty level of actual TCRN exam questions. More importantly, every question comes with a detailed explanation that teaches you the underlying concept.

45+ Clinical Scenarios: Real trauma nursing isn't about isolated facts. It's about applying knowledge to complex patient situations. These scenarios help you practice clinical reasoning and decision-making skills.

Strategic Test-Taking Guidance: Knowing the content is only half the battle. You'll learn proven strategies for approaching multiple-choice questions, managing your time, and maximizing your score.

Flexible Study Plans: Whether you have 30, 60, or 90 days to prepare, you'll find a structured study schedule that fits your timeline.

Who This Guide is For

This guide is designed for registered nurses who are preparing to take the TCRN exam. You might be:

- An emergency department nurse looking to formalize your trauma expertise
- A trauma center nurse seeking career advancement

- A nurse transitioning into trauma care from another specialty
- Someone who took the exam before and wants to improve your score

No matter where you're starting from, this guide meets you there and helps you reach your goal.

Your Path to Success

Preparing for a certification exam can feel overwhelming, but it doesn't have to be. Success comes from consistent, focused effort over time. This guide breaks down the massive amount of information you need to know into manageable pieces. Each study session builds on the previous one, helping you develop both knowledge and confidence.

Remember, you're not just studying to pass an exam. You're investing in your ability to provide excellent trauma care. The knowledge you gain here will serve your patients long after exam day.

Let's get started on this journey together. You've got this.

How to Use This Study Guide

Getting the most out of this guide requires a strategic approach. Here's how to use each component effectively.

Start With Assessment

Before you begin studying, take a few minutes with Chapter 2 to assess your current knowledge. This helps you identify your strong areas and topics that need more attention. Be honest with yourself about what you know and what you need to review. This assessment will help you personalize your study plan.

Choose Your Study Timeline

Look at your calendar and figure out how much time you have before your exam date. Then select the appropriate study schedule:

30-Day Plan: This intensive schedule works if you already have a strong foundation in trauma nursing and need focused review. You'll study 5-6 days per week with longer sessions.

60-Day Plan: This balanced approach gives you time to learn new material while reinforcing what you already know. Most nurses find this timeline manageable alongside work and personal commitments.

90-Day Plan: This comprehensive schedule allows for deeper learning with shorter, more frequent study sessions. It's ideal if you're transitioning into trauma nursing or want to build mastery gradually.

Work Through Content Systematically

Read each chapter thoroughly, not just skimming for highlights. The detailed explanations are where real learning happens. As you read:

- Take notes on concepts that are new to you
- Flag sections you find confusing to review later
- Try to connect new information to your clinical experience
- Think about how you would apply each concept in practice

Practice Actively

After reading each section, complete the practice questions right away. Don't wait until you've finished the entire chapter. This active practice helps cement the information in your memory.

When you answer questions:

1. Try to answer without looking back at the content first
2. If you get it wrong, that's fine. Wrong answers teach you what you need to review
3. Read every explanation, even for questions you answered correctly
4. Keep a log of topics where you consistently miss questions

Use Clinical Scenarios for Integration

The clinical scenarios at the end of each chapter are designed to help you think holistically about trauma care. They require you to pull together information from multiple sections. Work through these carefully, considering:

- What's your initial assessment priority?
- What findings are most critical?
- What interventions come first?
- How would you anticipate this patient's needs?

Build in Regular Review

Learning isn't linear. You'll forget things, and that's normal. The study schedules build in review time, but you should also:

- Review previous chapters before starting new ones
- Go back to questions you missed and try them again
- Use the quick reference charts in the appendices as memory aids
- Test yourself regularly on high-yield facts

Take the Practice Exams Under Realistic Conditions

When you're ready for the full practice exams:

- Set aside 2.5 hours of uninterrupted time
- Remove distractions (phone, TV, other people)
- Use scratch paper for notes, just like the real exam
- Time yourself to practice pacing
- Review your results thoroughly, focusing on patterns in your mistakes

Adjust Your Approach as Needed

Your study plan isn't set in stone. If you're finding certain topics particularly challenging, spend extra time there. If you're excelling in an area, you can move through it more quickly. The goal is mastery, not just completing the schedule.

Stay Consistent

The most important factor in your success is consistency. Studying for 45 minutes every day is far more effective than cramming for 5 hours once a week. Your brain needs time to process and consolidate new information. Regular, spaced practice is the key to long-term retention.

Take Care of Yourself

Finally, remember that your physical and mental wellbeing directly impacts your ability to learn. Get enough sleep, eat well, exercise, and take breaks. Burnout helps no one. You're preparing for an important exam, but your health comes first.

Study Planning Tools

Creating Your Personalized Study Schedule

The following pages contain three different study schedules: 30-day, 60-day, and 90-day plans. Each schedule is designed to help you cover all the material systematically while building in time for practice and review.

How to Choose Your Schedule:

Consider these factors:

Your Current Knowledge Level: If you work in trauma regularly and feel confident in most areas, the 30-day plan might work. If trauma nursing is newer to you, give yourself more time with the 60 or 90-day plan.

Your Available Study Time: Be realistic about how much time you can dedicate to studying each day. The 90-day plan requires less time per day but more days overall. The 30-day plan is more intensive.

Your Work Schedule: Consider your shift patterns and other commitments. It's better to choose a longer timeline and stick with it than to choose an aggressive schedule and fall behind.

Your Learning Style: Some people learn better with intensive, focused study periods. Others prefer spacing out learning over more time. Pick what works for your brain.

Study Session Guidelines

Regardless of which schedule you choose, make your study sessions effective:

Set Specific Goals: Don't just say "study trauma." Say "complete Chapter 3 sections on airway management and shock recognition."

Eliminate Distractions: Find a quiet space, silence your phone, and tell people you're not available during study time.

Use Active Learning: Don't just read passively. Take notes, answer questions, and explain concepts out loud.

Take Strategic Breaks: Use the Pomodoro Technique or similar. Study for 45-50 minutes, then take a 10-minute break.

Mix It Up: Alternate between reading new content, answering practice questions, and reviewing previous material.

Track Your Progress

Use the checkboxes in each study schedule to track your completed sessions. This visual progress can be motivating and helps you see how far you've come.

Keep a study log where you note:

- What you covered each session
- Topics you found challenging
- Questions you want to revisit
- Your practice question scores

When to Adjust Your Schedule

Life happens. If you miss a study session, don't panic. Just get back on track the next day. If you consistently can't keep up with your chosen schedule, it's okay to switch to a longer timeline. The goal is to be prepared for your exam, not to stick rigidly to a schedule that isn't working.

Maximizing Retention

To remember what you study:

Spaced Repetition: Review material multiple times over increasing intervals. The schedules build this in, but you can add extra reviews of challenging topics.

Active Recall: Test yourself frequently rather than just rereading. This is why the practice questions are so important.

Elaboration: Connect new information to things you already know. Think about how concepts relate to patients you've cared for.

Interleaving: Mix up topics rather than studying one thing for hours. This is built into the chapter structure but can be enhanced by reviewing multiple chapters in one session.

Teaching Others: If you can explain a concept to someone else, you truly understand it. Consider studying with a colleague or explaining topics to a non-medical friend.

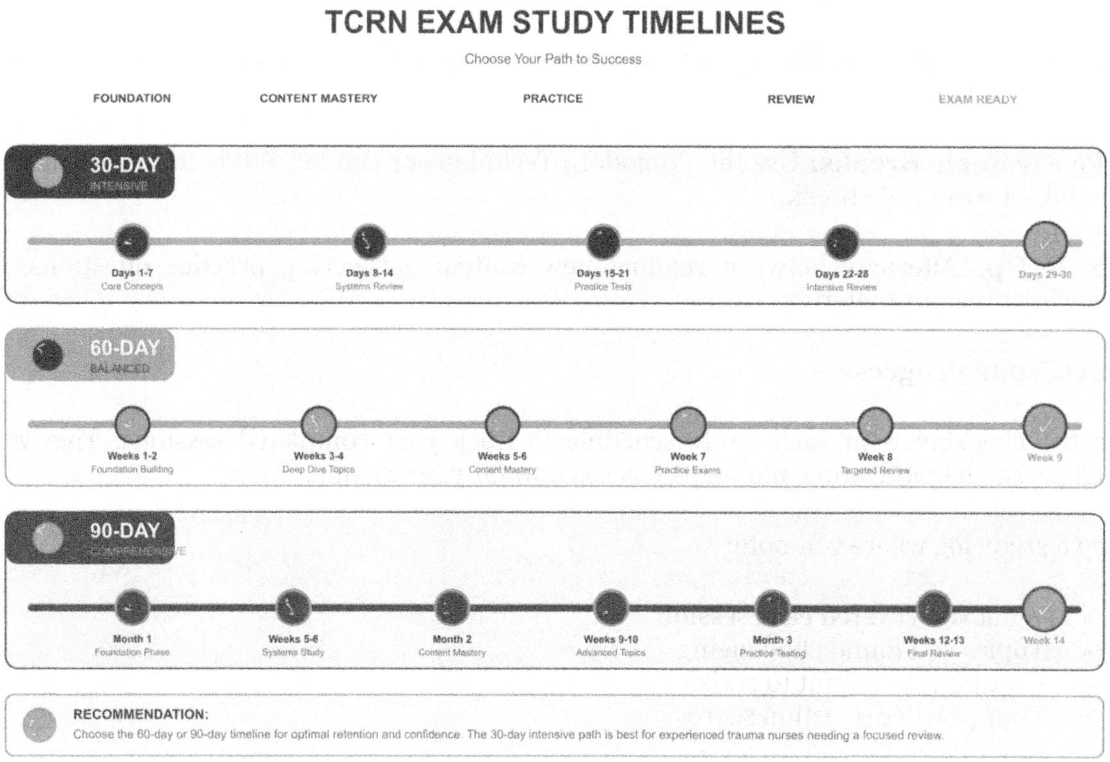

Your 30-Day Study Schedule

Week 1: Foundation and Assessment

Day 1:

- ☐ Read Front Matter and Study Planning Tools
- ☐ Complete Chapter 1: Exam Overview
- ☐ Register for your exam if you haven't already
- ☐ Set up your study space

Day 2:

- ☐ Complete Chapter 2: Creating Your Study Plan
- ☐ Take self-assessment
- ☐ Review Chapter 1 key points
- ☐ Begin Chapter 3: Initial Assessment and Resuscitation

Day 3:

- ☐ Complete Chapter 3 reading
- ☐ Answer Chapter 3 practice questions (45 questions)
- ☐ Review missed questions thoroughly

Day 4:

- ☐ Complete Chapter 3 clinical scenarios
- ☐ Review Chapter 3 weak areas
- ☐ Begin Chapter 4: Thoracic and Neck Trauma

Day 5:

- ☐ Complete Chapter 4 reading
- ☐ Answer Chapter 4 practice questions (40 questions)
- ☐ Review missed questions

Day 6:

- ☐ Complete Chapter 4 clinical scenarios
- ☐ Review Chapters 3-4 key concepts
- ☐ Begin Chapter 5: Abdominal and Genitourinary Trauma

Day 7:

- ☐ Review Week 1 material
- ☐ Redo missed questions from Chapters 3-4
- ☐ Rest and light review

Week 2: Core Body Systems

Day 8:

- ☐ Complete Chapter 5 reading
- ☐ Answer Chapter 5 practice questions (45 questions)
- ☐ Review missed questions

Day 9:

- ☐ Complete Chapter 5 clinical scenarios
- ☐ Begin Chapter 6: Orthopedic and Neurovascular Trauma
- ☐ Complete Chapter 6 reading

Day 10:

- ☐ Answer Chapter 6 practice questions (40 questions)
- ☐ Complete Chapter 6 clinical scenarios
- ☐ Review Chapters 5-6

Day 11:

- ☐ Begin Chapter 7: Neurological Trauma
- ☐ Complete Chapter 7 reading (this is a longer chapter)
- ☐ Review Appendix A: Quick Reference Charts

Day 12:

- ☐ Answer Chapter 7 practice questions (50 questions)
- ☐ Complete Chapter 7 clinical scenarios
- ☐ Review missed questions

Day 13:

- ☐ Begin Chapter 8: Burns and Environmental Trauma
- ☐ Complete Chapter 8 reading
- ☐ Answer Chapter 8 practice questions (35 questions)

Day 14:

- ☐ Complete Chapter 8 clinical scenarios
- ☐ Review Weeks 1-2 material
- ☐ Focus on consistently missed topics

Week 3: Specialized Topics and Practice

Day 15:

- ☐ Begin Chapter 9: Maxillofacial and Ocular Trauma
- ☐ Complete Chapter 9 reading
- ☐ Answer Chapter 9 practice questions (30 questions)
- ☐ Complete Chapter 9 clinical scenarios

Day 16:

- ☐ Begin Chapter 10: Special Populations
- ☐ Complete Chapter 10 reading
- ☐ Answer Chapter 10 practice questions (40 questions)

Day 17:

- ☐ Complete Chapter 10 clinical scenarios
- ☐ Begin Chapter 11: Psychosocial Aspects
- ☐ Complete Chapter 11 reading
- ☐ Answer Chapter 11 practice questions (25 questions)

Day 18:

- ☐ Complete Chapter 11 clinical scenarios
- ☐ Begin Chapter 12: Trauma Systems
- ☐ Complete Chapter 12 reading

Day 19:

- ☐ Answer Chapter 12 practice questions (30 questions)
- ☐ Complete Chapter 12 clinical scenarios
- ☐ Read Chapter 13: Mastering Multiple-Choice Questions

Day 20:

- ☐ Review all weak areas identified so far
- ☐ Create summary notes for high-yield topics
- ☐ Review Appendix B: Medication Quick Reference

Day 21:

- ☐ Take Practice Exam 1 (125 questions, timed)
- ☐ Score your exam

- ☐ Identify patterns in missed questions

Week 4: Final Review and Mastery

Day 22:

- ☐ Review Practice Exam 1 explanations thoroughly
- ☐ Study weak areas identified in Practice Exam 1
- ☐ Review corresponding chapters

Day 23:

- ☐ Comprehensive review of Chapters 3-6
- ☐ Redo missed questions from these chapters
- ☐ Review clinical scenarios

Day 24:

- ☐ Comprehensive review of Chapters 7-9
- ☐ Redo missed questions from these chapters
- ☐ Focus on neurological trauma

Day 25:

- ☐ Comprehensive review of Chapters 10-12
- ☐ Review special populations
- ☐ Study quick reference charts

Day 26:

- ☐ Take Practice Exam 2 (125 questions, timed)
- ☐ Score your exam
- ☐ Compare results with Practice Exam 1

Day 27:

- ☐ Review Practice Exam 2 explanations
- ☐ Focus on remaining weak areas
- ☐ Review test-taking strategies from Chapter 13

Day 28:

- ☐ Read Chapter 14: Final Week Preparation
- ☐ Review high-yield topics
- ☐ Study must-know facts and formulas
- ☐ Light review of all appendices

Day 29:

- ☐ Light review only (no new material)
- ☐ Review your personal summary notes
- ☐ Practice relaxation techniques
- ☐ Prepare materials for exam day

Day 30:

- ☐ REST - Minimal to no studying
- ☐ Review Day-Before Checklist
- ☐ Get everything ready for exam day
- ☐ Go to bed early
- ☐ **Exam Day Tomorrow - You've Got This!**

Your 60-Day Study Schedule

Weeks 1-2: Foundation and Understanding

Day 1:

- ☐ Read Front Matter and Study Planning Tools
- ☐ Complete Chapter 1: Exam Overview
- ☐ Register for exam if not done

Day 2:

- ☐ Complete Chapter 2: Creating Your Study Plan
- ☐ Take self-assessment
- ☐ Set up study routine

Day 3:

- ☐ Begin Chapter 3: Initial Assessment
- ☐ Read Primary and Secondary Survey sections

Day 4:

- ☐ Complete Chapter 3 reading
- ☐ Answer first 25 practice questions

Day 5:

- ☐ Answer remaining Chapter 3 questions (20 questions)
- ☐ Review all missed questions

Day 6:

- ☐ Complete Chapter 3 clinical scenarios
- ☐ Review Chapter 3 key points

Day 7:

- ☐ Rest day with light review of Chapter 3

Day 8:

- ☐ Begin Chapter 4: Thoracic and Neck Trauma
- ☐ Read through pneumothorax and hemothorax

Day 9:

- ☐ Complete Chapter 4 reading
- ☐ Answer Chapter 4 practice questions

Day 10:

- ☐ Complete Chapter 4 clinical scenarios
- ☐ Review Chapters 3-4

Day 11:

- ☐ Begin Chapter 5: Abdominal Trauma
- ☐ Read blunt and penetrating trauma sections

Day 12:

- ☐ Complete Chapter 5 reading
- ☐ Answer first 25 Chapter 5 questions

Day 13:

- ☐ Answer remaining Chapter 5 questions (20 questions)
- ☐ Review missed questions

Day 14:

- ☐ Complete Chapter 5 clinical scenarios
- ☐ Weekly review of Chapters 3-5

Weeks 3-4: Major Body Systems

Day 15:

- ☐ Begin Chapter 6: Orthopedic Trauma
- ☐ Read fractures and dislocations sections

Day 16:

- ☐ Complete Chapter 6 reading
- ☐ Answer Chapter 6 practice questions

Day 17:

- ☐ Complete Chapter 6 clinical scenarios
- ☐ Review compartment syndrome and vascular injuries

Day 18:

- ☐ Begin Chapter 7: Neurological Trauma
- ☐ Read TBI assessment and concussion sections

Day 19:

- ☐ Continue Chapter 7: intracranial hemorrhages
- ☐ Read ICP management section

Day 20:

- ☐ Complete Chapter 7: spinal cord injuries
- ☐ Answer first 25 Chapter 7 questions

Day 21:

- ☐ Rest day - light review of difficult concepts

Day 22:

- ☐ Answer remaining Chapter 7 questions (25 questions)
- ☐ Review all missed questions

Day 23:

- ☐ Complete Chapter 7 clinical scenarios
- ☐ Review neurological assessment tools

Day 24:

- ☐ Begin Chapter 8: Burns and Environmental
- ☐ Read burn classification and assessment

Day 25:

- ☐ Complete Chapter 8 reading
- ☐ Answer Chapter 8 practice questions

Day 26:

- ☐ Complete Chapter 8 clinical scenarios
- ☐ Review Chapters 6-8

Day 27:

- ☐ Comprehensive review Chapters 3-5
- ☐ Redo missed questions

Day 28:

- ☐ Comprehensive review Chapters 6-8
- ☐ Review Appendix A: Quick Reference Charts

Weeks 5-6: Specialized Topics

Day 29:

- ☐ Begin Chapter 9: Maxillofacial and Ocular
- ☐ Complete Chapter 9 reading

Day 30:

- ☐ Answer Chapter 9 practice questions
- ☐ Complete Chapter 9 clinical scenarios

Day 31:

- ☐ Begin Chapter 10: Special Populations
- ☐ Read pediatric trauma section

Day 32:

- ☐ Continue Chapter 10: geriatric trauma
- ☐ Read pregnancy-related trauma

Day 33:

- ☐ Complete Chapter 10 reading
- ☐ Answer first 20 Chapter 10 questions

Day 34:

- ☐ Answer remaining Chapter 10 questions (20 questions)
- ☐ Complete Chapter 10 clinical scenarios

Day 35:

- ☐ Rest day - review special populations

Day 36:

- ☐ Begin Chapter 11: Psychosocial Aspects
- ☐ Complete Chapter 11 reading

Day 37:

- ☐ Answer Chapter 11 practice questions
- ☐ Complete Chapter 11 clinical scenarios

Day 38:

- ☐ Begin Chapter 12: Trauma Systems
- ☐ Complete Chapter 12 reading

Day 39:

- ☐ Answer Chapter 12 practice questions
- ☐ Complete Chapter 12 clinical scenarios

Day 40:

- ☐ Read Chapter 13: Test-Taking Strategies
- ☐ Review all chapters completed so far

Day 41:

- ☐ Review Chapters 9-12
- ☐ Focus on weak areas

Day 42:

- ☐ Comprehensive review week
- ☐ Review Appendix B: Medications

Weeks 7-8: Practice and Refinement

Day 43:

- ☐ Take Practice Exam 1 (timed, 2.5 hours)
- ☐ Score exam

Day 44:

- ☐ Review Practice Exam 1 explanations (first half)
- ☐ Note weak areas

Day 45:

- ☐ Review Practice Exam 1 explanations (second half)
- ☐ Create list of topics to review

Day 46:

- ☐ Review weak areas from Practice Exam 1
- ☐ Revisit corresponding chapters

Day 47:

- ☐ Continue targeted review
- ☐ Redo missed questions from chapters

Day 48:

- ☐ Review Chapters 3-4 thoroughly
- ☐ Focus on initial assessment

Day 49:

- ☐ Rest day - light review only

Day 50:

- ☐ Review Chapters 5-7 thoroughly
- ☐ Focus on neurological trauma

Day 51:

- ☐ Review Chapters 8-10 thoroughly
- ☐ Focus on special populations

Day 52:

- ☐ Review Chapters 11-12
- ☐ Review all clinical scenarios

Day 53:

- ☐ Take Practice Exam 2 (timed, 2.5 hours)
- ☐ Score exam

Day 54:

- ☐ Review Practice Exam 2 explanations thoroughly
- ☐ Compare with Practice Exam 1 results

Day 55:

- ☐ Targeted review of remaining weak areas
- ☐ Focus on persistent problem topics

Day 56:

- ☐ Final comprehensive review
- ☐ Review all appendices

Week 9: Final Preparation

Day 57:

- ☐ Read Chapter 14: Final Week Preparation
- ☐ Review high-yield topics list
- ☐ Study must-know facts

Day 58:

- ☐ Light review of all quick reference charts
- ☐ Review medication quick reference
- ☐ Practice test-taking strategies

Day 59:

- ☐ Very light review - your personal notes only
- ☐ Prepare exam day materials
- ☐ Review Day-Before Checklist

Day 60:

- ☐ REST - Minimal studying
- ☐ Relax and prepare mentally
- ☐ Get everything ready for tomorrow
- ☐ **Exam Day Tomorrow - You're Prepared!**

Chapter 1: Exam Overview and Structure

Understanding what you're preparing for is the first step to success. This chapter gives you a complete picture of the TCRN exam, from registration to test day procedures.

What is the TCRN Certification?

The Trauma Certified Registered Nurse (TCRN) certification is a specialized credential offered by the Board of Certification for Emergency Nursing (BCEN). This certification validates your expertise in caring for trauma patients across all age groups and in various settings.

Why pursue TCRN certification? The certification demonstrates your commitment to professional excellence in trauma nursing. It shows employers, colleagues, and patients that you've met rigorous standards in trauma care knowledge. Many healthcare facilities recognize TCRN certification with salary increases, promotion opportunities, or specialized roles. Beyond professional benefits, the certification process deepens your understanding of trauma care, making you a more confident and effective nurse.

Who can benefit from TCRN certification? While the certification is most commonly pursued by emergency department nurses and trauma center staff, it's valuable for any nurse who cares for trauma patients. This includes:

- Emergency department nurses at all levels of trauma centers
- Flight nurses and critical care transport teams
- ICU nurses in trauma centers
- Operating room nurses who handle trauma cases
- Military nurses
- Nurses working in urgent care or trauma clinics

The knowledge you gain preparing for this exam applies directly to patient care, regardless of your specific work setting.

Exam Format and Scoring

The TCRN exam is a computer-based test consisting of 150 multiple-choice questions. You'll have 2.5 hours (150 minutes) to complete the exam. Out of these 150 questions, 125 are scored questions that count toward your final result. The remaining 25 are pilot questions being tested for future exams. You won't know which questions are pilot questions, so treat every question as if it counts.

Question format: Each question presents a scenario or asks about a specific concept, followed by four answer choices (A, B, C, D). Only one answer is correct. The questions test your ability to apply knowledge to clinical situations rather than simply recall facts.

Content distribution: The exam covers several major content areas:

- Initial assessment and resuscitation (approximately 18% of scored questions)
- Thoracic trauma (approximately 10%)
- Abdominal and genitourinary trauma (approximately 11%)
- Orthopedic trauma (approximately 14%)
- Neurological trauma (approximately 14%)
- Wound management and burns (approximately 8%)
- Maxillofacial, ocular, and ENT trauma (approximately 6%)
- Special populations (pediatric, geriatric, obstetric) (approximately 11%)
- Psychosocial and professional issues (approximately 8%)

These percentages guide the test's construction but can vary slightly from one exam administration to another.

Scoring: The TCRN exam uses a scaled scoring system. Your raw score (the number of questions you answered correctly out of 125 scored questions) is converted to a scaled score ranging from 0 to 150. The passing score is 106 on this scaled system.

You receive your pass/fail results immediately after completing the exam. If you pass, you'll see your scaled score. If you don't pass, you'll receive a diagnostic report showing your performance in each content area, helping you focus your study efforts for a retake.

What this means for your preparation: You need to answer approximately 75-80 questions correctly out of 125 to pass (about 60-64% correct). This might seem manageable, but remember that exam questions are designed to test clinical judgment and application, not just memorization. That's why thorough preparation is essential.

Eligibility Requirements

To take the TCRN exam, you must meet specific eligibility criteria:

Basic requirements:

- Hold a current, unrestricted Registered Nurse (RN) license in the United States or its territories, or internationally equivalent RN licensure
- Have at least two years of experience as a registered nurse (this doesn't have to be specifically in trauma nursing)

No additional requirements: Unlike some certifications, you don't need to complete specific courses, accumulate trauma-specific hours, or work in a particular setting. The two-year RN experience requirement ensures you have a foundation of clinical judgment and nursing practice to build upon.

International candidates: If you're licensed outside the United States, you need equivalent RN licensure recognized by your country's nursing regulatory body. Contact BCEN directly if you have questions about international eligibility.

Why these requirements exist: The two-year experience requirement reflects the reality that trauma nursing requires clinical judgment that develops with nursing experience. While you don't need trauma-specific experience to sit for the exam, you do need the foundational skills that come from practicing as an RN.

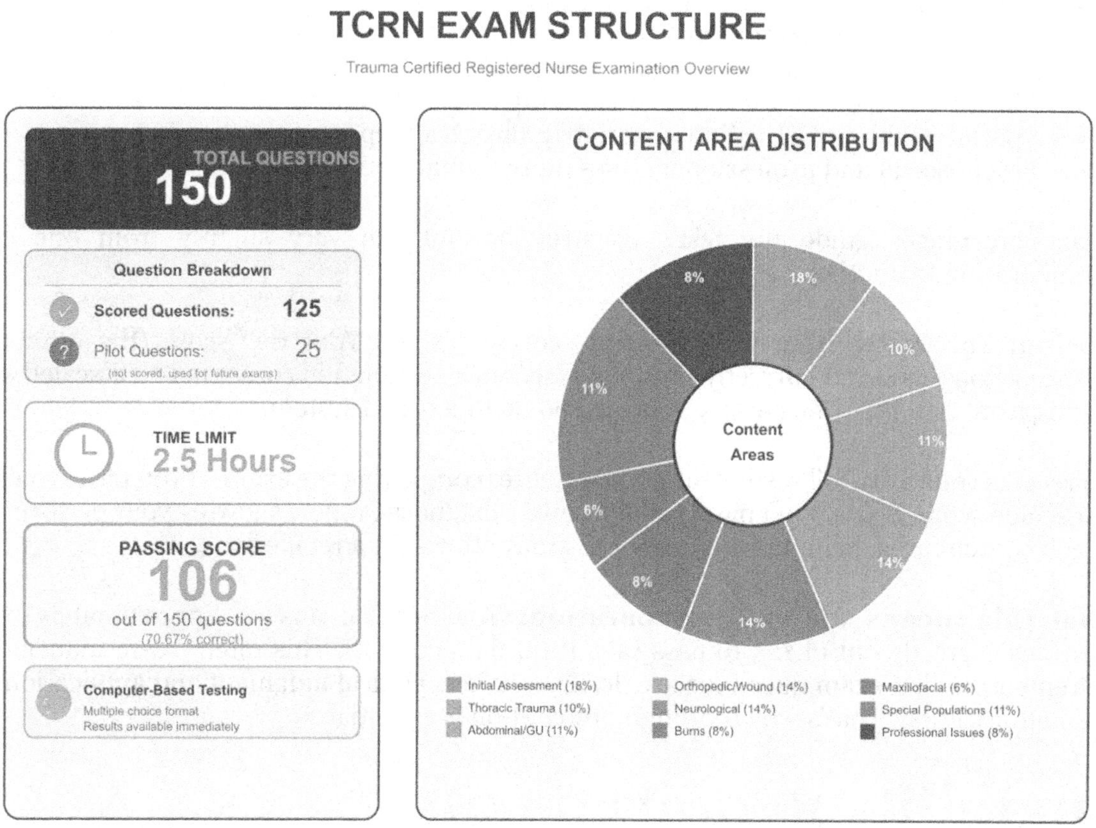

Registration Process

Registering for the TCRN exam involves several steps. Starting early helps you secure your preferred testing date and location.

Step 1: Create a BCEN account

Visit the BCEN website (bcen.org) and create an account if you don't already have one. You'll need to provide your basic contact information and RN license details.

Step 2: Submit your application

Complete the online application form, which asks about your nursing license, education, and experience. You'll need to:

- Verify your current RN licensure
- Attest that you meet the experience requirements
- Pay the exam fee (currently $370 for BCEN members, $470 for non-members)

Step 3: Wait for approval

BCEN processes applications within 2-3 business days. You'll receive an email notification once your application is approved. This email contains your authorization to test (ATT), which is valid for 90 days.

Step 4: Schedule your exam

Once you receive your ATT, you can schedule your exam at any Pearson VUE testing center. Visit the Pearson VUE website, log in using the information from your ATT email, and select your preferred date, time, and location. Testing appointments are available year-round, but popular times fill quickly, so schedule early.

Step 5: Receive confirmation

You'll get a confirmation email with your exam details. Print this confirmation or save it to your phone. You'll need it on test day.

Important timing considerations:

- Schedule your exam at least two weeks in advance to ensure availability
- Choose a test time when you're typically most alert
- Consider scheduling time off work before and after the exam to reduce stress
- Remember your ATT expires 90 days after approval, so don't wait too long to schedule

Cost considerations: The exam fee is non-refundable, but you can reschedule your appointment up to 24 hours before the exam for a rescheduling fee. If you don't pass, you can retake the exam after a 90-day waiting period by paying the full exam fee again.

What to Expect on Test Day

Knowing what to expect on test day helps reduce anxiety and lets you focus on the exam itself.

Arrival and check-in:

Arrive at the testing center at least 30 minutes before your scheduled exam time. This buffer handles any unexpected delays and gives you time to complete check-in procedures without rushing.

What to bring:

- Two forms of identification (one must be government-issued with photo and signature)
- Your test confirmation email (printed or on your phone)

What NOT to bring:

- Study materials, books, or notes
- Cell phones, smartwatches, or any electronic devices
- Bags, purses, or backpacks
- Food or drinks
- Calculators (not needed for the exam)
- Hats or outerwear with pockets

The testing center provides secure lockers for personal belongings. You cannot access these items during the exam or breaks.

Check-in procedures:

The testing center staff will verify your identity, take your photo, and have you review the testing center policies. You'll receive scratch paper and a pen for calculations or notes during the exam. Some centers provide a physical whiteboard and marker instead.

The testing room:

You'll be escorted to a computer station in a quiet room monitored by video cameras. The rooms typically have several testing stations, and other test-takers may be taking different exams. The environment is quiet but not silent. Some centers provide earplugs if needed.

Starting the exam:

Before the actual exam begins, you'll complete a brief tutorial explaining how to navigate the computer interface, mark questions for review, and access the calculator tool. This tutorial time doesn't count against your 150 minutes of exam time. Take your time with the tutorial to ensure you're comfortable with the system.

During the exam:

Once you start the actual exam, your 150 minutes begins. You can:

- Move forward through questions
- Mark questions to review later
- See how much time remains

- Take an optional break (though the clock continues running)
- Use the on-screen calculator if needed

You cannot go back to previous questions once you move forward past a certain point in some testing systems, so read the tutorial instructions carefully.

Breaks:

You can take breaks during the exam, but the clock keeps running. Most test-takers don't take breaks to maximize their available time. If you need to leave the testing room, you must follow the center's procedures, which include additional identity verification when you return.

After the exam:

Once you answer all questions, you'll see a brief survey about your testing experience. After completing the survey, your pass/fail results appear on the screen immediately. You can print this unofficial score report or have it emailed to you. Your official results and certificate (if you passed) arrive via email within 2-3 business days.

If you pass: Congratulations! Your TCRN certification is active for four years. BCEN will send your official certificate and information about maintaining your certification.

If you don't pass: Don't be discouraged. You'll receive a diagnostic report showing your performance in each content area. This report guides your studying for a retake. You must wait 90 days before retaking the exam.

Strategic Approach to Multiple-Choice Questions

Understanding how to approach multiple-choice questions strategically can improve your score even before you study specific content.

Read the question stem carefully:

The question stem is everything before the answer choices. It tells you what the question is really asking. Look for key words that indicate what type of answer is needed:

- "Priority," "first," or "initial" means you need to identify what comes before other actions
- "Most important" or "essential" asks you to prioritize among several correct actions
- "Indicates understanding" means you're looking for a correct statement
- "Requires follow-up" or "needs clarification" means you're looking for an incorrect statement

Identify the question type:

TCRN questions typically fall into several categories:

Knowledge questions test whether you know specific facts. Example: "What is the normal range for intracranial pressure in adults?"

Application questions ask you to apply knowledge to a situation. Example: "A patient presents with a Glasgow Coma Scale score of 6. What intervention is the priority?"

Analysis questions require you to interpret data or situations. Example: "Which finding suggests the patient is developing compartment syndrome?"

Evaluation questions ask you to determine if interventions were effective or if outcomes met expectations. Example: "Which finding indicates that fluid resuscitation has been adequate?"

Answer application questions using the nursing process:

For scenario-based questions, work through the nursing process systematically:

1. **Assessment:** What information do you have? What's missing?
2. **Diagnosis:** What's the likely problem or priority?
3. **Planning:** What outcome are you working toward?
4. **Implementation:** What action addresses the problem?
5. **Evaluation:** How do you know if it worked?

Most priority questions focus on assessment or implementation.

Use the ABCs:

When a question asks about priorities, think about ABCs (Airway, Breathing, Circulation). Interventions addressing airway problems take priority over breathing problems, which take priority over circulation problems. This hierarchy helps you choose between multiple correct answers.

However, remember that life-threatening circulation problems (like massive hemorrhage) might take precedence over non-life-threatening airway issues. Context matters.

Eliminate obviously wrong answers:

Even if you don't know the right answer immediately, you can often eliminate one or two clearly incorrect options. This improves your odds significantly.

Eliminate answers that:

- Contradict basic nursing principles
- Would harm the patient

- Aren't feasible in the described situation
- Use absolute terms like "always" or "never" (unless the answer is about safety or legal requirements)

Look for the "most correct" answer:

Many TCRN questions present multiple correct actions or true statements. Your job is to identify which is MOST correct or MOST important in the given situation. The question isn't asking "could this work?" but rather "what's the best choice here?"

Watch for distractors:

Test writers include plausible but incorrect answers called distractors. Common distractors include:

- Actions that are correct but not the priority
- Interventions appropriate for different conditions
- Steps that come later in the sequence
- Options that sound technical or complex but aren't relevant

Trust your clinical judgment:

If you have trauma nursing experience, trust your instincts about what makes sense in practice. Test questions reflect real-world situations. If an answer seems impractical or unsafe, it's probably not correct.

Manage your time:

With 150 questions and 150 minutes, you have one minute per question. This is generally sufficient, but some questions require more thought than others. If you're stuck on a question:

- Mark it for review
- Make your best guess
- Move on
- Come back if time permits

Never leave questions blank. There's no penalty for guessing, and you have a 25% chance of guessing correctly even if you have no idea.

Practice these strategies:

The practice questions throughout this guide give you opportunities to apply these strategies. As you work through questions, consciously practice:

- Identifying what the question is really asking
- Eliminating wrong answers
- Prioritizing among correct options
- Using the nursing process

- Managing your time

These skills improve with practice. The more questions you answer, the more comfortable you'll become with the question format and style.

Chapter 2: Creating Your Study Plan

Success on the TCRN exam doesn't happen by accident. It requires a thoughtful, organized approach to studying. This chapter helps you create a personalized study plan that fits your schedule, learning style, and knowledge level.

Assessing Your Current Knowledge

Before you start studying, figure out where you stand. This self-assessment helps you allocate study time efficiently, spending more time on weak areas and less on topics you already know well.

Conduct an honest self-inventory:

For each major content area covered on the TCRN exam, rate your current knowledge and confidence:

Initial Assessment and Resuscitation

- Primary and secondary survey
- Airway management
- Shock recognition and treatment
- Hemorrhage control
- Resuscitation principles

Rate yourself: Strong / Moderate / Needs Review / Weak

Thoracic Trauma

- Pneumothorax and hemothorax
- Cardiac tamponade
- Rib fractures and flail chest
- Great vessel injuries

Rate yourself: Strong / Moderate / Needs Review / Weak

Abdominal and Genitourinary Trauma

- Blunt vs. penetrating trauma assessment
- Solid organ injuries
- Hollow viscus injuries
- Pelvic fractures
- Genitourinary trauma

Rate yourself: Strong / Moderate / Needs Review / Weak

Orthopedic and Neurovascular Trauma

- Fracture management
- Dislocations
- Compartment syndrome
- Vascular injuries

Rate yourself: Strong / Moderate / Needs Review / Weak

Neurological Trauma

- Traumatic brain injury assessment
- Intracranial hemorrhages
- ICP management
- Spinal cord injuries

Rate yourself: Strong / Moderate / Needs Review / Weak

Burns and Environmental Trauma

- Burn assessment and classification
- Fluid resuscitation
- Inhalation injuries
- Hypothermia/hyperthermia

Rate yourself: Strong / Moderate / Needs Review / Weak

Maxillofacial and Ocular Trauma

- Facial fractures
- Eye injuries
- Dental trauma

Rate yourself: Strong / Moderate / Needs Review / Weak

Special Populations

- Pediatric trauma
- Geriatric trauma
- Pregnancy-related trauma

Rate yourself: Strong / Moderate / Needs Review / Weak

Professional Issues

- Forensic evidence
- Crisis intervention
- Trauma systems

Rate yourself: Strong / Moderate / Needs Review / Weak

Review your ratings:

Count how many areas you rated as "Needs Review" or "Weak." These are your priority study areas. You'll want to allocate more time to these topics in your study schedule.

Areas you rated as "Strong" still need review, but you can move through this content more quickly. The goal is mastery of all content areas, but efficient use of your study time means focusing where you need it most.

Identify your learning gaps:

Beyond rating whole content areas, think about specific gaps in your knowledge:

- Are there conditions you've never encountered clinically?
- Are there age groups you rarely work with?
- Are there procedures you assist with but don't fully understand?
- Are there theoretical concepts you know you should understand better?

Write these down. They're your specific learning targets.

Consider a baseline practice test:

If you want a more objective assessment, consider taking 20-30 practice questions from various content areas before you begin studying. Don't worry about your score. The goal is to identify patterns in what you know and don't know.

Look for:

- Content areas where you consistently miss questions
- Question types that give you trouble (priority questions, application questions, etc.)
- Whether you're missing questions because you don't know the content or because you're misreading questions

This diagnostic information shapes your study approach.

Setting Realistic Goals

With your self-assessment complete, set specific, achievable goals for your exam preparation.

Your ultimate goal: Pass the TCRN exam on your first attempt.

Supporting goals: Break this down into smaller, measurable goals:

Knowledge goals:

- "Master initial trauma assessment using the primary and secondary survey framework"
- "Understand the pathophysiology and management of all life-threatening thoracic injuries"
- "Accurately assess and manage traumatic brain injuries across severity levels"

Practice goals:

- "Answer all 650+ practice questions in this guide with 75% accuracy or higher"
- "Complete all clinical scenarios, identifying priority actions correctly"
- "Score 80% or higher on both practice exams"

Study process goals:

- "Complete all assigned reading according to my study schedule"
- "Study for at least 45 minutes per day, six days per week"
- "Review missed questions thoroughly, understanding why I got them wrong"

Write down your goals:

Research shows that written goals are more likely to be achieved. Write your goals somewhere visible. Review them weekly to track your progress and maintain motivation.

Make goals specific and time-bound:

Instead of "Study neurological trauma," say "Complete Chapter 7 on neurological trauma and answer all practice questions by [specific date]."

Instead of "Get better at answering questions," say "Improve my practice question accuracy from 65% to 80% over the next four weeks."

Set both outcome and process goals:

Outcome goals focus on results: "Pass the TCRN exam" or "Score 85% on the practice exam."

Process goals focus on actions: "Study for 45 minutes daily" or "Complete two chapters per week."

You have direct control over process goals, and achieving process goals leads to outcome goals. If you're feeling discouraged about outcome goals, refocus on your process goals. Consistent effort pays off.

Building Your Study Routine

Consistency matters more than intensity. Studying for 45 minutes every day is far more effective than studying for six hours once a week.

Choose your study time:

When are you most alert? Some people think best in the morning. Others are night owls. Schedule study time when your brain works best.

When is your schedule most consistent? Pick a time you can protect most days. Early morning before work, lunch breaks, or evenings after dinner are common choices.

How much time can you realistically commit? Be honest. If you can only study 30 minutes per day, that's fine. Plan accordingly and choose a longer timeline to cover all material.

Create a dedicated study space:

Find a quiet location free from distractions. This might be a home office, library, coffee shop, or quiet hospital break room.

Gather your materials so everything you need is in one place: this guide, notebook, pens, highlighters, computer or tablet for online resources.

Eliminate distractions: Turn off your phone or put it in another room. Close social media. Tell family members you're studying and shouldn't be interrupted.

Make the space comfortable but not too comfortable. You want to stay alert. Good lighting, comfortable seating, and proper temperature all matter.

Structure your study sessions:

Effective study sessions follow a pattern:

1. Review (5-10 minutes): Start each session by reviewing what you studied last time. This activates prior knowledge and creates connections.

2. New content (25-35 minutes): Read new material actively. Take notes, highlight key points, and think about how concepts apply to practice.

3. Practice (10-15 minutes): Answer practice questions related to what you just studied. This immediate application reinforces learning.

4. Reflect (5 minutes): End by summarizing what you learned. What are the key takeaways? What questions do you still have?

Use active learning strategies:

Passive reading isn't enough. Research shows that active engagement with material leads to better retention. Here are strategies that work:

Take handwritten notes: Writing by hand engages your brain more than typing. Summarize concepts in your own words rather than copying text verbatim. The act of translating information into your own language deepens understanding.

Teach the material: Explaining concepts out loud forces you to organize your thoughts and identify gaps in your understanding. Pretend you're teaching a new nurse about tension pneumothorax or explaining compartment syndrome to a nursing student. If you can teach it, you know it.

Create visual aids: Draw diagrams of anatomical injuries, create flowcharts for decision-making processes, or make concept maps showing relationships between ideas. Visual learning activates different parts of your brain and creates additional memory pathways.

Use mnemonics and memory tricks: Create acronyms or phrases to remember lists or sequences. For example, "SAMPLE" helps you remember what to ask during patient history: Signs/Symptoms, Allergies, Medications, Past medical history, Last oral intake, Events leading to injury. These memory tools make recall easier under pressure.

Practice spaced repetition: Review material at increasing intervals. Study a concept today, review it tomorrow, again in three days, then in a week. This spacing combats the natural forgetting curve and moves information into long-term memory.

Connect new to old: Link new information to concepts you already understand. If you're learning about flail chest, connect it to your existing knowledge of respiratory mechanics. These connections make new information easier to remember and retrieve.

Managing Test Anxiety

Test anxiety is normal, but it doesn't have to control your performance. Understanding and managing anxiety helps you think clearly on exam day.

Understand the physiology of anxiety:

When you're anxious, your sympathetic nervous system activates. Your heart races, palms sweat, and thinking becomes fuzzy. This "fight or flight" response evolved to help us escape danger, but it's not helpful when you're trying to remember trauma assessment priorities.

The good news is that you can influence this response through specific techniques that activate your parasympathetic nervous system, which promotes calm and clear thinking.

Practice relaxation techniques:

Deep breathing: When you feel anxious, your breathing becomes shallow and rapid. Consciously slowing your breath signals your nervous system to calm down. Try the 4-7-8 technique: inhale for 4 counts, hold for 7 counts, exhale for 8 counts. Repeat four times.

Progressive muscle relaxation: Systematically tense and release muscle groups, starting with your toes and working up to your face. This releases physical tension and focuses your mind on the present moment rather than anxious thoughts.

Visualization: Imagine yourself taking the exam calmly and successfully. Picture yourself reading questions carefully, recognizing concepts you've studied, and selecting correct answers confidently. Mental rehearsal builds confidence and familiarity.

Mindfulness meditation: Even five minutes of daily meditation can reduce baseline anxiety levels. Apps like Headspace or Calm offer guided meditations specifically for test anxiety.

Reframe negative thoughts:

Anxiety often comes from negative self-talk. Common thoughts include "I'm going to fail," "I don't know enough," or "Everyone else is more prepared than me."

Challenge these thoughts with evidence:

- Instead of "I'm going to fail," think "I've prepared systematically and am working to master this material."
- Instead of "I don't know enough," think "I'm identifying my weak areas and strengthening them through practice."

- Instead of "Everyone else is more prepared," think "I don't know what others have done. I'm focusing on my own preparation."

Prepare thoroughly:

The single best anxiety reducer is solid preparation. When you've covered the material systematically, answered hundreds of practice questions, and performed well on practice exams, you have concrete evidence that you're ready. This evidence counteracts anxious thoughts.

Develop test-day strategies:

Arrive early so you're not rushing. Build in extra time for traffic or parking issues.

Establish a pre-exam routine that calms you. This might include listening to specific music, eating a particular breakfast, or doing a short meditation. Familiar routines are comforting.

Use grounding techniques if anxiety hits during the exam. Focus on physical sensations: feel your feet on the floor, notice the temperature of the air, or describe the room to yourself. This anchors you in the present moment rather than anxious future thoughts.

Take micro-breaks during the exam if needed. Close your eyes for 10 seconds, take three deep breaths, and refocus. Even brief pauses can reset your nervous system.

Remember perspective:

This exam is important, but it's not the only thing that defines you as a nurse or as a person. If you don't pass on the first attempt, you can retake it. Many successful TCRN-certified nurses needed multiple attempts. What matters is persistence and commitment to learning, not perfection on the first try.

Last-Minute Preparation Tips

The final days before your exam require a different approach than your earlier study period. These strategies help you maintain your knowledge without burning out.

One week before:

Shift to review mode: Stop learning new content. Focus exclusively on reviewing what you've already studied. This isn't the time to discover new topics or tackle completely unfamiliar material.

Take your final practice exam: If you haven't taken both practice exams yet, complete the remaining one under test conditions. Use the results to guide your final review priorities.

Review your weak areas: Look at questions you've consistently missed throughout your preparation. Review the explanations and the related content sections. These persistent weak spots need attention.

Use the quick reference charts: The appendices contain condensed information about vital signs, scoring systems, and key formulas. Review these daily during your final week. They're high-yield material that's easy to reinforce.

Maintain healthy habits: Continue exercising, eating well, and getting adequate sleep. Your brain functions best when your body is well-cared for.

Two to three days before:

Do light review only: Spend no more than one hour per day studying. Focus on high-yield topics and concepts you find most challenging.

Practice test-taking strategies: Review the strategic approaches from Chapter 1. Remind yourself how to identify priority questions, eliminate wrong answers, and manage time.

Avoid cramming: Cramming creates stress and doesn't improve retention. Trust your preparation. At this point, you either know the material or you don't. Cramming won't change that, but it will increase anxiety.

Prepare your test-day materials: Gather your identification documents, print your confirmation email, and plan your route to the testing center. Eliminating these logistics reduces last-minute stress.

The day before:

Stop studying: Seriously. Close the books. Your brain needs rest to consolidate everything you've learned. One more day of study won't make a difference, but adequate rest will.

Do something enjoyable: Watch a favorite movie, spend time with friends or family, or engage in a hobby. Give your mind a break from trauma nursing.

Get light exercise: A walk, yoga session, or other gentle exercise helps release tension and promotes good sleep.

Eat a good dinner: Choose foods that make you feel satisfied and energized, but avoid anything that might upset your stomach.

Pack for tomorrow: Lay out comfortable clothes for test day. Dress in layers so you can adjust if the testing room is too warm or cold. Put your ID and confirmation in a safe, obvious place.

Set multiple alarms: Don't trust a single alarm clock. Set two or three to ensure you wake up on time.

Go to bed at a reasonable hour: Aim for 7-9 hours of sleep. If you're too anxious to sleep, try the relaxation techniques described earlier. Even resting quietly is better than worrying.

Test day morning:

Eat a balanced breakfast: Choose familiar foods that provide sustained energy. Include protein, complex carbohydrates, and some healthy fat. Avoid excessive caffeine, which can increase anxiety.

Do a brief review of one page: If you must look at study material, limit yourself to one page of key facts or formulas. Then put the materials away.

Use positive self-talk: Remind yourself that you've prepared well and are ready for this challenge.

Arrive early: Give yourself plenty of time to get to the testing center without rushing.

During the exam:

Read each question completely: Don't jump to conclusions based on the first few words.

Answer systematically: Work through questions in order. Don't spend too much time on any single question.

Trust your preparation: If you're torn between answers, your first instinct is often correct unless you have a clear reason to change it.

Stay calm: If you encounter difficult questions, remember that everyone does. Some questions are pilot questions that don't count toward your score. Do your best and move on.

After the exam:

Whether you pass or not, acknowledge that you've worked hard and completed a significant professional challenge. If you pass, celebrate your achievement. If you don't pass, use the diagnostic report to guide your next attempt. Either way, give yourself credit for pursuing professional development and working to improve your practice.

PART II: Core Content Review

Chapter 3: Initial Assessment and Resuscitation

The initial assessment and resuscitation phase is the foundation of trauma care. This is where you identify and address life-threatening conditions before they lead to death or permanent disability. Understanding these principles isn't just important for the TCRN exam—it's essential for saving lives.

This chapter covers the systematic approach to trauma assessment using the primary and secondary survey methodology, along with critical interventions for airway management, shock, hemorrhage control, and resuscitation. Every trauma nurse must master these concepts because they apply to virtually every trauma patient you'll encounter.

Primary and Secondary Survey (ABCDE Approach)

The primary and secondary survey provides a systematic framework for assessing trauma patients. This approach ensures you don't miss critical injuries while managing the chaos that often accompanies trauma situations.

The Primary Survey: Identifying Immediate Threats to Life

The primary survey focuses on identifying and immediately treating conditions that will kill the patient within minutes if not addressed. It follows the ABCDE sequence: Airway, Breathing, Circulation, Disability, and Exposure.

This sequence is prioritized because you can't breathe without an airway, circulation doesn't matter if you're not breathing, and you can't assess neurological function if the patient is dying from airway or circulatory problems. Each step must be addressed before moving to the next.

A - Airway with Cervical Spine Protection

The first question you ask about any trauma patient is: "Is the airway patent?" Without a patent airway, the patient will die within minutes from hypoxia.

Assessment: Look, listen, and feel. Can the patient speak clearly? Speaking requires air movement, so a patient who's talking has at least a partially patent airway, though this can change quickly. Listen for abnormal sounds like stridor (upper airway obstruction), gurgling (blood or secretions), or snoring (tongue obstruction). Look for signs of obstruction like accessory muscle use, retractions, or paradoxical chest movement.

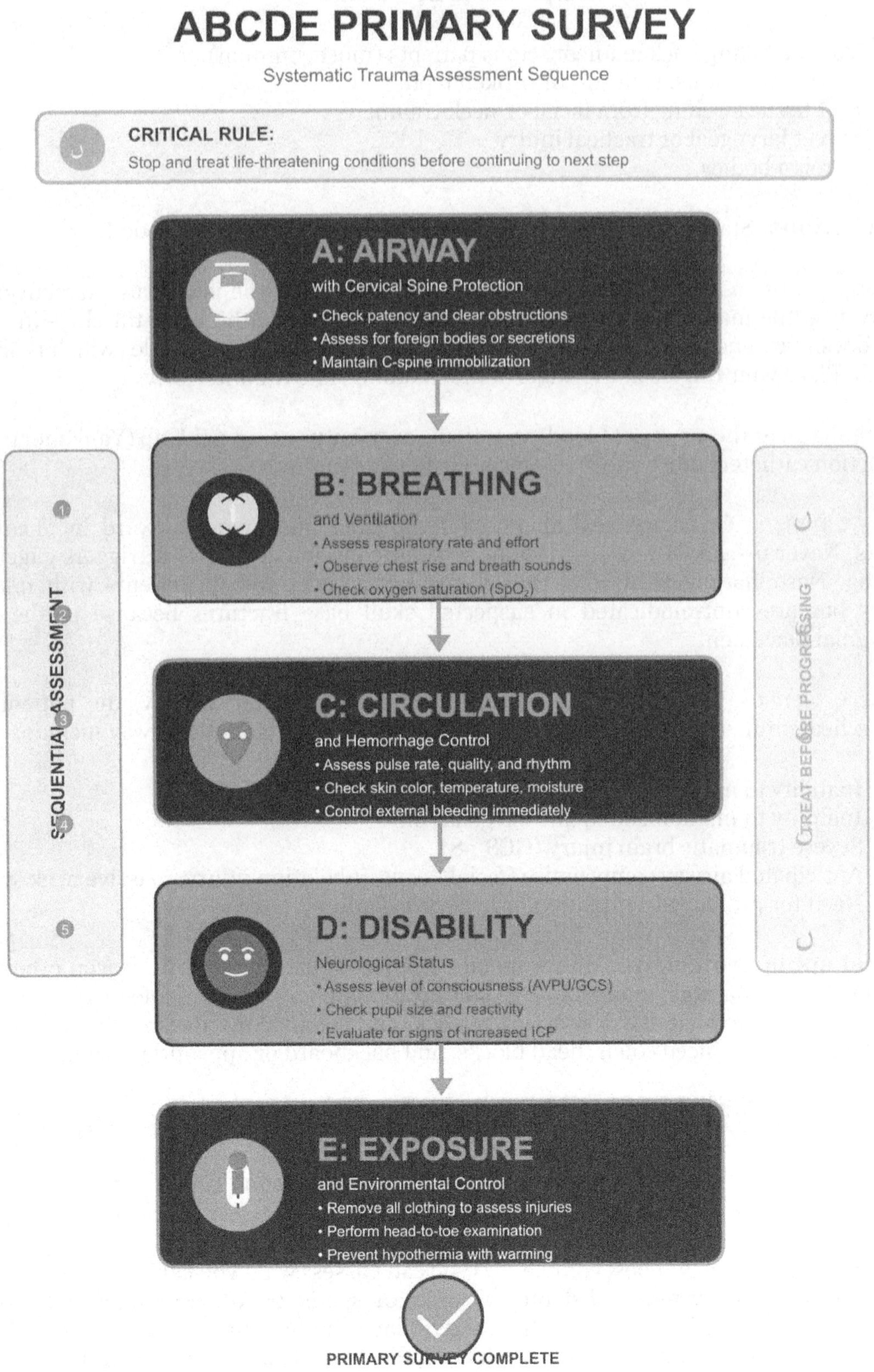
ABCDE PRIMARY SURVEY
Systematic Trauma Assessment Sequence
CRITICAL RULE:
Stop and treat life-threatening conditions before continuing to next step
A: AIRWAY
with Cervical Spine Protection
• Check patency and clear obstructions
• Assess for foreign bodies or secretions
• Maintain C-spine immobilization
B: BREATHING
and Ventilation
• Assess respiratory rate and effort
• Observe chest rise and breath sounds
• Check oxygen saturation (SpO_2)
C: CIRCULATION
and Hemorrhage Control
• Assess pulse rate, quality, and rhythm
• Check skin color, temperature, moisture
• Control external bleeding immediately
D: DISABILITY
Neurological Status
• Assess level of consciousness (AVPU/GCS)
• Check pupil size and reactivity
• Evaluate for signs of increased ICP
E: EXPOSURE
and Environmental Control
• Remove all clothing to assess injuries
• Perform head-to-toe examination
• Prevent hypothermia with warming
SEQUENTIAL ASSESSMENT
1
2
3
4
5
TREAT BEFORE PROGRESSING
PRIMARY SURVEY COMPLETE

Common causes of airway compromise in trauma:

- Tongue falling back in unconscious patients (most common)
- Blood, secretions, vomitus, or broken teeth
- Soft tissue swelling from facial or neck trauma
- Direct laryngeal or tracheal injury
- Foreign bodies

Interventions: Start with the simplest interventions and escalate as needed:

Positioning and basic maneuvers: For unconscious patients, the jaw thrust maneuver opens the airway while maintaining cervical spine alignment. Unlike the head-tilt chin-lift, the jaw thrust doesn't extend the neck, making it safe when spinal injury is possible (which is always in trauma). Place your fingers at the angle of the mandible and lift anteriorly.

Suctioning: Clear the airway of blood, secretions, or vomitus using rigid-tip (Yankauer) suction. Soft suction catheters don't effectively clear particulate matter.

Airway adjuncts: Oropharyngeal airways (OPAs) hold the tongue forward in unconscious patients. Never use an OPA in a conscious or semi-conscious patient—it triggers gagging and vomiting. Nasopharyngeal airways (NPAs) are better tolerated in patients with intact gag reflexes but are contraindicated in suspected skull base fractures because of the risk of intracranial placement.

Definitive airway: If basic maneuvers don't maintain a patent airway, the patient needs endotracheal intubation or a surgical airway. Indications for definitive airway include:

- Inability to maintain airway patency
- Inability to maintain adequate oxygenation
- Severe traumatic brain injury (GCS ≤8)
- Anticipated airway compromise (facial burns, inhalation injury, massive neck swelling)
- Need for prolonged ventilation or hyperventilation

Cervical spine protection: Always assume cervical spine injury until proven otherwise in trauma patients. Maintain manual in-line stabilization during airway maneuvers, then apply a rigid cervical collar once the airway is secured. The collar alone doesn't provide adequate immobilization—you need collar, head blocks, and backboard or appropriate padding.

B - Breathing and Ventilation

Having an open airway doesn't guarantee adequate ventilation. The second step addresses whether the patient is breathing effectively.

Assessment: Expose the chest completely (you can't assess what you can't see). Look for chest rise, assess respiratory rate and depth, observe for symmetry of movement, and note any paradoxical motion. Listen for breath sounds bilaterally, comparing side to side. Feel for subcutaneous emphysema (crepitus), which indicates air escaping from the lungs into surrounding tissue.

Critical breathing problems in trauma:

Tension pneumothorax: This is an immediately life-threatening condition where air accumulates in the pleural space under pressure, collapsing the lung and shifting mediastinal structures. The affected side can't expand, venous return to the heart decreases, and cardiac output drops.

Signs include respiratory distress, absent breath sounds on one side, hyperresonance to percussion, tracheal deviation away from the affected side (late sign), and hemodynamic instability. Don't wait for a chest X-ray if you suspect tension pneumothorax—it's a clinical diagnosis requiring immediate treatment.

Treatment is needle decompression: insert a large-bore (14-gauge) needle or catheter into the second intercostal space at the midclavicular line on the affected side. You should hear a rush of air. This converts the tension pneumothorax to a simple pneumothorax, buying time until you can place a chest tube.

Open pneumothorax (sucking chest wound): A chest wall defect allows air to enter the pleural space with each breath, collapsing the lung. The wound "sucks" air with inspiration.

Signs include an obvious chest wall wound, respiratory distress, and decreased breath sounds on the affected side.

Treatment involves immediately covering the wound with an occlusive dressing taped on three sides, creating a flutter valve effect. Air can escape during exhalation but can't enter during inhalation. Then place a chest tube away from the wound itself.

Flail chest: Multiple rib fractures create a free-floating chest wall segment that moves paradoxically (inward during inspiration, outward during expiration). The paradoxical motion impairs ventilation, and there's usually underlying pulmonary contusion.

Signs include visible paradoxical chest wall movement, severe chest pain, and respiratory distress. The patient splints their breathing to avoid pain, leading to hypoventilation and atelectasis.

Treatment focuses on pain control (to allow deeper breathing), oxygen supplementation, and possibly positive pressure ventilation for severe cases. The rib fractures themselves aren't typically surgically fixed—internal stabilization through positive pressure ventilation provides support while healing occurs.

Massive hemothorax: Blood accumulation in the pleural space (≥1500 mL or one-third of blood volume) can compromise ventilation and circulation simultaneously.

Signs include decreased breath sounds, dullness to percussion (versus hyperresonance in pneumothorax), respiratory distress, and shock.

Treatment requires large-bore chest tube placement for drainage, fluid resuscitation for the blood loss, and possible surgical intervention if bleeding continues (>200 mL/hour for 2-4 hours).

Interventions for inadequate breathing:

- Supplemental oxygen for all trauma patients initially (15L via non-rebreather mask)
- Assisted ventilation with bag-valve-mask if respiratory effort is inadequate
- Chest tube placement for pneumothorax or hemothorax
- Pain management to facilitate breathing (intercostal blocks or systemic analgesics)
- Endotracheal intubation and mechanical ventilation for severe cases

C - Circulation and Hemorrhage Control

The third priority is identifying and controlling bleeding while maintaining adequate perfusion to vital organs.

Assessment: Check level of consciousness (brain perfusion indicator), skin color and temperature (peripheral perfusion indicator), pulse quality and rate (cardiac output indicator), and blood pressure (late indicator—blood pressure stays normal until significant volume loss has occurred).

Understanding shock in trauma:

Shock is inadequate tissue perfusion and oxygenation. In trauma, shock is usually hypovolemic (from blood loss), though other types can occur.

Classes of hemorrhagic shock: The body has compensatory mechanisms that maintain blood pressure initially, making early shock difficult to detect. Classification helps estimate blood loss and guide treatment:

Class I (up to 15% blood loss, <750 mL):

- Minimal symptoms
- Slight anxiety
- Normal vital signs (compensatory mechanisms handle this easily)
- No specific treatment needed beyond observation

Class II (15-30% blood loss, 750-1500 mL):

- Subtle signs: mild tachycardia (100-120 bpm), slight tachypnea
- Narrowed pulse pressure (compensatory vasoconstriction increases diastolic pressure)
- Delayed capillary refill, cool extremities
- Mild anxiety or restlessness
- Treatment: crystalloid fluid resuscitation usually sufficient

Class III (30-40% blood loss, 1500-2000 mL):

- Obvious shock: significant tachycardia (>120 bpm), tachypnea (30-40 breaths/min)
- Hypotension develops (systolic <90 mmHg)
- Altered mental status (confusion, agitation)
- Decreased urine output (<0.5 mL/kg/hr)
- Treatment: aggressive fluid resuscitation and likely blood transfusion

Class IV (>40% blood loss, >2000 mL):

- Life-threatening: severe tachycardia (>140 bpm) or bradycardia (pre-terminal)
- Severe hypotension
- Minimal or absent urine output
- Profound confusion or unresponsiveness
- Treatment: immediate massive transfusion protocol, surgical hemorrhage control

Key concept: In trauma, if a patient is in shock, assume it's from bleeding until proven otherwise. The most common mistake is attributing hypotension to other causes (neurogenic shock, cardiac problems) when the patient is simply bleeding.

Sources of major hemorrhage:

External: Visible bleeding from wounds. Often dramatic but usually controllable with direct pressure.

Chest: Each hemithorax can hold 3000+ mL of blood (more than half the patient's blood volume). Massive hemothorax shows decreased breath sounds and dullness to percussion.

Abdomen: The peritoneal cavity can accommodate massive blood loss without obvious external signs. Patients with blunt abdominal trauma and shock need immediate imaging or surgical exploration.

Pelvis: Pelvic fractures can cause life-threatening bleeding from fractured bone surfaces and torn vessels. Bleeding into the retroperitoneal space can be massive and difficult to control. Unstable pelvic fractures need emergent stabilization (pelvic binder or external fixation).

Long bones: Femur fractures can cause 1000-1500 mL blood loss per fracture into the thigh. Multiple long bone fractures compound this effect.

Hemorrhage control interventions:

Direct pressure: The first and most effective intervention for external bleeding. Apply firm, continuous pressure directly on the wound. Don't keep lifting the dressing to "check" —this disrupts clot formation.

Pressure dressings: Once bleeding slows, apply a pressure dressing to maintain compression while freeing your hands for other interventions.

Tourniquets: For severe extremity hemorrhage not controlled by direct pressure, apply a commercial tourniquet proximal to the wound. Note the time of application. Modern evidence from military medicine shows that properly applied tourniquets are safe for several hours and save lives. Don't hesitate to use one when needed.

Hemostatic agents: Combat Gauze and similar products contain substances that promote clotting. Pack deep wounds firmly with hemostatic dressing, then apply direct pressure.

Pelvic binder: For suspected pelvic fractures, apply a binder around the greater trochanters (not the iliac crests) to compress the pelvis and reduce the pelvic volume, tamponading bleeding.

Surgical control: Some bleeding requires operative intervention—thoracotomy for chest hemorrhage, laparotomy for abdominal bleeding, orthopedic fixation for long bone fractures, or angiography with embolization for pelvic bleeding.

Fluid resuscitation principles:

Traditional teaching emphasized aggressive crystalloid resuscitation for hemorrhagic shock. Current evidence supports a more balanced approach:

Permissive hypotension: For patients with uncontrolled bleeding (especially penetrating trauma), maintaining systolic blood pressure around 80-90 mmHg until hemorrhage is surgically controlled prevents clot disruption from aggressive resuscitation. This doesn't apply to traumatic brain injury patients, who need normal blood pressure for cerebral perfusion.

Balanced resuscitation: When blood products are needed, use a balanced ratio of packed red blood cells, plasma, and platelets (1:1:1 ratio) rather than crystalloid alone. This replaces both volume and clotting factors.

Damage control resuscitation: For severely injured patients, limit crystalloid fluids, use blood products early, correct hypothermia and acidosis, and get the patient to surgery quickly rather than trying to "fully resuscitate" them in the ED.

D - Disability (Neurological Assessment)

Once airway, breathing, and circulation are addressed, assess neurological status. This quick assessment identifies severe brain injury and establishes a baseline for monitoring.

Glasgow Coma Scale (GCS):

The GCS quantifies level of consciousness using three components:

Eye opening:

- 4: Spontaneous
- 3: To verbal command
- 2: To pain
- 1: None

Verbal response:

- 5: Oriented

- 4: Confused conversation
- 3: Inappropriate words
- 2: Incomprehensible sounds
- 1: None

Motor response:

- 6: Obeys commands
- 5: Localizes to pain
- 4: Withdraws from pain
- 3: Flexion to pain (decorticate posturing)
- 2: Extension to pain (decerebrate posturing)
- 1: None

Total score ranges from 3 (completely unresponsive) to 15 (fully alert). Score of 8 or less indicates severe brain injury and typically requires intubation and mechanical ventilation.

Pupil assessment:

Check pupil size, symmetry, and reaction to light. Unilateral dilated, non-reactive pupil suggests increased intracranial pressure with herniation on that side—a neurosurgical emergency. Bilateral pinpoint pupils might indicate drug intoxication. Bilateral dilated, non-reactive pupils are an ominous sign of severe brain injury or brain death.

E - Exposure and Environmental Control

The final step of the primary survey involves completely undressing the patient to identify all injuries while preventing hypothermia.

Complete exposure:

Cut away all clothing to visualize the entire body, front and back. Hidden injuries are common—you can't find what you don't look for. Check the back by log-rolling the patient while maintaining spinal precautions.

Environmental control (prevent hypothermia):

Trauma patients develop hypothermia from multiple factors: exposure to environment, cold IV fluids, open body cavities, and impaired thermoregulation from shock or brain injury.

Hypothermia worsens outcomes by:

- Impairing coagulation (clotting factors work poorly when cold)
- Causing cardiac arrhythmias
- Worsening acidosis
- Decreasing immune function

Prevention strategies:

- Keep the room warm (yes, even though staff find it uncomfortable)
- Cover the patient with warm blankets once the examination is complete
- Use fluid warmers for all IV fluids
- Consider warming devices (forced-air warming blankets)

- Warm blood products before transfusion

The Secondary Survey: Comprehensive Head-to-Toe Assessment

Once immediate life threats are addressed, conduct a thorough head-to-toe examination to identify all injuries. This systematic approach ensures nothing is missed.

The secondary survey uses the mnemonic "SAMPLE" for history:

- **S**igns and symptoms
- **A**llergies
- **M**edications
- **P**ast medical history
- **L**ast oral intake
- **E**vents surrounding the injury

Head-to-toe examination:

Head: Palpate the entire skull for depressions, crepitus, lacerations. Inspect ears for blood or cerebrospinal fluid (CSF) leak (halo sign on gauze). Check nose for bleeding or CSF. Examine eyes for pupil response, foreign bodies, hemorrhage. Assess facial bones for stability and symmetry.

Neck: Palpate cervical spine for tenderness (maintain immobilization). Check jugular veins (distended suggests cardiac tamponade or tension pneumothorax if associated with shock; flat suggests hypovolemia). Inspect for wounds, tracheal deviation, subcutaneous emphysema.

Chest: Inspect for wounds, bruising, paradoxical movement. Palpate ribs and sternum for tenderness, crepitus, instability. Auscultate breath sounds and heart sounds. Note any muffled heart sounds (suggests tamponade).

Abdomen: Inspect for bruising (seatbelt sign suggests internal injury), distension, wounds. Palpate all four quadrants for tenderness, rigidity, guarding. A tender, distended abdomen in a shock patient needs immediate surgical evaluation. Note that abdominal examination can be unreliable—some patients with significant injuries have minimal findings, while others with minor injuries have impressive tenderness.

Pelvis: Compress gently from the sides to assess stability. Never "rock" the pelvis vigorously—this can disrupt clots and worsen bleeding. Pelvic instability or severe tenderness requires pelvic binder application and stabilization.

Extremities: Inspect each limb for deformity, swelling, wounds. Palpate for tenderness, crepitus, pulses. Assess motor and sensory function. Check capillary refill. Splint obvious fractures. Any extremity with absent pulses needs immediate evaluation for vascular injury.

Back: Log-roll the patient (maintaining spinal precautions) to examine the entire posterior surface. Palpate spinous processes for tenderness or step-offs. Inspect for wounds, especially entry/exit wounds in penetrating trauma.

Rectal/genitourinary: Check for blood at urethral meatus (suggests urethral injury—don't insert catheter). Assess for scrotal hematoma, vaginal bleeding, rectal blood. Digital rectal exam assesses sphincter tone (decreased suggests spinal cord injury) and prostate position (high-riding prostate suggests urethral disruption).

Adjuncts to the secondary survey:

Laboratory tests, imaging studies, and monitoring equipment provide additional information:

- Focused Assessment with Sonography for Trauma (FAST exam) identifies free fluid in abdomen/pericardium
- Chest and pelvic X-rays identify major fractures and hemopneumothorax
- CT scanning (once stable) provides detailed injury identification
- Blood work (CBC, type and crossmatch, coagulation studies, lactate, blood gas)

The secondary survey repeats throughout the patient's care as conditions change and additional information becomes available.

Airway Management and Oxygen Therapy

Effective airway management prevents hypoxia, the leading preventable cause of death in trauma. This section expands on primary survey concepts with practical details.

Oxygen Delivery Devices

All trauma patients initially receive supplemental oxygen. Different devices deliver different oxygen concentrations:

Nasal cannula (1-6 L/min): Delivers 24-44% oxygen. Appropriate only for stable patients with minor injuries and normal respiratory effort. Not adequate for trauma patients in the acute phase.

Simple face mask (5-10 L/min): Delivers 35-60% oxygen. Better than nasal cannula but still not optimal for acute trauma.

Non-rebreather mask (10-15 L/min): Delivers 80-95% oxygen when properly fitted with reservoir bag fully inflated. This is the standard oxygen delivery device for trauma patients initially. The one-way valve prevents exhaled air from entering the reservoir bag, maximizing inspired oxygen concentration.

Bag-valve-mask (BVM): Provides assisted or controlled ventilation with high oxygen concentration. Used when patient's respiratory effort is inadequate. Effective BVM ventilation requires:

- Proper mask seal using two-handed technique when possible
- Adequate tidal volume (chest rise visible but not excessive)
- Appropriate rate (10-12 breaths/min for adults)
- Supplemental oxygen connected to reservoir (providing nearly 100% oxygen)

Common errors: inadequate seal (air leaks reduce effectiveness), hyperventilation (too fast or too large breaths), and single-handed mask hold (less effective seal).

Advanced Airway Management

When basic airway maneuvers don't provide adequate oxygenation and ventilation, the patient needs a definitive airway.

Endotracheal intubation:

This is the gold standard definitive airway. The tube passes through the vocal cords into the trachea, providing:

- Secure airway that won't obstruct
- Protection from aspiration
- Route for mechanical ventilation
- Ability to suction secretions
- Access for medication administration if needed

Intubation techniques in trauma:

Rapid sequence intubation (RSI): The standard approach in trauma. It uses medications to sedate and paralyze the patient, facilitating intubation while minimizing aspiration risk. Steps include:

1. **Preparation:** Equipment ready, monitoring in place, personnel assigned roles
2. **Preoxygenation:** 100% oxygen for 3-5 minutes (or 8 deep breaths)
3. **Pretreatment:** Medications to blunt physiologic responses (optional, controversial)
4. **Paralysis with induction:** Sedative and paralytic given in rapid succession
5. **Protection and positioning:** Maintain cervical spine precautions, position for intubation
6. **Placement with proof:** Insert tube, confirm placement
7. **Post-intubation management:** Secure tube, continue sedation/analgesia, mechanical ventilation

Medications commonly used:

Induction agents (sedation):

- Etomidate: Most hemodynamically stable, preferred in shock patients
- Ketamine: Provides sedation and analgesia, maintains blood pressure, useful in trauma
- Propofol: Can cause hypotension, use cautiously in hemodynamically unstable patients

Paralytics:

- Succinylcholine: Rapid onset (45 seconds), short duration, traditional choice
- Rocuronium: Alternative to succinylcholine, slightly slower onset but no contraindications related to hyperkalemia

Confirmation of tube placement:

Never assume the tube is correctly placed. Always confirm:

Clinical confirmation:

- Direct visualization of tube passing through cords (best)
- Chest rise with ventilation
- Breath sounds present bilaterally
- Absent sounds over epigastrium
- Condensation in tube with exhalation

Objective confirmation:

- End-tidal CO_2 detection (most reliable—sustained waveform confirms tracheal placement)
- Esophageal detector device
- Chest X-ray (shows tube position, but don't delay other confirmations waiting for X-ray)

Unrecognized esophageal intubation (tube in esophagus instead of trachea) causes hypoxia and death. Always confirm placement using multiple methods.

Surgical Airway

When you can't intubate and can't ventilate, the patient needs a surgical airway. This is rare but life-saving when necessary.

Indications:

- Cannot intubate, cannot ventilate scenario
- Severe maxillofacial trauma preventing oral/nasal intubation
- Laryngeal fracture or severe airway edema
- Massive hemorrhage in upper airway

Cricothyrotomy (surgical airway through cricothyroid membrane):

Anatomy: The cricothyroid membrane is the soft space between the thyroid cartilage (Adam's apple) and cricoid cartilage below it. It's relatively superficial and avascular, making it the ideal site for emergency surgical airway.

Technique:

1. Identify landmarks (thyroid cartilage, cricoid cartilage, cricothyroid membrane between them)
2. Stabilize the larynx with non-dominant hand
3. Make vertical skin incision over the membrane
4. Make horizontal incision through the cricothyroid membrane
5. Insert tracheal hook to stabilize and pull upward, or use hemostat to dilate opening
6. Insert appropriately sized tracheostomy or endotracheal tube (6.0 or 6.5 typically)
7. Confirm placement
8. Secure tube

Contraindications: Children under 12 years old (needle cricothyrotomy preferred due to small anatomy and risk of subglottic stenosis).

This is a high-stress procedure performed in crisis situations, but the technique is straightforward when anatomy is understood and equipment is ready.

Shock Recognition and Management

Shock is inadequate tissue perfusion and oxygenation at the cellular level. When cells don't receive enough oxygen and nutrients, they shift from aerobic to anaerobic metabolism, producing lactic acid and eventually dying if perfusion isn't restored. Understanding shock physiology and recognizing its signs early can mean the difference between life and death for your trauma patient.

Understanding the Pathophysiology of Shock

To recognize and treat shock effectively, you need to understand what's happening inside the body when perfusion fails.

Normal cellular metabolism requires oxygen delivered by red blood cells in adequate blood volume, pumped by a functioning heart through patent blood vessels. When this system fails at any point, shock develops.

The shock cascade progresses through predictable stages:

Stage 1: Initial/compensated shock The body recognizes decreased perfusion and activates compensatory mechanisms. The sympathetic nervous system releases catecholamines (epinephrine and norepinephrine), which cause:

- Increased heart rate (to maintain cardiac output)

- Peripheral vasoconstriction (to maintain blood pressure and shunt blood to vital organs)
- Increased contractility (to pump blood more forcefully)

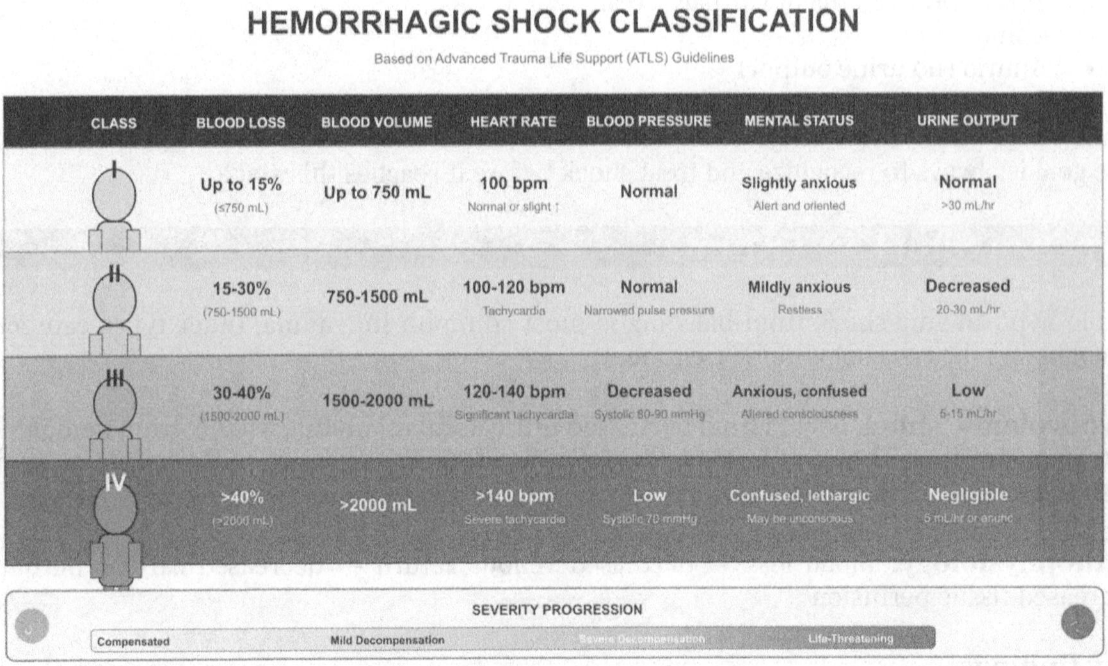

HEMORRHAGIC SHOCK CLASSIFICATION

Based on Advanced Trauma Life Support (ATLS) Guidelines

CLASS	BLOOD LOSS	BLOOD VOLUME	HEART RATE	BLOOD PRESSURE	MENTAL STATUS	URINE OUTPUT
I	Up to 15% (≤750 mL)	Up to 750 mL	100 bpm Normal or slight ↑	Normal	Slightly anxious Alert and oriented	Normal >30 mL/hr
II	15-30% (750-1500 mL)	750-1500 mL	100-120 bpm Tachycardia	Normal Narrowed pulse pressure	Mildly anxious Restless	Decreased 20-30 mL/hr
III	30-40% (1500-2000 mL)	1500-2000 mL	120-140 bpm Significant tachycardia	Decreased Systolic 80-90 mmHg	Anxious, confused Altered consciousness	Low 5-15 mL/hr
IV	>40% (>2000 mL)	>2000 mL	>140 bpm Severe tachycardia	Low Systolic 70 mmHg	Confused, lethargic May be unconscious	Negligible 5 mL/hr or anuric

SEVERITY PROGRESSION

Compensated — Mild Decompensation — Severe Decompensation — Life-Threatening

During this stage, blood pressure remains normal or near-normal because compensation works. However, subtle signs appear: mild tachycardia, cool extremities, delayed capillary refill, and anxiety or restlessness. Many nurses miss shock at this stage because the patient "looks okay" and vital signs seem acceptable.

Clinical pearl: A patient who's anxious, tachycardic, and has cool, pale skin is in shock even if their blood pressure is normal. Don't wait for hypotension to act.

Stage 2: Progressive/decompensated shock Compensatory mechanisms begin failing. The body can no longer maintain adequate perfusion to all tissues. Blood pressure drops as vasoconstriction reaches its maximum and cardiac output decreases. Lactic acid accumulates from anaerobic metabolism, causing metabolic acidosis.

Signs include:

- Hypotension (systolic BP <90 mmHg)
- Tachycardia and tachypnea worsen
- Altered mental status (confusion, agitation, combativeness)
- Decreased urine output (<0.5 mL/kg/hr)
- Metabolic acidosis on blood gas

This stage requires immediate aggressive intervention. Without treatment, progression to irreversible shock occurs rapidly.

Stage 3: Irreversible shock Cellular death is so widespread that recovery becomes impossible even with treatment. Multiple organ systems fail simultaneously. Signs include:

- Profound hypotension unresponsive to treatment
- Severe bradycardia or cardiac arrest
- Coma
- Anuria (no urine output)
- Severe lactic acidosis

The goal is always to recognize and treat shock before it reaches this stage.

Types of Shock in Trauma

While hypovolemic shock from bleeding is most common in trauma, other types can occur. Recognizing the type helps guide treatment.

Hypovolemic shock results from decreased intravascular volume, usually from hemorrhage in trauma patients. The heart has insufficient preload (blood returning to the heart), so cardiac output drops.

Pathophysiology: Blood loss → decreased venous return → decreased cardiac output → decreased tissue perfusion

Key findings:

- Flat neck veins (low central venous pressure)
- Cool, clammy skin
- Tachycardia
- Narrowed pulse pressure (systolic-diastolic difference <30 mmHg)

Treatment: Stop the bleeding and replace lost volume with blood products.

Cardiogenic shock occurs when the heart can't pump effectively. In trauma, this usually results from cardiac contusion, cardiac tamponade, or myocardial infarction (from stress or pre-existing disease).

Pathophysiology: Pump failure → decreased cardiac output → decreased tissue perfusion despite adequate blood volume

Key findings:

- Distended neck veins (blood backs up because heart can't pump it forward)
- Cool, clammy skin
- Tachycardia
- Pulmonary edema (crackles on auscultation)
- Chest pain (if MI is cause)

Treatment: Depends on cause. Cardiac tamponade needs pericardiocentesis. Cardiogenic shock from contusion needs inotropic support.

Distributive shock occurs when blood vessels dilate inappropriately, causing relative hypovolemia (blood volume is normal but vascular space has expanded).

Neurogenic shock is a type of distributive shock caused by spinal cord injury above T6, disrupting sympathetic nervous system control. Without sympathetic tone, blood vessels dilate and heart rate can't increase appropriately.

Pathophysiology: Spinal cord injury → loss of sympathetic tone → vasodilation → relative hypovolemia

Key findings (the classic triad):

- Hypotension
- Bradycardia (not tachycardia like other shock types)
- Warm, dry skin below the injury level (vessels are dilated, not constricted)

This presentation is opposite to hypovolemic shock. If a trauma patient has a mechanism suggesting spinal injury (fall, diving accident, motor vehicle crash) and presents with hypotension, bradycardia, and warm skin, think neurogenic shock. However, always rule out hemorrhage first because missing bleeding is more immediately life-threatening.

Treatment: Fluid resuscitation (carefully, because these patients can't compensate for fluid overload), vasopressors to restore vascular tone, and spinal cord injury management.

Obstructive shock occurs when blood flow is physically obstructed. In trauma, causes include tension pneumothorax and cardiac tamponade.

Tension pneumothorax: Air under pressure in the pleural space compresses the vena cava, preventing blood return to the heart.

Cardiac tamponade: Blood in the pericardial sac compresses the heart, preventing ventricular filling.

Key findings for obstructive shock:

- Distended neck veins (blood can't return to heart)
- Hypotension
- Tachycardia
- Specific findings for the cause (decreased breath sounds for pneumothorax, muffled heart sounds for tamponade)

Treatment: Remove the obstruction (needle decompression for tension pneumothorax, pericardiocentesis for tamponade).

Recognizing Shock: Systematic Assessment

Early recognition of shock saves lives. Use a systematic approach to identify shock before it progresses to late stages.

Vital signs:

- **Heart rate:** Tachycardia is often the first sign. Normal range is 60-100 bpm in adults. In shock, expect >100 bpm and climbing. However, some patients (athletes, those on beta-blockers, patients with neurogenic shock) may not show tachycardia despite being in shock.
- **Blood pressure:** This is a late indicator. Compensatory mechanisms maintain blood pressure until 30% blood volume is lost. A patient can be in significant shock with normal blood pressure. When hypotension develops (systolic <90 mmHg in adults), shock is already advanced.
- **Pulse pressure:** The difference between systolic and diastolic pressure. Normal is 40-60 mmHg. Narrowing pulse pressure (difference <30 mmHg) indicates vasoconstriction and early shock. For example, a patient with BP 110/90 (pulse pressure 20) is more concerning than one with BP 100/60 (pulse pressure 40).
- **Respiratory rate:** Tachypnea develops as the body tries to compensate for metabolic acidosis and maintain oxygenation. Normal is 12-20 breaths per minute. Rates >20 suggest shock or respiratory compromise.
- **Temperature:** Trauma patients become hypothermic from environmental exposure and decreased perfusion. Core temperature <36°C (96.8°F) worsens shock by impairing coagulation.

Clinical assessment:

- **Mental status:** The brain is sensitive to decreased perfusion. Anxiety, restlessness, confusion, or decreased responsiveness all suggest inadequate cerebral blood flow. A patient who's "acting weird" may be showing the first signs of shock.
- **Skin:** Assess color, temperature, and moisture. Pale, cool, clammy skin indicates vasoconstriction (hypovolemic, cardiogenic, obstructive shock). Warm, dry skin in a hypotensive trauma patient suggests neurogenic shock. Capillary refill >2 seconds indicates poor peripheral perfusion.
- **Urine output:** The kidneys receive 20-25% of cardiac output, and decreased renal perfusion quickly reduces urine production. Normal output is 0.5-1 mL/kg/hr (about 30-50 mL/hr for average adult). Decreased output indicates shock. Insert a Foley catheter early in resuscitation to monitor this important parameter.
- **Jugular veins:** Flat neck veins suggest hypovolemia. Distended neck veins with shock suggest cardiogenic or obstructive shock.

Laboratory indicators:

- **Lactate:** Elevated lactate (>2 mmol/L) indicates anaerobic metabolism from inadequate tissue perfusion. Rising lactate confirms shock even when vital signs seem acceptable. Lactate that decreases with treatment shows successful resuscitation.
- **Base deficit:** Negative base excess (base deficit >-6) on arterial blood gas indicates metabolic acidosis from shock. Like lactate, this confirms tissue hypoperfusion.

- **Hemoglobin/hematocrit:** These lag behind acute blood loss because plasma and red cells are lost proportionally. Early in hemorrhagic shock, hemoglobin may be normal. As the body compensates by moving fluid from interstitial space into vessels, and as IV fluids are given, hemodilution occurs and hemoglobin drops.

Managing Shock: Priority Interventions

Shock treatment follows a logical sequence based on the type and severity. For trauma patients, assume hemorrhagic shock until proven otherwise.

Step 1: Control obvious hemorrhage You can't resuscitate someone who's actively bleeding. Apply direct pressure, pressure dressings, tourniquets, or pelvic binders as indicated. Get surgical consultation immediately for injuries requiring operative control.

Step 2: Establish IV access Large-bore peripheral IV access is essential for rapid fluid administration. Place two 18-gauge or larger IV catheters. Larger catheters allow faster flow rates because flow is proportional to the radius to the fourth power (a 16-gauge catheter allows vastly more flow than an 18-gauge).

Preferred sites: Antecubital (inside elbow) veins are large and easy to access. Avoid hand or wrist veins for resuscitation—they're too small.

If peripheral access fails: Consider intraosseous (IO) access, which provides rapid, reliable access through bone marrow. IO can deliver fluids and medications effectively. Central venous access (internal jugular, subclavian, or femoral lines) is an option but takes longer to place.

Step 3: Initiate fluid resuscitation Crystalloid solutions (normal saline or lactated Ringer's) are the initial resuscitation fluid. Give 1-2 liters rapidly (wide open) to adults. Reassess after each liter.

Fluid warming: Use fluid warmers or rapid infusion devices to prevent hypothermia from cold IV fluids.

Balanced resuscitation approach: Current evidence supports limiting crystalloid to 1-2 liters before starting blood products. Excessive crystalloid causes:

- Dilution of clotting factors (dilutional coagulopathy)
- Decreased oxygen-carrying capacity (fewer red cells per volume)
- Increased bleeding (elevated blood pressure disrupts clots)
- Tissue edema (crystalloid distributes throughout body, not just in vessels)

Step 4: Transfuse blood products For hemorrhagic shock not responding to initial crystalloid, start blood products immediately.

Massive Transfusion Protocol (MTP): Most trauma centers have protocols for rapid delivery of blood products in predictable ratios. Typical MTP includes:

- Packed red blood cells (PRBCs)

- Fresh frozen plasma (FFP)
- Platelets
- Sometimes cryoprecipitate (for fibrinogen replacement)

Balanced ratio: Give products in approximately 1:1:1 ratio (PRBCs:FFP:Platelets). This replaces both volume and clotting factors, preventing coagulopathy.

Type O negative blood is the universal donor type, given when the patient's blood type is unknown and no time exists for crossmatch. Men and post-menopausal women can receive type O positive blood (which is more readily available) without risk of Rh sensitization.

Tranexamic acid (TXA): This antifibrinolytic medication reduces mortality in bleeding trauma patients when given within 3 hours of injury. Dose is 1 gram IV over 10 minutes, followed by 1 gram infused over 8 hours. TXA works by preventing clot breakdown, giving the body time to control bleeding.

Step 5: Correct coagulopathy, hypothermia, and acidosis These three factors (the "lethal triad") worsen each other and dramatically increase mortality. Address them aggressively:

Hypothermia: Keep patient warm, use fluid warmers, increase room temperature, apply forced-air warming devices.

Acidosis: Results from poor perfusion and anaerobic metabolism. The treatment is restoring perfusion, not giving sodium bicarbonate. As shock resolves, the body clears lactic acid naturally.

Coagulopathy: Blood doesn't clot properly due to dilution of clotting factors, hypothermia, acidosis, and consumption of clotting factors. Treatment includes:

- Maintaining temperature >35°C (95°F)
- Transfusing FFP and platelets with PRBCs
- Giving calcium (citrate in blood products binds calcium needed for clotting)
- Considering factor VIIa or prothrombin complex concentrate for severe coagulopathy

Step 6: Vasopressors if needed Most trauma patients in hemorrhagic shock don't need vasopressors—they need blood and bleeding control. However, vasopressors may be used:

- In neurogenic shock (after adequate fluid resuscitation)
- To maintain perfusion pressure temporarily until definitive bleeding control
- In refractory hypotension despite adequate resuscitation

Common vasopressors include norepinephrine (first-line), phenylephrine, and vasopressin.

Step 7: Monitor response to treatment Continuously reassess effectiveness of resuscitation:

- Vital signs improving (heart rate decreasing, blood pressure stabilizing)

- Mental status clearing
- Skin warming, improving color
- Urine output improving (target 0.5-1 mL/kg/hr)
- Lactate decreasing
- Base deficit improving

Failure to respond to resuscitation suggests either ongoing bleeding or inadequate resuscitation. Escalate treatment and get surgical consultation immediately.

Hemorrhage Control

Controlling bleeding is the most critical intervention in trauma care. All other treatments are futile if the patient continues to hemorrhage.

Principles of Hemorrhage Control

External hemorrhage is usually obvious and controllable at the bedside. **Internal hemorrhage** is insidious and may require operative intervention.

The sequence of hemorrhage control:

1. Direct pressure
2. Pressure dressing
3. Tourniquets (extremity hemorrhage only)
4. Hemostatic agents
5. Surgical intervention

External Hemorrhage Management

Direct pressure is the first and most effective method for controlling external bleeding. Apply firm, continuous pressure directly over the wound. Use your gloved hand, gauze, or any clean cloth. The pressure mechanically compresses bleeding vessels and allows clot formation.

How to apply direct pressure correctly:

- Use enough pressure to stop or significantly slow bleeding
- Hold pressure for at least 5-10 minutes without removing it to check (checking disrupts clot formation)
- If bleeding soaks through initial dressing, add more material on top rather than removing the saturated dressing

Common mistake: Repeatedly removing dressings to "check if it's still bleeding." Each time you lift the dressing, you disrupt clot formation and restart the clock. Apply pressure and leave it there.

Pressure dressings maintain compression once initial bleeding is controlled. Wrap the wound firmly (but not so tightly as to obstruct distal circulation) with elastic bandages or commercial pressure dressings. This frees your hands for other interventions while maintaining hemorrhage control.

Tourniquet application is appropriate for severe extremity hemorrhage not controlled by direct pressure. Modern evidence from military medicine demonstrates that tourniquets save lives and, when properly applied, rarely cause complications.

When to use a tourniquet:

- Severe extremity hemorrhage with active spurting
- Bleeding not controlled by direct pressure
- Multiple casualties requiring hemorrhage control (tourniquets allow you to control one patient's bleeding and move to the next)
- Partial or complete amputation

How to apply a tourniquet:

1. Place the tourniquet 2-3 inches proximal to the wound (toward the trunk from the injury)
2. Never place directly over a joint
3. Tighten until bleeding stops
4. Note the time of application clearly
5. Don't cover the tourniquet—leave it visible for reassessment
6. Don't release a tourniquet to "check" if still needed—leave it until surgical evaluation

Commercial tourniquets (Combat Application Tourniquet, SOF Tactical Tourniquet) are more effective than improvised ones. However, if no commercial tourniquet is available, improvise using a wide cloth band and windlass (stick for twisting).

Misconceptions about tourniquets:

- **Myth:** Tourniquets cause limb loss. **Reality:** Properly applied tourniquets rarely cause lasting damage. Uncontrolled hemorrhage definitely causes death.
- **Myth:** You must loosen tourniquets every 20-30 minutes. **Reality:** Don't loosen tourniquets unnecessarily. They're safe for several hours.

Hemostatic agents promote rapid clot formation in wounds. Products like Combat Gauze contain substances (kaolin, chitosan) that activate clotting cascades.

How to use hemostatic dressings:

1. Expose the wound completely
2. Pack the hemostatic gauze directly into the wound, filling the entire wound cavity
3. Pack firmly—loose packing doesn't work
4. Apply direct pressure over the packed wound for 3-5 minutes
5. Apply pressure dressing to maintain compression

Hemostatic agents work best when:

- Applied directly to the bleeding source (deep packing is often necessary)
- Used with firm, sustained pressure
- The patient isn't already severely coagulopathic

Internal Hemorrhage Recognition and Management

Internal bleeding is more challenging because you can't see it. High suspicion based on mechanism of injury and shock signs is essential.

Common sites of internal hemorrhage in trauma:

Chest: Each hemithorax can hold >3000 mL of blood (half the patient's blood volume or more). Massive hemothorax presents with decreased breath sounds, dullness to percussion, and shock.

Management: Place large-bore (36-40 French) chest tube. If drainage is immediately >1500 mL or continues >200 mL/hr, the patient needs thoracotomy for surgical hemorrhage control.

Abdomen: The peritoneal cavity can accommodate massive blood loss. Free intraperitoneal blood from liver, spleen, or mesenteric injuries may cause shock with minimal physical findings initially.

Assessment: FAST (Focused Assessment with Sonography for Trauma) exam identifies free fluid in the peritoneum. CT scan (in stable patients) shows specific injuries. Peritoneal lavage (rarely used now) can confirm intraperitoneal blood.

Management: Hemodynamically unstable patients with positive FAST go directly to the operating room. Stable patients can undergo CT for detailed injury assessment. Many solid organ injuries (especially spleen and liver) can be managed non-operatively in stable patients with serial exams and monitoring.

Pelvis: Pelvic fractures can cause life-threatening retroperitoneal hemorrhage. Blood accumulates in the retroperitoneal space, which can hold several liters. Bleeding comes from fractured bone surfaces and torn pelvic vessels.

Assessment: Pelvic instability on exam, pelvic fracture on X-ray, shock without another obvious source.

Management:

- Immediate pelvic binder application (around the greater trochanters)
- Stabilize the pelvis to decrease pelvic volume and tamponade bleeding
- Massive transfusion protocol
- Angiography with embolization for arterial bleeding
- External fixation or open reduction internal fixation for unstable fractures

Long bones: Femur fractures cause 1000-1500 mL blood loss into the thigh. Tibial and humeral fractures each cause 500-750 mL loss. Multiple long bone fractures compound this effect.

Management:

- Early splinting or traction to stabilize fractures and reduce ongoing bleeding
- Resuscitation for blood loss
- Surgical fixation when patient is stable

Retroperitoneum: Kidney injuries, major vascular injuries (aorta, vena cava), and pancreatic injuries can cause significant retroperitoneal bleeding.

Management: Depends on specific injury identified on CT. Some kidney injuries can be managed non-operatively. Vascular injuries usually require surgical repair.

Resuscitation Principles

Trauma resuscitation has evolved significantly based on military experience and civilian research. Current best practices balance restoring perfusion with avoiding complications of overly aggressive resuscitation.

Damage Control Resuscitation

This strategy aims to keep the patient alive long enough to control bleeding surgically while minimizing the complications that worsen outcomes.

Key principles:

1. Permissive hypotension (until hemorrhage control) Traditional resuscitation targeted normal blood pressure. However, raising blood pressure before controlling bleeding can:

- Increase bleeding by disrupting formed clots
- Cause dilutional coagulopathy
- Lead to worse outcomes

Permissive hypotension accepts lower than normal blood pressure (systolic 80-90 mmHg) until surgical bleeding control is achieved. This maintains perfusion to vital organs without increasing hemorrhage.

When NOT to use permissive hypotension:

- Traumatic brain injury (brain needs adequate perfusion pressure)
- Elderly patients (may have hypertension at baseline, so 80-90 is severely low for them)
- After bleeding is surgically controlled

2. Limit crystalloid Crystalloid dilutes clotting factors and red blood cells. It also extravasates into tissues, causing edema. Current recommendations limit crystalloid to 1-2 liters before starting blood products.

3. Early blood product administration Start blood products early rather than trying to fully resuscitate with crystalloid first. Use balanced ratios (1:1:1) to replace both oxygen-carrying capacity and clotting factors.

4. Correct coagulopathy aggressively Monitor coagulation status (PT/INR, PTT, fibrinogen, platelets) and transfuse appropriate products to maintain hemostasis:

- FFP for clotting factor replacement
- Platelets when count <50,000 or <100,000 with ongoing bleeding
- Cryoprecipitate or fibrinogen concentrate when fibrinogen <150-200 mg/dL

5. Prevent and treat hypothermia Maintain patient temperature >35°C (95°F):

- Warm room temperature
- Warm all IV fluids
- Use forced-air warming devices
- Minimize exposure time during exams

6. Minimize acidosis The treatment for acidosis in trauma is restoring perfusion, not giving bicarbonate. Adequate resuscitation allows the body to clear lactate naturally.

Massive Transfusion Protocols

Massive transfusion is defined as replacing one blood volume (approximately 10 units of PRBCs) in 24 hours, or transfusing >4 units in 1 hour with expectation of continued need.

Massive Transfusion Protocol activation criteria (vary by institution, but generally include):

- Hemodynamically unstable trauma patient
- Obvious major hemorrhage
- Positive FAST with shock
- Penetrating torso trauma with shock

How MTP works: Once activated, the blood bank prepares pre-packaged "coolers" containing PRBCs, FFP, and platelets in balanced ratios. These are delivered rapidly to the ED or OR without waiting for individual orders. This system dramatically reduces time to blood product delivery.

Monitoring during massive transfusion:

- Vital signs continuously
- Laboratory tests every 30-60 minutes (CBC, coagulation studies, electrolytes, lactate, ABG)

- Thromboelastography (TEG or ROTEM where available) for real-time coagulation assessment
- Calcium levels (citrate in blood products binds calcium)

Complications of massive transfusion:

- Hypothermia (from cold blood products)
- Citrate toxicity/hypocalcemia
- Hyperkalemia (from stored red blood cells)
- Acid-base disturbances
- Transfusion reactions
- Transfusion-related acute lung injury (TRALI)

When to stop massive transfusion:

- Bleeding surgically controlled
- Hemodynamic stability achieved
- Coagulation parameters normalized
- Lactate clearing

Chapter 3 Practice Questions

Now that you've learned the content, test your understanding with these practice questions. Remember to read each question carefully, identify what it's really asking, and use the principles you've learned to select the best answer.

Question 1: A trauma patient arrives with respiratory distress, absent breath sounds on the right side, hyperresonance to percussion, and tracheal deviation to the left. What is the priority intervention?

A) Obtain a chest X-ray to confirm the diagnosis
B) Prepare for chest tube insertion
C) Perform needle decompression of the right chest
D) Intubate the patient immediately

Answer: C

Explanation: This patient has a tension pneumothorax, which is a clinical diagnosis requiring immediate treatment. The signs (absent breath sounds, hyperresonance, tracheal deviation, respiratory distress) are classic for tension pneumothorax. Needle decompression is the immediate life-saving intervention that converts the tension pneumothorax to a simple pneumothorax. Waiting for a chest X-ray (option A) delays life-saving treatment. Chest tube insertion (option B) will be needed but takes longer to perform than needle decompression. Intubation (option D) may be needed but doesn't address the underlying problem of air under pressure in the chest.

Question 2: During the primary survey, you assess a patient's airway and find it patent. The patient is speaking in full sentences. What is the next priority assessment?

A) Assess for spinal cord injury
B) Assess breathing and ventilation
C) Obtain vital signs
D) Assess pupillary response

Answer: B

Explanation: The primary survey follows the ABCDE sequence: Airway, Breathing, Circulation, Disability, Exposure. After confirming airway patency (A), you immediately move to assessing breathing (B). While the patient is speaking (indicating air movement), you must still assess adequacy of ventilation by examining chest rise, respiratory rate, breath sounds, and work of breathing. Spinal cord assessment (option A) is part of Disability (D). Vital signs (option C) are obtained during the assessment but aren't a specific step in the sequence.

Pupillary response (option D) is also part of Disability assessment.

Question 3: A patient presents with hypotension, bradycardia, and warm, dry skin below the waist following a fall from height. What type of shock is most likely?

A) Hypovolemic shock
B) Cardiogenic shock
C) Neurogenic shock
D) Septic shock

Answer: C

Explanation: This is the classic triad of neurogenic shock: hypotension, bradycardia, and warm/dry skin. Neurogenic shock results from spinal cord injury (likely from the fall) disrupting sympathetic nervous system control. This causes vasodilation (warm skin) and prevents compensatory tachycardia (bradycardia instead). Hypovolemic shock (option A) would present with tachycardia and cool, clammy skin. Cardiogenic shock (option B) would have cool, clammy skin and possibly signs of heart failure. Septic shock (option D) is unlikely immediately after trauma and typically presents with warm skin but tachycardia, not bradycardia.

Question 4: A trauma patient has received 2 liters of crystalloid fluid without improvement in blood pressure or heart rate. What is the priority intervention?

A) Administer another liter of normal saline
B) Start a vasopressor infusion
C) Initiate massive transfusion protocol
D) Perform a FAST exam

Answer: C

Explanation: A trauma patient in hemorrhagic shock not responding to 2 liters of crystalloid needs blood products immediately. Current evidence supports limiting crystalloid and starting blood products early. The massive transfusion protocol ensures rapid delivery of balanced blood products. Giving more crystalloid (option A) causes dilutional coagulopathy and doesn't address the fundamental problem of blood loss. Vasopressors (option B) aren't appropriate for hypovolemic shock—the patient needs volume, not artificially elevated blood pressure. FAST exam (option D) might be helpful to identify bleeding source but shouldn't delay resuscitation with blood products.

Question 5: Which finding best indicates adequate fluid resuscitation in a trauma patient?

A) Blood pressure 120/80 mmHg
B) Urine output 40 mL/hour
C) Heart rate 70 bpm
D) Capillary refill 2 seconds

Answer: B

Explanation: Urine output is one of the best indicators of adequate end-organ perfusion. Normal urine output (0.5-1 mL/kg/hr, or approximately 30-50 mL/hr for an average adult) indicates the kidneys are adequately perfused. While blood pressure (option A), heart rate (option C), and capillary refill (option D) are all important parameters, urine output most directly reflects tissue perfusion. A patient can have normal vital signs but still have inadequate perfusion, but adequate urine output confirms that resuscitation is effective at the tissue level.

Question 6: During the primary survey, when should you expose the patient completely?

A) During the Airway assessment
B) During the Breathing assessment
C) During the Circulation assessment
D) During the Exposure step

Answer: D

Explanation: Complete exposure of the patient occurs during the E (Exposure) step of the primary survey, which is the final step. While you expose specific areas during earlier assessments (chest for breathing assessment, for example), complete exposure—including log-rolling to examine the back—occurs during the Exposure step. This systematic approach ensures life-threatening conditions are addressed in order of priority before spending time on complete physical examination. Environmental control (preventing hypothermia) is also addressed during this step.

Question 7: A patient with a Glasgow Coma Scale score of 7 requires which immediate intervention?

A) CT scan of the head
B) Endotracheal intubation
C) Administration of mannitol
D) Neurosurgical consultation

Answer: B

Explanation: GCS of 8 or less indicates severe brain injury and inability to protect the airway. This patient needs immediate endotracheal intubation to secure the airway, prevent aspiration, and allow controlled ventilation (important for managing intracranial pressure). While head CT (option A), mannitol for elevated ICP (option C), and neurosurgery consultation (option D) may all be needed, securing the airway is the immediate priority. Remember the primary survey priorities: airway problems will kill the patient faster than anything else.

Question 8: Which mechanism of injury has the highest risk for cervical spine injury?

A) Fall from standing height
B) Rear-end motor vehicle collision at low speed
C) Diving accident in shallow water
D) Ground-level fall in elderly patient

Answer: C

Explanation: Diving into shallow water commonly causes cervical spine injury due to axial loading (compression force directly down the spine) when the head strikes the bottom. This mechanism frequently causes fractures or dislocations in the cervical spine. Fall from standing (option A), low-speed rear-end collision (option B), and ground-level fall (option D) carry lower risk for cervical spine injury, though spinal precautions should still be maintained until injury is ruled out in any trauma patient.

Question 9: A patient has a suspected open pneumothorax with a sucking chest wound. What is the appropriate initial management?

A) Apply an occlusive dressing taped on all four sides
B) Apply an occlusive dressing taped on three sides
C) Insert a chest tube immediately
D) Pack the wound with gauze

Answer: B

Explanation: An open pneumothorax (sucking chest wound) should be covered with an occlusive dressing taped on three sides, creating a flutter valve. This allows air to escape during exhalation but prevents air entry during inhalation. Taping all four sides (option A) could create a tension pneumothorax by trapping air in the chest. A chest tube (option C) will be needed but should be placed away from the wound itself after applying the occlusive dressing. Packing the wound with gauze (option D) doesn't seal the defect and doesn't address the pneumothorax.

Question 10: What is the primary purpose of applying a pelvic binder?

A) Stabilize the pelvis for patient transfer
B) Reduce pain from pelvic fractures
C) Decrease pelvic volume to tamponade

hemorrhage
D) Prevent further fracture displacement

Answer: C

Explanation: The primary purpose of a pelvic binder is to decrease pelvic volume and tamponade internal hemorrhage from pelvic fractures. By compressing the pelvis, the binder reduces the space where blood can accumulate, helping control life-threatening bleeding. While it does stabilize the pelvis and reduce pain, these are secondary benefits—the main goal is hemorrhage control.

Question 11: A trauma patient has a heart rate of 120 bpm, blood pressure 110/85 mmHg, and cool, clammy skin. What class of hemorrhagic shock is most likely?

A) Class I
B) Class II
C) Class III
D) Class IV

Answer: B

Explanation: This patient demonstrates Class II hemorrhagic shock (15-30% blood loss). Signs include tachycardia (100-120 bpm), narrowed pulse pressure (25 mmHg in this case), and cool extremities, while blood pressure remains relatively normal. Class I has minimal symptoms with normal vitals. Class III would show hypotension. Class IV would present with severe shock and altered mental status.

Question 12: Which intervention should be performed first during rapid sequence intubation?

A) Administer paralytic medication
B) Preoxygenate with 100% oxygen
C) Position the patient for intubation
D) Administer sedative medication

Answer: B

Explanation: Preoxygenation is the first step in RSI after preparation. It provides an oxygen reservoir that allows several minutes of apnea during intubation without desaturation. This safety margin is critical in trauma patients who may be difficult to intubate. Positioning occurs after preoxygenation, and medications are given only after adequate preoxygenation is achieved.

Question 13: A patient has absent breath sounds on the left with dullness to percussion and shock. What condition is most likely?

A) Tension pneumothorax
B) Massive hemothorax
C) Pulmonary contusion
D) Flail chest

Answer: B

Explanation: Massive hemothorax presents with absent breath sounds, dullness to percussion (blood in chest cavity), and shock from blood loss. Tension pneumothorax would show hyperresonance, not dullness. Pulmonary contusion doesn't typically cause complete absence of breath sounds or immediate shock. Flail chest presents with paradoxical chest wall movement.

Question 14: What is the correct placement location for a tourniquet on an extremity?

A) Directly over the wound
B) 2-3 inches distal to the wound
C) 2-3 inches proximal to the wound
D) Over the nearest joint

Answer: C

Explanation: Tourniquets should be placed 2-3 inches proximal to the wound (toward the trunk). This placement ensures the tourniquet occludes blood flow before it reaches the injury. Placing it distal to the wound doesn't stop bleeding. Placing it directly over the wound is ineffective, and placement over joints can be less effective and more damaging.

Question 15: Which assessment finding indicates adequate organ perfusion during resuscitation?

A) Systolic blood pressure >90 mmHg
B) Heart rate <100 bpm
C) Lactate level decreasing from 6 to 3 mmol/L
D) Temperature 36°C

Answer: C

Explanation: Decreasing lactate levels indicate improved tissue perfusion and resolution of anaerobic metabolism. This is one of the best markers of successful resuscitation. Blood pressure and heart rate can be misleading—a patient can have acceptable vital signs but still have poor tissue perfusion. Temperature is important but doesn't directly measure perfusion.

Question 16: During the secondary survey, you note blood at the urethral meatus. What is the appropriate action?

A) Insert a Foley catheter immediately
B) Perform a digital rectal exam
C) Do not insert a Foley catheter until urethral injury is ruled out
D) Obtain a urinalysis

Answer: C

Explanation: Blood at the urethral meatus indicates possible urethral injury. Inserting a Foley catheter could worsen the injury or create a false passage. Urethral injury must be ruled out with a retrograde urethrogram before catheter insertion. If urethral injury is confirmed, a suprapubic catheter may be needed instead.

Question 17: A patient requires massive transfusion. What is the recommended ratio of blood products?

A) PRBCs only until hemoglobin improves
B) 2:1:1 (PRBCs:FFP:Platelets)
C) 1:1:1 (PRBCs:FFP:Platelets)
D) PRBCs and FFP only, no platelets

Answer: C

Explanation: Current evidence supports balanced 1:1:1 ratio of packed red blood cells, fresh frozen plasma, and platelets during massive transfusion. This approach replaces both oxygen-carrying capacity and clotting factors, preventing dilutional coagulopathy and improving survival compared to PRBC-heavy transfusion strategies.

Question 18: What is the primary compensatory mechanism in early hemorrhagic shock?

A) Decreased respiratory rate
B) Vasodilation to increase blood flow
C) Peripheral vasoconstriction and tachycardia
D) Bradycardia to reduce cardiac workload

Answer: C

Explanation: The body compensates for early blood loss through sympathetic nervous system activation, causing peripheral vasoconstriction (maintaining blood pressure and shunting blood to vital organs) and tachycardia (maintaining cardiac output despite reduced volume). Respiratory rate increases, not decreases. Vasodilation would worsen shock. Bradycardia is not a compensatory mechanism in hemorrhagic shock.

Question 19: Which patient requires immediate needle decompression?

A) Respiratory distress with equal breath sounds bilaterally
B) Absent breath sounds on one side with hyperresonance and hypotension
C) Decreased breath sounds bilaterally with subcutaneous emphysema

D) Paradoxical chest wall movement with severe pain

Answer: B

Explanation: Absent breath sounds on one side with hyperresonance and hypotension indicates tension pneumothorax requiring immediate needle decompression. This is a clinical diagnosis that shouldn't wait for imaging. Option A suggests other respiratory problems. Option C might indicate pneumothorax but without signs of tension. Option D describes flail chest.

Question 20: What is the correct hand position for the jaw thrust maneuver?

A) Place hands on the forehead and chin, tilting the head back
B) Place fingers at the angle of the mandible and lift anteriorly
C) Place thumbs under the chin and push upward
D) Place one hand on the forehead and lift the chin with the other

Answer: B

Explanation: The jaw thrust involves placing fingers at the angle of the mandible and lifting anteriorly (forward), which opens the airway without extending the neck. This makes it safe for trauma patients with potential cervical spine injury. Options A and D describe head-tilt chin-lift, which extends the neck and is contraindicated in trauma. Option C is not an effective airway maneuver.

Question 21: A patient has a GCS of 12 (E3, V4, M5). This indicates:

A) Severe brain injury requiring immediate intubation
B) Moderate brain injury requiring close monitoring
C) Mild brain injury with minimal intervention needed
D) Normal neurological function

Answer: B

Explanation: GCS 9-12 indicates moderate brain injury. These patients require close neurological monitoring, serial assessments, and often CT imaging, but don't necessarily need immediate intubation. GCS ≤8 indicates severe injury requiring intubation. GCS 13-15 indicates mild injury. GCS 15 is normal.

Question 22: Which fluid is preferred for initial trauma resuscitation?

A) D5W (5% dextrose in water)
B) 0.45% sodium chloride
C) Lactated Ringer's solution
D) Albumin

Answer: C

Explanation: Lactated Ringer's solution or normal saline are the preferred crystalloid solutions for trauma resuscitation. Lactated Ringer's is slightly preferred because it more closely matches plasma electrolyte composition and doesn't cause hyperchloremic acidosis. D5W is hypotonic and inappropriate for resuscitation. 0.45% saline is also hypotonic. Albumin is expensive and offers no survival benefit over crystalloid.

Question 23: A patient with suspected spinal cord injury has hypotension and bradycardia. After ruling out hemorrhage, what is the appropriate treatment?

A) Aggressive fluid boluses only
B) Atropine for the bradycardia
C) Cautious fluid resuscitation and vasopressors
D) Immediate surgical intervention

Answer: C

Explanation: Neurogenic shock requires careful fluid resuscitation (these patients can't compensate for fluid overload) combined with vasopressors to restore vascular tone. Aggressive fluid boluses alone can cause pulmonary edema. Atropine addresses bradycardia but not the underlying vasodilation and hypotension. Surgery isn't the immediate priority for managing hemodynamics.

Question 24: What does a narrowing pulse pressure indicate in a trauma patient?

A) Adequate fluid resuscitation
B) Neurogenic shock
C) Early compensated shock
D) Cardiac tamponade

Answer: C

Explanation: Narrowing pulse pressure (difference between systolic and diastolic pressures <30 mmHg) indicates peripheral vasoconstriction, a compensatory mechanism in early shock. It's one of the earliest signs of hemorrhagic shock, often appearing before hypotension. Adequate resuscitation would show normal or widening pulse pressure. Cardiac tamponade shows narrowing but with other specific signs.

Question 25: When should tranexamic acid (TXA) be administered to a bleeding trauma patient?

A) Only after hemorrhage is surgically controlled
B) Within 3 hours of injury
C) Only if coagulopathy is confirmed by lab tests
D) After transfusing 10 units of blood products

Answer: B

Explanation: TXA is most effective when given within 3 hours of injury and is proven to reduce mortality in bleeding trauma patients. It works by preventing clot breakdown (antifibrinolytic). Administration after 3 hours may actually increase mortality. It's given based on clinical suspicion of significant bleeding, not waiting for lab confirmation of coagulopathy.

Question 26: A flail chest is defined as:

A) Single rib fracture with severe pain
B) Two or more ribs fractured in two or more places
C) Sternal fracture with respiratory distress
D) Rib fractures with associated pneumothorax

Answer: B

Explanation: Flail chest occurs when two or more adjacent ribs are fractured in two or more places, creating a free-floating segment of chest wall that moves paradoxically with respiration. Single rib fractures don't create flail segments. Sternal fractures alone aren't flail chest. Rib fractures with pneumothorax describe a different injury pattern.

Question 27: What is the priority intervention for an open pneumothorax?

A) Immediate chest tube insertion
B) Apply occlusive dressing taped on three sides
C) Endotracheal intubation
D) Needle decompression

Answer: B

Explanation: The immediate priority for an open pneumothorax is covering the wound with an occlusive dressing taped on three sides, creating a flutter valve that allows air to escape but not enter. Chest tube insertion will be needed but should be placed away from the wound. Intubation may be needed but doesn't address the open defect. Needle decompression is for tension pneumothorax.

Question 28: Which site can hold the largest volume of blood loss in trauma?

A) Chest (each hemithorax)
B) Abdomen

C) Pelvis/retroperitoneum
D) Thigh (from femur fracture)

Answer: A

Explanation: Each hemithorax can hold 3000+ mL of blood (more than half of total blood volume), making it the largest potential site for blood loss. The abdomen and pelvis can also hold large volumes but typically less than the chest. A femur fracture causes 1000-1500 mL loss, which is significant but less than chest capacity.

Question 29: A patient's lactate level is 5 mmol/L (normal <2). This indicates:

A) Adequate tissue perfusion
B) Anaerobic metabolism from inadequate perfusion
C) Respiratory alkalosis
D) Hyperglycemia

Answer: B

Explanation: Elevated lactate indicates tissue hypoperfusion leading to anaerobic metabolism. When cells don't receive adequate oxygen, they produce lactate as a byproduct. Lactate >2 mmol/L confirms shock even when vital signs appear stable. Adequate perfusion would show normal lactate. It doesn't directly indicate respiratory alkalosis or hyperglycemia.

Question 30: What is permissive hypotension in trauma resuscitation?

A) Allowing blood pressure to drop below 60 mmHg systolic
B) Maintaining systolic pressure around 80-90 mmHg until bleeding is controlled
C) Avoiding all fluid resuscitation until surgery
D) Accepting hypotension in all trauma patients

Answer: B

Explanation: Permissive hypotension involves maintaining systolic BP around 80-90 mmHg (rather than targeting normal BP) until surgical hemorrhage control is achieved. This prevents clot disruption from elevated pressure while maintaining vital organ perfusion. It's not used in traumatic brain injury patients who need higher perfusion pressure, and doesn't mean avoiding all resuscitation.

Question 31: During the primary survey, you note distended neck veins in a hypotensive trauma patient. This suggests:

A) Hypovolemic shock
B) Neurogenic shock
C) Obstructive shock (tension pneumothorax or cardiac tamponade)
D) Adequate fluid resuscitation

Answer: C

Explanation: Distended neck veins with hypotension indicate obstructive shock, most commonly from tension pneumothorax or cardiac tamponade. Both conditions prevent blood from returning to or leaving the heart, causing backup and jugular venous distension. Hypovolemic shock would show flat neck veins. Neurogenic shock typically shows flat veins. This doesn't indicate adequate resuscitation in a shock patient.

Question 32: What is the most reliable method to confirm endotracheal tube placement?

A) Seeing the tube pass through the vocal cords
B) Hearing breath sounds bilaterally
C) Sustained end-tidal CO2 waveform
D) Chest X-ray confirmation

Answer: C

Explanation: End-tidal CO2 detection showing sustained waveform is the most reliable objective confirmation of tracheal placement. While visualizing tube passage through cords is excellent, it's not always possible. Breath sounds can be misleading (esophageal sounds can transmit to chest). Chest X-ray confirms position but shouldn't delay other immediate confirmation methods. Multiple methods should be used together.

Question 33: A patient with a pelvic fracture is bleeding severely. Which intervention provides the fastest hemorrhage control?

A) External pelvic fixation
B) Pelvic binder application
C) Angiography with embolization
D) Immediate laparotomy

Answer: B

Explanation: Pelvic binder application is the fastest bedside intervention for pelvic hemorrhage control and should be done immediately. It reduces pelvic volume and provides tamponade. External fixation requires OR time. Angiography is excellent for arterial bleeding but requires transport to IR and procedural time. Laparotomy doesn't address pelvic or retroperitoneal bleeding effectively.

Question 34: Which blood type should be given to a trauma patient when immediate transfusion is needed and blood type is unknown?

A) Type A positive
B) Type B negative
C) Type O negative
D) Type AB positive

Answer: C

Explanation: Type O negative is the universal donor blood type and should be given when immediate transfusion is needed and the patient's blood type is unknown. It lacks A, B, and Rh antigens, so it won't cause reaction in any blood type. Type O positive can be given to males and post-menopausal females if O negative is unavailable.

Question 35: A trauma patient becomes agitated and combative. What should you assess first?

A) Blood alcohol level
B) Need for physical restraints
C) Oxygenation and perfusion status
D) Psychiatric history

Answer: C

Explanation: Agitation and combativeness in trauma patients often indicate hypoxia or hypoperfusion (shock) affecting brain function. Always assess and correct physiologic causes first—check airway patency, oxygenation, ventilation, and perfusion before attributing behavior to intoxication or psychiatric causes. Assume altered mental status is from trauma until proven otherwise.

Question 36: What is the recommended tidal volume for bag-valve-mask ventilation in adults?

A) 300-400 mL
B) 500-600 mL
C) 800-1000 mL
D) 1200-1500 mL

Answer: B

Explanation: Appropriate tidal volume for BVM ventilation in adults is 500-600 mL (approximately 6-7 mL/kg), delivered over 1 second. This volume produces visible chest rise without excessive pressure that could cause gastric inflation and aspiration. Smaller volumes don't provide adequate ventilation. Larger volumes increase risk of barotrauma and gastric distension.

Question 37: Which assessment finding most reliably indicates a complete airway obstruction?

A) Stridor
B) Snoring respirations
C) Inability to speak or cough with no air movement
D) Decreased breath sounds

Answer: C

Explanation: Complete airway obstruction presents with inability to speak, cough, or move any air, often with the universal choking sign (hands clutching throat). Stridor indicates partial obstruction with some air movement. Snoring suggests tongue obstruction but partial patency. Decreased breath sounds could have multiple causes and don't necessarily mean complete obstruction.

Question 38: A trauma patient has a blood pressure of 88/64 mmHg, heart rate 134 bpm, and respiratory rate 32/min. These findings most likely indicate:

A) Class I hemorrhagic shock
B) Class II hemorrhagic shock
C) Class III hemorrhagic shock
D) Class IV hemorrhagic shock

Answer: C

Explanation: This presentation indicates Class III hemorrhagic shock (30-40% blood loss): hypotension, significant tachycardia (>120), and tachypnea (30-40). Class I and II maintain blood pressure. Class IV would show more severe hypotension, possible bradycardia, and decreased consciousness. This patient needs immediate aggressive resuscitation with blood products.

Question 39: What is the most common cause of airway obstruction in an unconscious trauma patient?

A) Blood or secretions
B) Foreign body
C) Tongue falling backward
D) Laryngeal edema

Answer: C

Explanation: The tongue falling backward is the most common cause of airway obstruction in unconscious patients. Loss of muscle tone allows the tongue to block the posterior pharynx. This is why jaw thrust or chin lift are effective first interventions—they move the mandible and tongue forward. While blood, foreign bodies, and edema occur, tongue obstruction is most common.

Question 40: Which finding during the secondary survey requires immediate intervention?

A) Abrasions on both knees
B) Rigid, tender abdomen in a hypotensive patient
C) Bruising on the chest wall
D) Tenderness over the ribs

Answer: B

Explanation: A rigid, tender abdomen in a hypotensive patient indicates likely intraperitoneal hemorrhage requiring immediate surgical intervention. This patient needs emergency laparotomy. The other findings require treatment but aren't immediately life-threatening. Abrasions need cleaning, chest bruising needs monitoring for underlying injury, and rib tenderness needs pain management, but none require immediate intervention like intra-abdominal bleeding.

Question 41: What intervention should be avoided in a patient with suspected increased intracranial pressure?

A) Elevating the head of bed 30 degrees
B) Maintaining adequate blood pressure

C) Hyperventilation to PCO_2 of 25 mmHg
D) Administering pain medication

Answer: C

Explanation: Aggressive hyperventilation to very low PCO_2 (<30 mmHg) should be avoided except as a temporizing measure for acute herniation because it causes cerebral vasoconstriction and can worsen ischemia. Mild hyperventilation targeting PCO_2 of 30-35 mmHg may be appropriate. Elevating the head, maintaining adequate BP, and managing pain are all appropriate for ICP management.

Question 42: A hemothorax is best detected by which assessment finding?

A) Hyperresonance to percussion
B) Dullness to percussion
C) Increased breath sounds
D) Tracheal deviation toward affected side

Answer: B

Explanation: Hemothorax (blood in pleural space) causes dullness to percussion because percussion sound is dampened by fluid. Pneumothorax would cause hyperresonance. Hemothorax decreases (not increases) breath sounds. Tracheal deviation away from (not toward) the affected side occurs in tension pneumothorax, not hemothorax.

Question 43: What is the purpose of the SAMPLE mnemonic in trauma assessment?

A) To guide the primary survey
B) To obtain patient history during secondary survey
C) To prioritize interventions
D) To assess neurological status

Answer: B

Explanation: SAMPLE guides history-taking during the secondary survey: Signs/Symptoms, Allergies, Medications, Past medical history, Last oral intake, Events/Environment. This systematic approach ensures important information isn't missed. The primary survey uses ABCDE. Intervention prioritization follows the primary survey sequence. Neurological assessment uses GCS and pupil checks.

Question 44: Which laboratory value best indicates successful resuscitation from shock?

A) Hemoglobin returning to normal
B) Lactate decreasing toward normal
C) White blood cell count normalizing
D) Sodium level stabilizing

Answer: B

Explanation: Decreasing lactate levels indicate improving tissue perfusion and resolution of anaerobic metabolism, making it the best marker of successful shock resuscitation. Hemoglobin may remain low even with adequate perfusion if blood loss hasn't been fully replaced. WBC changes don't directly reflect perfusion. Sodium levels aren't markers of shock resolution.

Question 45: A patient requires cricothyrotomy. Where should the incision be made?

A) Through the thyroid cartilage
B) Through the cricothyroid membrane
C) Through the cricoid cartilage
D) Between the second and third tracheal rings

Answer: B

Explanation: Cricothyrotomy is performed through the cricothyroid membrane, the space between the thyroid cartilage (above) and cricoid cartilage (below). This location is relatively avascular and accessible, making it ideal for emergency surgical airway. Cutting through cartilage or lower tracheal rings would be more difficult and potentially more damaging.

Clinical Scenarios

These scenarios integrate multiple concepts and require you to think through complete patient management. Read each carefully and consider what priorities guide your decision-making.

Clinical Scenario 1:

A 28-year-old male arrives after a motorcycle crash. He is alert but anxious, with visible road rash on his left side. Initial vital signs: HR 118, BP 108/82, RR 24, SpO2 94% on room air. He complains of left-sided chest pain and difficulty breathing deeply.

On examination, you note decreased breath sounds on the left side, tenderness over multiple left ribs, and crepitus in the left chest wall. His abdomen is soft and non-tender. Pelvis is stable. He has a deformed left forearm.

Questions:

1. What is your primary concern based on the initial assessment?
2. What immediate interventions should be performed?
3. What diagnostic studies are priorities?
4. The patient's BP drops to 88/58 and HR increases to 138. What has likely occurred and what is your intervention?

Answers:

1. Primary concern is potential pneumothorax or hemothorax given decreased breath sounds, chest pain, difficulty breathing, and rib fractures. The mechanism (motorcycle crash) and findings suggest significant thoracic trauma.
2. Immediate interventions: Apply high-flow oxygen via non-rebreather mask, establish two large-bore IV lines, initiate cardiac monitoring, obtain chest X-ray urgently, assess for tension pneumothorax signs, splint the forearm fracture, provide pain control.
3. Priority diagnostics: Chest X-ray (to confirm pneumo/hemothorax), FAST exam (to assess for intra-abdominal bleeding given mechanism), pelvis X-ray, left forearm X-ray. Blood work including CBC, type and crossmatch, lactate.
4. The deterioration suggests progression to tension pneumothorax or development of hemothorax with ongoing bleeding. If tension pneumothorax signs present (tracheal deviation, jugular venous distension, worsening respiratory distress), perform immediate needle decompression. If massive hemothorax suspected, place chest tube. Initiate fluid resuscitation and prepare for possible blood transfusion.

Clinical Scenario 2:

A 62-year-old female fell down a flight of stairs. She is confused and combative. Initial vitals: HR 52, BP 92/58, RR 16, SpO2 98% on room air, temperature 36.8°C. She has bruising on her forehead and abrasions on her back. Her skin is warm and dry below the waist.

1. What type of shock does this presentation suggest?
2. What key assessment must be performed immediately?
3. What findings would you expect on neurological examination?
4. What are your priorities for this patient?

Answers:

1. This presentation suggests neurogenic shock: bradycardia (not tachycardia), hypotension, warm/dry skin below waist. Combined with fall mechanism and confusion, spinal cord injury above T6 is likely.
2. Complete neurological examination including assessment of motor and sensory function in all extremities, GCS scoring, pupil examination, and evaluation for spinal tenderness/step-offs. Full spinal precautions must be maintained.
3. Neurological findings would likely show decreased or absent motor and sensory function below the level of spinal injury, decreased or absent reflexes below the injury, possible decreased rectal tone, and warm/dry skin below injury level from loss of sympathetic tone.
4. Priorities: Maintain spinal immobilization, secure airway (may need intubation if declining), careful fluid resuscitation (avoid overload—these patients can't compensate), likely need for vasopressors to maintain adequate perfusion pressure, urgent neurosurgical consultation, CT of head and complete spine imaging, manage hypothermia risk, treat other injuries identified.

Clinical Scenario 3:

A 19-year-old male presents after a stab wound to the left upper quadrant of his abdomen. He appears pale and diaphoretic. Vitals: HR 128, BP 84/54, RR 28, SpO2 92% on room air. He is alert but restless. The wound is approximately 3 cm long and appears deep. There is minimal external bleeding currently.

Questions:

1. What class of hemorrhagic shock is this patient in?
2. What is the most likely source of bleeding?
3. What immediate interventions should be performed?
4. Does this patient need operative intervention? Why or why not?

Answers:

1. This patient is in Class III hemorrhagic shock (30-40% blood loss): hypotension, significant tachycardia (>120), altered mental status (restlessness), tachypnea. The minimal external bleeding with shock signs indicates significant internal hemorrhage.

2. Most likely source is intra-abdominal bleeding from injury to spleen, stomach, or other left upper quadrant organs. Penetrating trauma to this area frequently injures the spleen. The diaphragm could also be injured, potentially causing hemothorax.
3. Immediate interventions: Apply high-flow oxygen, establish two large-bore IV lines, initiate massive transfusion protocol (don't wait—this patient needs blood now), limit crystalloid to 1-2 liters, perform FAST exam, chest X-ray (to rule out hemothorax if diaphragm injured), activate surgical team immediately, maintain permissive hypotension until OR, cover wound with sterile dressing (don't explore or pack), keep patient NPO.
4. Yes, this patient needs immediate operative intervention. He is hemodynamically unstable from penetrating torso trauma, indicating ongoing hemorrhage that won't stop without surgical control. The combination of mechanism (penetrating left upper quadrant), shock state, and lack of response to initial resuscitation mandates emergency laparotomy. Don't delay for CT imaging—this patient needs surgery now.

Clinical Scenario 4:

A 45-year-old construction worker was struck by a falling beam. He has obvious chest trauma with a segment of chest wall moving paradoxically. He is in severe distress. Vitals: HR 118, BP 128/88, RR 32 and labored, SpO2 88% on room air. He has bilateral breath sounds but they are decreased on the right.

Questions:

1. What injury does the paradoxical chest wall movement indicate?
2. What is the priority intervention?
3. What underlying injury commonly accompanies this chest wall injury?
4. How should pain be managed and why is it important?

Answers:

1. Paradoxical chest wall movement indicates flail chest—multiple ribs fractured in multiple places creating a free-floating segment. The segment moves inward during inspiration (when chest expands) and outward during expiration (opposite of normal chest wall movement).
2. Priority interventions: Immediate high-flow oxygen via non-rebreather (hypoxia must be corrected), position patient on injured side if possible (stabilizes flail segment), prepare for possible positive pressure ventilation if hypoxia doesn't improve, establish IV access, obtain chest X-ray, monitor closely for deterioration requiring intubation and mechanical ventilation.
3. Pulmonary contusion commonly accompanies flail chest. The force required to create flail chest also contuses underlying lung tissue, impairing gas exchange. This combination of chest wall instability and underlying lung injury causes the severe respiratory distress. Pulmonary contusion typically worsens over 24-48 hours.
4. Pain management is critical because severe chest pain causes splinting (shallow breathing), leading to atelectasis, pneumonia, and respiratory failure. Adequate analgesia allows deeper breathing and coughing. Options include IV opioids, epidural analgesia, or intercostal nerve blocks. Pain control may prevent need for mechanical ventilation by allowing effective spontaneous breathing.

Clinical Scenario 5:

A 35-year-old female was the restrained driver in a high-speed frontal collision. She complains of abdominal pain. Vitals: HR 102, BP 118/76, RR 20, SpO2 97%. She has bruising across her lower abdomen in a seatbelt pattern. Abdomen is tender but soft. FAST exam is negative. She is alert and oriented.

Two hours later, her vitals change: HR 118, BP 98/68, RR 24. She reports worsening abdominal pain. Repeat FAST exam shows free fluid in Morrison's pouch.

Questions:

1. What does the seatbelt sign indicate?
2. Why was the initial FAST exam negative?
3. What injury has likely occurred?
4. What is the appropriate management now?

Answers:

1. Seatbelt sign (bruising across abdomen from seatbelt) indicates significant force transmission to abdominal contents and is associated with high rates of intra-abdominal injury, particularly hollow viscus (bowel and mesentery) injuries and solid organ injuries. This sign should prompt thorough evaluation even if patient appears stable initially.
2. The initial FAST exam was negative because either insufficient blood had accumulated yet to be visible on ultrasound, or the bleeding was slow and contained initially. Some injuries (particularly hollow viscus injuries) don't initially cause significant free fluid. FAST sensitivity is limited for small amounts of blood or early in injury evolution.
3. Likely injury is spleen or liver laceration that was initially bleeding slowly but has now progressed, or delayed rupture of an injured organ. The mechanism (frontal impact), seatbelt sign, and progression from stable to shock with new free fluid strongly suggest solid organ injury with evolving hemorrhage.
4. Appropriate management: The patient was initially stable but now shows clinical deterioration with new free fluid on FAST—this requires immediate surgical consultation.

Options include:

If patient becomes hemodynamically unstable: Emergency laparotomy for hemorrhage control
If patient remains relatively stable: Urgent CT scan to define injury (shows specific organ injuries, grades them, identifies active bleeding), followed by either operative management or close observation with serial exams depending on findings

Chapter 4: Thoracic and Neck Trauma

Thoracic injuries account for approximately 25% of trauma deaths, with many being potentially survivable if recognized and treated promptly. The chest contains vital structures—heart, great vessels, lungs, trachea, esophagus—and injuries to these can rapidly become fatal. Understanding thoracic trauma requires knowledge of anatomy, injury patterns, and immediate life-saving interventions.

This chapter covers both immediately life-threatening injuries (addressed during the primary survey) and potentially life-threatening injuries (identified during secondary survey). We'll also address neck trauma, which shares anatomical proximity and similar management principles.

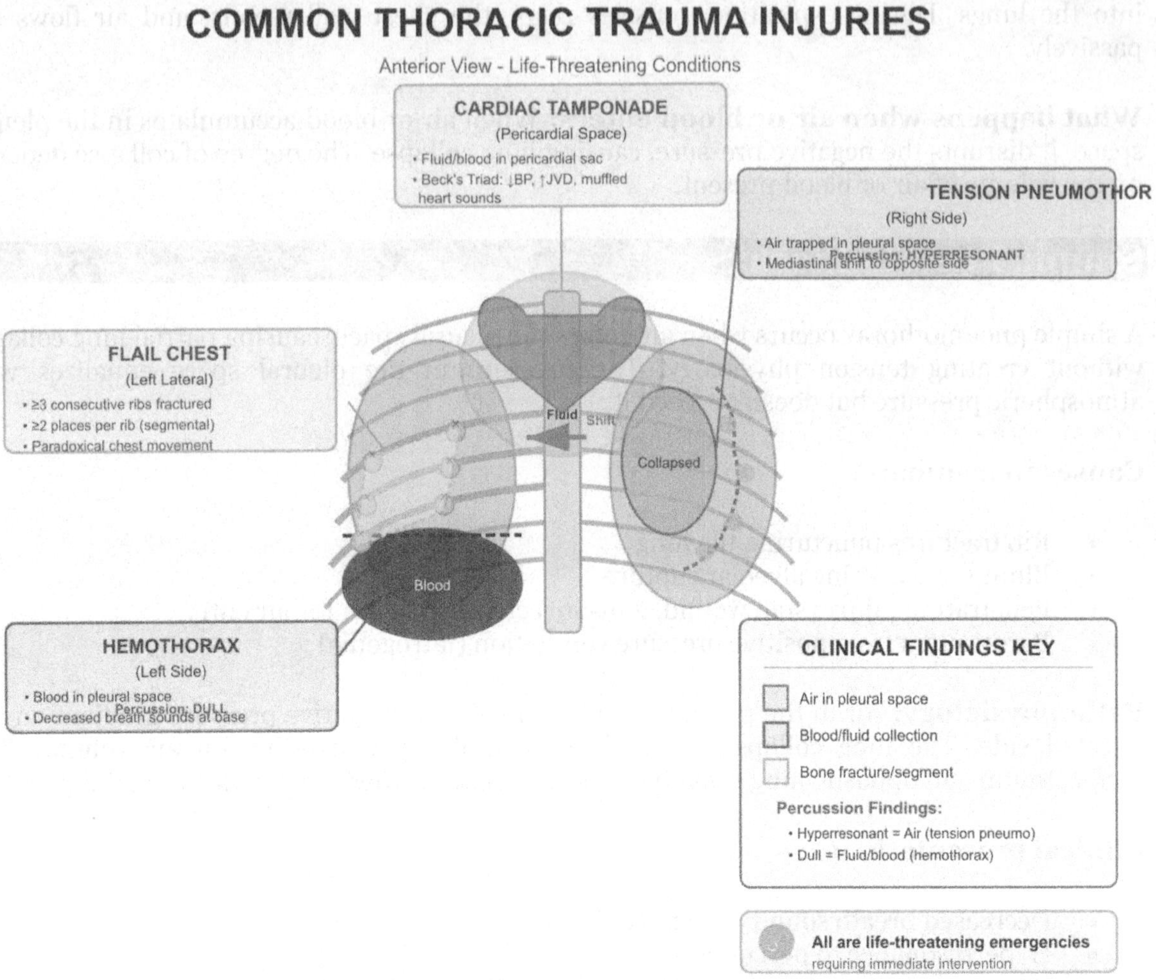

Semi-transparent overlay showing internal lung and heart structures with injury locations

Pneumothorax and Hemothorax

Air or blood in the pleural space disrupts normal respiratory mechanics and can compromise both breathing and circulation. Understanding the spectrum from simple to tension pneumothorax, and recognizing massive hemothorax, is fundamental to trauma nursing.

Understanding Pleural Space Physiology

The pleural space is the potential space between the visceral pleura (covering the lung) and parietal pleura (lining the chest wall). Normally, this space contains only a thin layer of lubricating fluid and has negative pressure relative to atmospheric pressure. This negative pressure keeps the lungs expanded against the chest wall.

Normal breathing mechanics: During inspiration, the diaphragm contracts and chest wall expands, creating more negative pressure in the pleural space. This pressure gradient pulls air into the lungs. During expiration, muscles relax, the chest wall recoils, and air flows out passively.

What happens when air or blood enters: When air or blood accumulates in the pleural space, it disrupts the negative pressure, causing lung collapse. The degree of collapse depends on the volume of air or blood present.

Simple Pneumothorax

A simple pneumothorax occurs when air enters the pleural space, causing partial lung collapse without creating tension physiology. The pressure in the pleural space equalizes with atmospheric pressure but doesn't exceed it.

Causes in trauma:

- Rib fractures puncturing the lung
- Blunt force causing alveolar rupture
- Penetrating injury (stab wound, gunshot) creating a path for air entry
- Barotrauma from positive pressure ventilation (iatrogenic)

Pathophysiology: Air in the pleural space eliminates the negative pressure gradient on the affected side. The lung collapses partially or completely depending on air volume. The mediastinum and opposite lung remain unaffected because there's no pressure buildup.

Clinical presentation:

- Decreased breath sounds on affected side
- Hyperresonance to percussion
- Chest pain (often pleuritic—worse with breathing)
- Dyspnea (mild to moderate depending on size)
- May be asymptomatic if small (<15% lung volume)

Diagnosis: Chest X-ray shows:

- Visible pleural line (edge of collapsed lung)
- Absence of lung markings peripheral to this line
- Lung appears collapsed toward the hilum

Management:

- Small pneumothorax (<15%) without respiratory distress: May observe with supplemental oxygen and serial chest X-rays
- Large pneumothorax or any pneumothorax with respiratory compromise: Chest tube insertion
- Positive pressure ventilation: Always requires chest tube (converts to tension risk)

Tension Pneumothorax

Tension pneumothorax is a life-threatening emergency where air continuously enters the pleural space but cannot escape, creating a one-way valve effect. Pressure builds progressively, causing complete lung collapse, mediastinal shift, and compression of the great vessels.

Mechanism: Often develops when:

- Chest wall injury creates a one-way valve (air enters during inspiration, can't escape during expiration)
- Positive pressure ventilation forces air into pleural space through lung injury
- Simple pneumothorax progresses under certain conditions

Pathophysiology cascade:

1. Air accumulates under increasing pressure
2. Lung collapses completely on affected side
3. Mediastinum shifts away from affected side
4. Vena cava gets kinked/compressed
5. Venous return to heart decreases
6. Cardiac output drops
7. Patient develops obstructive shock

Clinical presentation (classic signs):

- Severe respiratory distress
- Absent breath sounds on affected side
- Hyperresonance to percussion
- Tracheal deviation away from affected side (late sign)
- Jugular venous distension (may not be present if hypovolemic)
- Hypotension and shock
- Tachycardia
- Decreased oxygen saturation

Critical point: This is a clinical diagnosis. Never wait for chest X-ray confirmation if you suspect tension pneumothorax. The patient will die while you wait for imaging.

Immediate management:

1. **Needle decompression:** Insert 14-gauge or larger needle/catheter into the second intercostal space at the midclavicular line on the affected side. Insert just above the rib (avoiding neurovascular bundle that runs below ribs). You should hear a rush of air. This converts tension pneumothorax to simple pneumothorax, buying time for chest tube placement.
2. **Chest tube insertion:** Definitive treatment. Place large-bore chest tube (typically 36-40 French) in the "safe triangle" (bounded by lateral border of pectoralis major, lateral border of latissimus dorsi, line superior to horizontal level of nipple, and apex below axilla). This location avoids major muscles and breast tissue.

Technique considerations: Needle decompression may fail if:

- Needle too short to reach pleural space (obesity, muscular chest wall)
- Needle placed incorrectly
- Needle/catheter kinks
- Blood clot blocks catheter

If patient doesn't improve after needle decompression, proceed immediately to chest tube or consider repeating needle decompression.

Open Pneumothorax (Sucking Chest Wound)

An open pneumothorax occurs when a chest wall defect allows air to enter the pleural space directly with each breath. If the defect is larger than two-thirds the diameter of the trachea, air preferentially enters through the wound rather than the trachea because it's the path of least resistance.

Pathophysiology: Air flows in and out of the chest wound with breathing, creating a "sucking" sound. The affected lung can't expand properly because air enters the pleural space instead of the lung.

Clinical presentation:

- Obvious chest wall wound
- Audible sucking sound with breathing
- Blood bubbling from wound
- Decreased breath sounds on affected side
- Respiratory distress

Management:

1. **Immediate:** Cover wound with occlusive dressing (sterile plastic, petroleum gauze) taped on three sides only. This creates a flutter valve—air can escape during exhalation but can't enter during inhalation.
2. **Why three sides?** If you tape all four sides, you risk creating a tension pneumothorax as air that's already in the chest (or continuing to leak from lung injury) can't escape.
3. **Definitive:** Place chest tube away from the wound itself, then clean and close the wound surgically.

Monitoring: Watch for tension pneumothorax development. If patient deteriorates after dressing application, remove the dressing temporarily to release trapped air, then reapply.

Hemothorax

Hemothorax is blood accumulation in the pleural space. Massive hemothorax (≥1500 mL or one-third of blood volume) is immediately life-threatening from both impaired ventilation and hemorrhagic shock.

Sources of bleeding:

- Intercostal vessels (from rib fractures)
- Internal mammary artery
- Lung parenchyma (usually self-limiting)
- Great vessels (aorta, vena cava, subclavian)—massive, rapidly fatal if not quickly treated
- Heart (rarely—usually immediately fatal)

Pathophysiology: Blood in pleural space compresses the lung, preventing expansion. If volume is large, it also shifts mediastinum and compresses the opposite lung. Unlike air, blood doesn't expand with pressure, but large volumes still cause significant respiratory and circulatory compromise.

Clinical presentation:

- Decreased or absent breath sounds on affected side
- Dullness to percussion (blood dampens sound, opposite of pneumothorax)
- Decreased chest wall movement
- Signs of shock if massive (tachycardia, hypotension, pale/cool skin)
- Neck veins may be flat (hypovolemia) or distended (if mediastinal shift affects venous return)

Diagnosis:

- Chest X-ray shows white opacity (blood is radiopaque) usually at lung base initially
- Requires 200-500 mL to be visible on upright chest X-ray
- Supine chest X-ray (common in trauma) less sensitive—blood layers posteriorly

Management:

1. **Large-bore chest tube** (36-40 French) for drainage and monitoring
2. **Autotransfusion** if available—blood drained from chest can be collected and reinfused
3. **Massive transfusion protocol** if patient in shock
4. **Monitor drainage:**
    - Initial drainage >1500 mL: Consider thoracotomy
    - Ongoing drainage >200 mL/hr for 2-4 hours: Likely needs operative intervention
    - Decreasing drainage with improving vital signs: Continue monitoring

Complications:

- Retained hemothorax leading to fibrothorax (scarring) or empyema (infection)
- Coagulopathy from massive blood loss
- Need for early thoracotomy if bleeding doesn't stop

Hemopneumothorax

Both air and blood in pleural space—combines features of pneumothorax and hemothorax. Management is chest tube drainage with monitoring for both continued air leak (persistent pneumothorax) and continued bleeding (ongoing hemorrhage).

Cardiac Tamponade

Cardiac tamponade occurs when blood accumulates in the pericardial sac, compressing the heart and preventing adequate filling. This is an obstructive shock emergency.

Understanding pericardial anatomy: The pericardium is a fibrous sac surrounding the heart. It normally contains 15-50 mL of serous fluid for lubrication. The pericardium is relatively inelastic, so it can't stretch rapidly to accommodate additional fluid.

Pathophysiology: Blood entering the pericardial sac (from cardiac or great vessel injury) compresses all cardiac chambers. The compression prevents ventricular filling during diastole. Without adequate filling, cardiac output drops precipitously regardless of heart rate or contractility.

How much blood causes tamponade? This depends on rate of accumulation:

- Acute tamponade: As little as 150-200 mL can be fatal if it accumulates rapidly
- Chronic accumulation: Pericardium can stretch to accommodate larger volumes if accumulation is slow

In trauma, accumulation is acute, so small volumes cause critical compromise quickly.

Causes in trauma:

- Penetrating chest trauma (most common—stab wounds to chest, especially near sternum)
- Blunt cardiac injury with myocardial rupture (rare, usually fatal at scene)
- Great vessel injury with blood tracking into pericardium

Clinical presentation (Beck's triad):

1. **Hypotension** (from decreased cardiac output)
2. **Jugular venous distension** (blood backs up because heart can't accept incoming volume)
3. **Muffled heart sounds** (fluid in pericardium dampens sound transmission)

Additional signs:

- Pulsus paradoxus: Systolic blood pressure drops >10 mmHg during inspiration (compression prevents normal ventricular filling response to respiratory changes)
- Narrow pulse pressure
- Tachycardia (compensatory attempt to maintain cardiac output)
- Shock despite no obvious external bleeding

Diagnosis:

- **Clinical diagnosis:** High suspicion based on mechanism and presentation
- **FAST exam:** Shows fluid in pericardial sac (black stripe around heart)
- **ECG:** May show low voltage, electrical alternans (alternating QRS amplitude)
- **Chest X-ray:** May show enlarged cardiac silhouette if sufficient volume (not reliable acutely)

Management:

Temporizing measure—Pericardiocentesis:

- Insert needle below xiphoid process, directed toward left shoulder
- Aspirate fluid (even 20-30 mL can dramatically improve hemodynamics)
- This is a temporizing measure only—buys time until definitive surgical repair

Definitive treatment:

- Emergency thoracotomy (in ED if patient deteriorating)
- Operative repair of cardiac injury in OR if time permits transport

Key point: Aggressive fluid resuscitation before pericardiocentesis can temporarily improve cardiac output by increasing filling pressure, but definitive treatment is pericardial drainage and repair of the cardiac injury.

Flail Chest and Rib Fractures

Rib fractures are the most common thoracic injury. Flail chest—multiple ribs fractured in multiple places—is a severe injury with significant morbidity and mortality.

Simple Rib Fractures

Mechanism: Direct impact to chest wall (motor vehicle crash, fall, assault, crush injury).

Clinical presentation:

- Point tenderness at fracture site
- Pain with breathing, coughing, or movement
- Crepitus (bone ends grinding) sometimes palpable
- Patient splints breathing (takes shallow breaths to avoid pain)

Significance: The fracture itself isn't usually life-threatening, but complications are:

- **Hypoventilation:** Pain causes splinting, leading to atelectasis and pneumonia
- **Associated injuries:** First and second rib fractures (protected by clavicle and shoulder) require tremendous force and suggest possible great vessel injury. Lower rib fractures (9-12) suggest possible liver or spleen injury.
- **Elderly patients:** Higher mortality from rib fractures due to limited respiratory reserve and higher pneumonia risk

Diagnosis: Chest X-ray, though may not show all fractures. CT is more sensitive.

Management:

- **Pain control is priority:** Adequate analgesia allows deeper breathing and coughing, preventing complications
  - Oral or IV analgesics (NSAIDs, opioids)
  - Intercostal nerve blocks (local anesthetic injected around affected nerves)
  - Epidural analgesia for multiple fractures (excellent pain control)
- **Incentive spirometry:** Encourages deep breathing to prevent atelectasis
- **Pulmonary hygiene:** Coughing, deep breathing exercises
- **Avoid rib belts/chest wrapping:** These restrict breathing and increase pneumonia risk

Flail Chest

Definition: Two or more adjacent ribs fractured in two or more places, creating a free-floating segment of chest wall.

Mechanism: Significant blunt force to chest (high-speed motor vehicle crash, pedestrian struck, crushing injury).

Pathophysiology: The flail segment moves paradoxically:

- **Inspiration:** Negative intrathoracic pressure pulls flail segment inward while rest of chest expands outward
- **Expiration:** Positive pressure pushes flail segment outward while rest of chest contracts inward

This paradoxical motion impairs ventilation. However, the more significant problem is usually underlying pulmonary contusion (discussed below), which develops in most flail chest patients.

Clinical presentation:

- Visible paradoxical chest wall movement
- Severe pain
- Respiratory distress
- Decreased breath sounds on affected side
- Patient in severe distress, often splinting the area

Diagnosis: Clinical observation of paradoxical movement, confirmed by chest X-ray or CT showing multiple rib fractures.

Management:

Initial:

- Oxygen supplementation
- Aggressive pain control (often requires epidural for adequate relief)
- Fluid management (careful—risk of pulmonary contusion progression)

Definitive:

- **Internal pneumatic stabilization:** Positive pressure ventilation (non-invasive like BiPAP, or intubation with mechanical ventilation) acts as an internal splint, stabilizing the chest wall from inside
- **Duration:** May need ventilatory support for days to weeks until fractures begin healing
- **Surgical fixation:** Some centers now surgically repair flail segments with plates/screws in select patients, reducing ventilator days and improving outcomes

Complications:

- Pulmonary contusion progression
- Pneumonia (from splinting and impaired secretion clearance)
- Respiratory failure requiring prolonged ventilation
- Chronic pain and chest wall deformity

Tracheal and Laryngeal Injuries

Airway injuries from trauma are uncommon but immediately life-threatening. The trachea and larynx can be injured by blunt or penetrating mechanisms.

Mechanisms of Injury

Blunt trauma:

- Direct anterior neck impact (steering wheel, clothesline injury, hanging)
- Sudden deceleration with hyperextension (shearing forces)

Penetrating trauma:

- Stab wounds to neck
- Gunshot wounds traversing neck

Clinical Presentation

Cardinal signs suggesting airway injury:

- **Hoarseness or voice changes:** Vocal cord injury or laryngeal fracture
- **Subcutaneous emphysema:** Air escaping from airway into tissues (crepitus palpable in neck)
- **Hemoptysis:** Coughing blood from airway injury
- **Respiratory distress:** Partial airway obstruction or inadequate ventilation
- **Stridor:** High-pitched breath sound indicating upper airway narrowing
- **Dysphagia:** Difficulty swallowing may accompany laryngeal injury

Examination findings:

- Visible neck trauma
- Loss of thyroid cartilage prominence (suggests crush injury)
- Palpable crepitus
- Air bubbling from neck wound
- Hematoma compressing airway

Management

Immediate priorities:

1. **Secure airway:** This is challenging because:
    - Normal anatomy may be disrupted
    - Intubation attempts might create false passage
    - Bleeding may obscure view
    - Hematoma may compress airway

2. **Approach options:**
    - **If patient maintaining airway:** Position patient upright, give supplemental oxygen, prepare for emergency airway intervention, keep patient calm (agitation worsens dyspnea)
    - **If immediate intervention needed:** Consider awake fiberoptic intubation (allows visualization of anatomy), surgical airway (cricothyrotomy or tracheostomy) may be necessary
3. **Definitive:** Surgical exploration and repair in OR

Key principle: Never attempt blind intubation in patients with suspected laryngotracheal injury. If intubation is necessary and anatomy unclear, have surgical airway equipment immediately available.

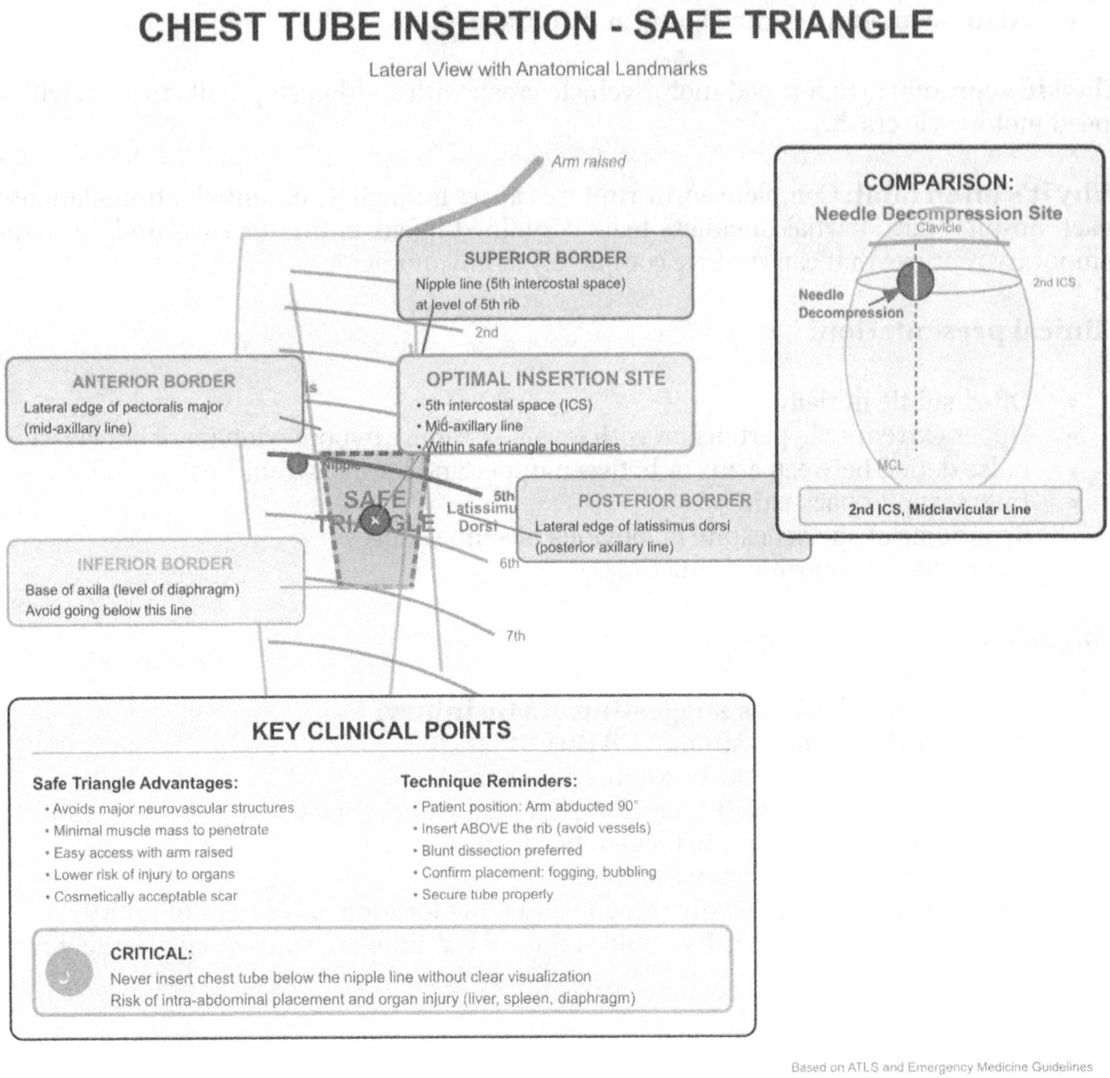

Great Vessel Injuries

Injuries to the aorta, vena cava, or other major thoracic vessels are often immediately fatal at the scene. Those who survive to hospital arrival require rapid diagnosis and intervention.

Traumatic Aortic Disruption

Mechanism: Sudden deceleration causes shearing forces at points where mobile aorta becomes fixed:

- **Most common site:** Aortic isthmus (just distal to left subclavian artery where aorta is tethered by ligamentum arteriosum)
- **Also occurs:** Ascending aorta, at diaphragm

Classic scenario: High-speed motor vehicle crash with sudden stop, falls from height, high-speed motorcycle crash.

Why it's often fatal: Complete aortic rupture causes immediate exsanguination. Patients who reach hospital have partial thickness tears contained by adventitia or surrounding tissues—a temporary reprieve that can rupture completely at any moment.

Clinical presentation:

- Often subtle initially
- Upper extremity hypertension with lower extremity hypotension (rare but classic)
- Pulse deficit between arms or between upper and lower extremities
- Interscapular back pain
- Symptoms of shock despite no obvious bleeding source
- Harsh systolic murmur (sometimes)

Diagnosis:

- **Chest X-ray findings suggesting aortic injury:**
    - Widened mediastinum (>8 cm)
    - Obliteration of aortic knob
    - Deviation of trachea or nasogastric tube to the right
    - Depression of left mainstem bronchus
    - Left pleural effusion (hemothorax)
- **CT angiography:** Definitive diagnosis, shows location and extent of injury
- **Traditional angiography:** Gold standard but time-consuming, now largely replaced by CT angiography

Management:

- **Blood pressure control:** Keep systolic <100-120 mmHg (reduces shear stress on injured vessel while maintaining perfusion)
- **Beta blockers:** Reduce heart rate and force of contraction

- **Surgical or endovascular repair:**
    - Traditional open repair (thoracotomy with graft placement)
    - Endovascular stent graft (less invasive, increasingly common)
- **Timing:** Emergency repair if unstable or expanding hematoma; may delay repair hours if patient stable and other life-threatening injuries need attention

Other Great Vessel Injuries

Injuries to subclavian vessels, innominate artery, or vena cava present with:

- Massive hemorrhage (external if penetrating neck injury, internal if intrathoracic)
- Expanding hematoma
- Shock out of proportion to visible injuries
- Absent or decreased pulses distal to injury
- Neurological deficits if brachial plexus compressed by hematoma

Management principles:

- Control external bleeding with direct pressure (never blindly clamp bleeding vessels in neck—risks nerve damage)
- Immediate vascular surgery consultation
- Prepare for operative repair
- Massive transfusion protocol if needed

Neck zones (for penetrating trauma): Understanding anatomical zones helps predict injury patterns:

- **Zone I:** Base of neck (clavicles to cricoid cartilage)—contains great vessels, thoracic outlet structures. Highest mortality. Difficult surgical access.
- **Zone II:** Mid-neck (cricoid to angle of mandible)—contains carotid arteries, jugular veins, trachea, esophagus. Most common injury site. Best surgical access.
- **Zone III:** Upper neck (angle of mandible to skull base)—contains distal carotid, vertebral arteries. Difficult surgical access.

Penetrating neck injury management:

- Zone II with hard signs of vascular injury (expanding hematoma, active bleeding, absent pulse, bruit): Immediate operative exploration
- Other zones or soft signs: CT angiography to identify specific injuries before surgery

Chapter 4 Practice Questions

Question 1: A patient presents with absent breath sounds on the right, hyperresonance to percussion, severe respiratory distress, hypotension, and tracheal deviation to the left. What is the priority intervention?

A) Obtain stat chest X-ray
B) Prepare for chest tube insertion
C) Perform immediate needle decompression
D) Intubate the patient

Answer: C

Explanation: This presentation indicates tension pneumothorax requiring immediate needle decompression. This is a clinical diagnosis that should never wait for imaging. Needle decompression converts tension to simple pneumothorax, stabilizing the patient until chest tube placement.

Question 2: Where should a chest tube be inserted for pneumothorax or hemothorax?

A) Second intercostal space, midclavicular line
B) Fourth or fifth intercostal space in the "safe triangle"
C) Sixth intercostal space, posterior axillary line
D) Third intercostal space, midaxillary line

Answer: B

Explanation: The safe triangle (bordered by lateral pectoralis major, lateral latissimus dorsi, and horizontal nipple line) in the fourth or fifth intercostal space is the standard location for chest tube placement. This avoids major muscles and breast tissue while providing good drainage. The second intercostal space is for needle decompression, not chest tube placement.

Question 3: An open pneumothorax should be initially managed by:

A) Immediate chest tube insertion
B) Occlusive dressing taped on all four sides
C) Occlusive dressing taped on three sides
D) Packing the wound with gauze

Answer: C

Explanation: An occlusive dressing taped on three sides creates a flutter valve effect, allowing air to escape during exhalation but preventing entry during inhalation. Taping all four sides risks creating tension pneumothorax. Chest tube placement follows initial dressing application but isn't the immediate first step.

Question 4: What assessment finding differentiates hemothorax from pneumothorax?

A) Absent breath sounds
B) Dullness to percussion
C) Respiratory distress
D) Decreased chest wall movement

Answer: B

Explanation: Hemothorax produces dullness to percussion because blood in the pleural space dampens the percussion sound. Pneumothorax produces hyperresonance. Both cause absent breath sounds, respiratory distress, and decreased chest wall movement, making dullness versus hyperresonance the key differentiating feature.

Question 5: A chest tube drains 1800 mL of blood immediately upon insertion. What is the appropriate action?

A) Continue monitoring and observe
B) Remove and reinsert the chest tube
C) Clamp the chest tube
D) Prepare for immediate thoracotomy

Answer: D

Explanation: Immediate drainage of >1500 mL indicates massive hemothorax with ongoing hemorrhage that likely requires surgical control. This patient needs thoracotomy for hemorrhage control. Simply monitoring allows continued blood loss. Never clamp a chest tube except briefly for tube changes.

Question 6: Beck's triad of cardiac tamponade includes:

A) Hypotension, muffled heart sounds, jugular venous distension
B) Hypotension, tachycardia, decreased breath sounds
C) Bradycardia, hypertension, irregular respirations
D) Tachycardia, hypertension, chest pain

Answer: A

Explanation: Beck's triad consists of hypotension (decreased cardiac output), muffled heart sounds (fluid in pericardium dampens sounds), and jugular venous distension (blood backs up because heart can't fill properly). This triad suggests cardiac tamponade, though all three signs may not always be present.

Question 7: What is the immediate management for cardiac tamponade in a deteriorating trauma patient?

A) Aggressive IV fluid resuscitation
B) Pericardiocentesis
C) Emergency thoracotomy
D) Stat echocardiogram

Answer: B

Explanation: Pericardiocentesis is the immediate intervention for cardiac tamponade, removing fluid from the pericardial sac to restore cardiac filling. Even small volumes (20-30 mL) can dramatically improve hemodynamics. Emergency thoracotomy may be needed for definitive repair, but pericardiocentesis is the initial stabilizing intervention. Don't delay for echocardiogram in a deteriorating patient.

Question 8: Flail chest is defined as:

A) Single rib fracture with severe pain
B) Multiple rib fractures on one side
C) Two or more ribs fractured in two or more places
D) Sternal fracture with costochondral separation

Answer: C

Explanation: Flail chest occurs when two or more adjacent ribs are fractured in two or more places each, creating a free-floating segment that moves paradoxically with breathing. This requires significant force and is associated with underlying pulmonary contusion.

Question 9: What is the most significant underlying injury associated with flail chest?

A) Pneumothorax
B) Hemothorax
C) Pulmonary contusion
D) Cardiac contusion

Answer: C

Explanation: Pulmonary contusion occurs in most flail chest patients and is often more problematic than the chest wall injury itself. The force required to create flail chest also contuses underlying lung tissue, impairing gas exchange. Contusion typically worsens over 24-48 hours.

Question 10: The primary goal of pain management in rib fractures is to:

A) Make the patient comfortable
B) Allow adequate ventilation and prevent complications
C) Facilitate early discharge
D) Reduce inflammation

Answer: B

Explanation: While patient comfort is important, the primary clinical goal of pain management in rib fractures is enabling adequate ventilation. Pain causes splinting (shallow breathing), leading to atelectasis and pneumonia. Adequate analgesia allows deeper breathing and effective coughing, preventing respiratory complications.

Question 11: Which rib fracture location suggests possible great vessel injury?

A) Ribs 3-5
B) Ribs 6-8
C) Ribs 1-2
D) Ribs 9-12

Answer: C

Explanation: First and second rib fractures require tremendous force because these ribs are protected by the clavicle and shoulder girdle. The force needed to fracture them suggests possible injury to underlying great vessels (subclavian artery and vein, aorta). Lower rib fractures (9-12) suggest possible liver or spleen injury.

Question 12: A patient with subcutaneous emphysema, hoarseness, and respiratory distress after blunt neck trauma most likely has:

A) Cervical spine fracture
B) Esophageal injury
C) Tracheal or laryngeal injury
D) Carotid artery injury

Answer: C

Explanation: This triad (subcutaneous emphysema, voice changes, respiratory distress) indicates tracheal or laryngeal injury. Air escaping from the damaged airway creates subcutaneous emphysema. Vocal cord or laryngeal damage causes hoarseness. This is an airway emergency requiring careful management.

Question 13: What is the most common site of traumatic aortic disruption?

A) Ascending aorta
B) Aortic arch
C) Aortic isthmus (just distal to left subclavian artery)
D) Descending aorta at the diaphragm

Answer: C

Explanation: The aortic isthmus (just distal to the left subclavian artery) is the most common site of traumatic aortic disruption. This location is where the mobile aortic arch transitions to the fixed descending aorta, creating shear forces during deceleration injuries. The aorta is tethered here by the ligamentum arteriosum.

Question 14: Which chest X-ray finding suggests possible traumatic aortic injury?

A) Pulmonary edema
B) Widened mediastinum (>8 cm)
C) Pleural effusion on the right
D) Elevated hemidiaphragm

Answer: B

Explanation: Widened mediastinum (>8 cm) on chest X-ray suggests mediastinal hematoma, which may indicate aortic or great vessel injury. Other suggestive findings include obliterated aortic knob, tracheal deviation to the right, and depression of the left mainstem bronchus. CT angiography confirms the diagnosis.

Question 15: Initial management of suspected traumatic aortic injury includes:

A) Immediate surgical repair
B) Blood pressure control to keep systolic 100-120 mmHg

C) Aggressive fluid resuscitation
D) Prophylactic antibiotics

Answer: B

Explanation: Blood pressure control is crucial in suspected aortic injury to reduce shear stress on the injured vessel while maintaining adequate organ perfusion. Target systolic BP 100-120 mmHg using beta-blockers to reduce both blood pressure and heart rate/contractility. This prevents rupture of the contained injury while preparing for definitive repair.

Question 16: A patient has paradoxical chest wall movement with severe respiratory distress. The most appropriate initial ventilatory support is:

A) Nasal cannula oxygen
B) Non-rebreather mask
C) Positive pressure ventilation (BiPAP or mechanical ventilation)
D) Simple face mask

Answer: C

Explanation: Flail chest with severe respiratory distress requires positive pressure ventilation, which acts as an internal pneumatic splint stabilizing the chest wall from inside. This may be non-invasive (BiPAP) or require intubation and mechanical ventilation. Simple oxygen delivery devices don't address the mechanical ventilation problem.

Question 17: What is the recommended size chest tube for hemothorax drainage?

A) 20-24 French
B) 28-32 French
C) 36-40 French
D) 12-16 French

Answer: C

Explanation: Large-bore chest tubes (36-40 French) are needed for adequate hemothorax drainage because blood is viscous and can clot. Smaller tubes may clog with clots, preventing effective drainage. Small tubes are appropriate for simple pneumothorax but inadequate for blood drainage.

Question 18: A tension pneumothorax that doesn't respond to needle decompression may be due to:

A) Incorrect diagnosis
B) Needle too short to reach pleural space
C) Needle placed in wrong location
D) All of the above

Answer: D

Explanation: Needle decompression can fail for multiple reasons: the diagnosis was wrong, the needle is too short (especially in obese or muscular patients), incorrect placement, or catheter kinking. If the patient doesn't improve, proceed immediately to chest tube insertion or consider repeating needle decompression in a different location.

Question 19: Pericardiocentesis is performed by inserting a needle:

A) Below the xiphoid process directed toward the left shoulder
B) At the cardiac apex directed superiorly
C) In the left fifth intercostal space
D) At the right sternal border

Answer: A

Explanation: The subxiphoid approach is standard for pericardiocentesis. Insert the needle just below and to the left of the xiphoid process, advancing at a 45-degree angle toward the left shoulder. This approach avoids coronary arteries and minimizes risk of myocardial puncture. ECG monitoring during the procedure helps detect ventricular contact.

Question 20: Which finding indicates that chest tube output requires surgical intervention?

A) 50 mL/hour for 4 hours
B) 200 mL/hour for 3 hours
C) Total output of 800 mL over 8 hours
D) Serosanguinous drainage

Answer: B

Explanation: Ongoing drainage of >200 mL/hour for 2-4 hours indicates continued bleeding requiring surgical intervention. Initial drainage >1500 mL also suggests need for surgery. Options A and C show manageable drainage rates. Serosanguinous drainage is normal as blood mixes with pleural fluid.

Question 21: A patient with multiple rib fractures develops increasing oxygen requirements and infiltrates on chest X-ray over 24 hours. This most likely represents:

A) Pneumonia
B) Pulmonary contusion progression
C) Acute respiratory distress syndrome
D) Pulmonary embolism

Answer: B

Explanation: Pulmonary contusion typically evolves over 24-48 hours after injury, with increasing infiltrates on imaging and worsening gas exchange. This pattern after chest trauma with rib fractures is classic for contusion progression. Pneumonia would be unlikely this early. ARDS typically develops later. PE wouldn't cause infiltrates.

Question 22: What intervention should be avoided in a patient with suspected laryngeal fracture?

A) Supplemental oxygen
B) Keeping patient calm and upright
C) Blind nasotracheal intubation attempts
D) Having surgical airway equipment ready

Answer: C

Explanation: Blind intubation attempts in suspected laryngeal injury risk creating a false passage, complete airway obstruction, or worsening the injury. If intubation is necessary, use fiberoptic guidance to visualize anatomy, or proceed directly to surgical airway. Oxygen, upright positioning, and surgical airway preparation are all appropriate.

Question 23: The purpose of autotransfusion in hemothorax management is to:

A) Prevent infection
B) Reinfuse the patient's own blood drained from the chest
C) Measure exact blood loss
D) Test for esophageal injury

Answer: B

Explanation: Autotransfusion collects blood drained from the chest tube and reinfuses it to the patient, providing immediate volume replacement with the patient's own blood. This avoids transfusion reactions, conserves blood bank resources, and replaces volume quickly. Blood must be collected in special autotransfusion systems and reinfused within 4-6 hours.

Question 24: A widened pulse pressure in a trauma patient with chest injury may indicate:

A) Cardiac tamponade
B) Tension pneumothorax
C) Aortic regurgitation from valve injury
D) Hypovolemic shock

Answer: C

Explanation: Widened pulse pressure (large difference between systolic and diastolic) can indicate aortic regurgitation from blunt cardiac injury affecting the aortic valve. Cardiac tamponade and tension pneumothorax cause narrowed pulse pressure. Hypovolemic shock also causes narrowed pulse pressure from vasoconstriction.

Question 25: Zone II penetrating neck injuries with hard signs of vascular injury require:

A) CT angiography before surgery
B) Immediate operative exploration
C) Observation for 24 hours
D) Angiography in interventional radiology

Answer: B

Explanation: Zone II injuries with hard signs (expanding hematoma, active bleeding, absent pulse, shock, airway compromise) require immediate operative exploration without delay for imaging. The neck has excellent surgical access in Zone II, and delays risk death from exsanguination or airway loss. Imaging is appropriate for soft signs or injuries in Zones I and III.

Question 26: What is the immediate concern with first and second rib fractures?

A) Severe pain limiting breathing
B) High risk of pneumothorax
C) Possible underlying great vessel injury
D) Delayed healing time

Answer: C

Explanation: First and second ribs are protected by the shoulder girdle and require tremendous force to fracture. This force level suggests possible injury to underlying structures, particularly great vessels (subclavian vessels, aorta). These patients need vascular imaging to rule out life-threatening vascular injuries.

Question 27: Muffled heart sounds in a trauma patient with hypotension suggest:

A) Hypovolemic shock
B) Tension pneumothorax
C) Cardiac tamponade
D) Pulmonary embolism

Answer: C

Explanation: Muffled heart sounds with hypotension strongly suggest cardiac tamponade. Fluid in the pericardial sac dampens sound transmission. Combined with hypotension and possibly jugular venous distension (Beck's triad), this indicates obstructive shock from tamponade requiring immediate pericardiocentesis.

Question 28: The definitive treatment for flail chest with respiratory failure is:

A) Surgical rib fixation
B) Chest tube placement
C) Positive pressure ventilation
D) Epidural analgesia

Answer: C

Explanation: Positive pressure ventilation (mechanical ventilation after intubation) is the definitive treatment for flail chest with respiratory failure. It provides internal pneumatic stabilization of the chest wall while the ribs heal. Surgical fixation is increasingly used but isn't universally standard. Pain control and chest tubes address specific issues but don't treat the flail segment itself.

Question 29: Subcutaneous emphysema in the neck after chest trauma indicates:

A) Cervical spine fracture
B) Esophageal rupture
C) Air leak from lung or airway injury
D) Venous air embolism

Answer: C

Explanation: Subcutaneous emphysema (crepitus from air in tissues) indicates air escaping from lung parenchyma, trachea, or bronchi into surrounding tissues. In chest trauma, this typically means pneumothorax with air tracking into neck tissues, or direct airway injury. It doesn't indicate spine fracture or esophageal injury specifically.

Question 30: A patient requires emergency cricothyrotomy. This procedure is performed through:

A) The thyroid cartilage
B) The cricothyroid membrane
C) Between the first and second tracheal rings
D) The cricoid cartilage

Answer: B

Explanation: Cricothyrotomy is performed through the cricothyroid membrane, which is the space between the thyroid cartilage (above) and cricoid cartilage (below). This membrane is relatively avascular and superficial, making it the ideal location for emergency surgical airway access. Don't cut through cartilage—find the membrane between cartilages.

Clinical Scenarios

Clinical Scenario 1:

A 32-year-old male arrives after a stab wound to the left chest at the fourth intercostal space, anterior axillary line. He is anxious and tachypneic. Vitals: HR 118, BP 96/62, RR 28, SpO2 90% on room air. The wound is approximately 2 cm, with blood bubbling from it with each breath. Breath sounds are decreased on the left.

Questions:

1. What injury does the bubbling blood from the wound indicate?
2. What is your immediate intervention?
3. What additional injury must be ruled out given the wound location?
4. The patient's oxygen saturation doesn't improve after your intervention. What should you consider?

Answers:

1. Bubbling blood from a chest wound indicates an open pneumothorax (sucking chest wound). Air is moving in and out of the pleural space through the chest wall defect with each breath, preventing effective lung expansion.
2. Immediate intervention: Apply an occlusive dressing taped on three sides to create a flutter valve, apply high-flow oxygen, establish IV access, and prepare for chest tube insertion away from the wound. The three-sided dressing allows air to escape during exhalation but prevents entry during inhalation.
3. Given the wound location (fourth intercostal space, anterior), cardiac injury must be ruled out. The heart extends to approximately the fourth or fifth intercostal space, making cardiac laceration possible with this mechanism. Perform FAST exam to assess for pericardial fluid and monitor closely for tamponade signs.
4. If oxygen saturation doesn't improve: Consider tension pneumothorax development (the occlusive dressing may have trapped air), ongoing bleeding causing hemothorax,

or cardiac tamponade. Remove the dressing temporarily if tension is suspected, proceed urgently to chest tube placement, and reassess for tamponade signs.

Clinical Scenario 2:

A 58-year-old female was the driver in a head-on collision at highway speed. She is awake but appears anxious. Vitals: HR 108, BP 142/96, RR 22, SpO2 96%. She complains of chest pain. Chest X-ray shows widened mediastinum (9.5 cm), obliterated aortic knob, and left pleural effusion.

Questions:

1. What injury do these chest X-ray findings suggest?
2. What is the priority intervention?
3. What medication management is indicated?
4. The patient's BP increases to 168/102. Why is this concerning and what should you do?

Answers:

1. These findings suggest traumatic aortic disruption. Widened mediastinum, obliterated aortic knob, and left pleural effusion (likely hemothorax) after high-speed deceleration are classic for aortic injury at the isthmus.
2. Priority interventions: Maintain strict blood pressure control (target systolic 100-120 mmHg), administer beta-blockers to reduce heart rate and contractility (decreasing shear forces on the injured aorta), keep patient calm and at rest, arrange for CT angiography to confirm diagnosis and locate injury, and consult vascular or cardiothoracic surgery immediately.
3. Beta-blockers (esmolol or labetalol) are first-line to reduce heart rate, contractility, and blood pressure. If BP remains elevated, add additional antihypertensives as needed. Avoid pure vasodilators alone as they can cause reflex tachycardia. The goal is reducing both pressure and force of cardiac contraction.
4. Elevated BP increases shear stress on the injured aorta, risking complete rupture and death. Immediately increase beta-blocker dosing, add additional antihypertensive medications if needed, ensure adequate analgesia (pain increases BP), and prepare for urgent operative or endovascular repair. Uncontrolled hypertension in aortic injury is an emergency requiring immediate aggressive treatment.

Clinical Scenario 3:

A 25-year-old male presents after a motorcycle crash. He has obvious chest trauma with visible paradoxical movement of the right chest wall. Vitals: HR 122, BP 118/78, RR 34 and labored, SpO2 85% on non-rebreather mask. He's in severe distress, unable to speak in complete sentences due to pain and dyspnea.

Questions:

1. What injury causes paradoxical chest wall movement?
2. What is your immediate management priority?
3. What underlying injury commonly accompanies this chest wall injury?

4. The patient's respiratory status continues to deteriorate despite oxygen and pain management. What intervention is needed?

Answers:

1. Paradoxical chest wall movement indicates flail chest—multiple ribs fractured in multiple places creating a free-floating segment. This requires significant blunt force trauma.
2. Immediate priorities: High-flow oxygen (already in place but clearly inadequate), aggressive pain control (IV opioids or prepare for epidural analgesia—pain prevents effective breathing), position patient on affected side if possible (uses weight to stabilize flail segment), prepare for possible intubation and mechanical ventilation given severe distress, establish IV access, obtain chest X-ray and ABG, assess for other injuries (pneumothorax, hemothorax).
3. Pulmonary contusion almost always accompanies flail chest. The force that creates the chest wall injury also contuses underlying lung tissue, impairing gas exchange. Contusion typically worsens over 24-48 hours, explaining why some flail chest patients deteriorate despite adequate chest wall stabilization and pain control.
4. Continued deterioration despite oxygen and pain management indicates need for intubation and mechanical ventilation. Positive pressure ventilation provides internal pneumatic stabilization of the flail segment while supporting gas exchange through the contused lung. This patient has failed non-invasive management and needs immediate airway control and ventilatory support.

Clinical Scenario 4:

A 40-year-old construction worker was struck in the anterior neck by a swinging beam. He arrives sitting upright, leaning forward, with obvious neck swelling and bruising. He's anxious, speaks in short phrases with a hoarse voice. You palpate crepitus in the neck. Vitals: HR 108, BP 132/86, RR 24, SpO2 94% on room air.

Questions:

1. What injuries do the hoarseness, crepitus, and mechanism suggest?
2. What is your primary concern?
3. Should you attempt to intubate this patient? Why or why not?
4. The patient's respiratory distress worsens suddenly. What is your action?

Answers:

1. Hoarseness, subcutaneous emphysema (crepitus), and direct anterior neck trauma suggest laryngeal or tracheal injury. Air escaping from the damaged airway creates the crepitus. Vocal cord or laryngeal damage causes voice changes.
2. Primary concern is airway. This patient currently maintains his airway but is at high risk for sudden complete obstruction from expanding hematoma, worsening edema, or complete structural disruption. The airway could be lost at any moment, requiring immediate intervention.
3. Blind intubation should NOT be attempted because normal anatomy may be disrupted, intubation attempts could create a false passage or worsen injury, or could cause

complete obstruction. If intubation is necessary: Keep patient upright and calm, consider awake fiberoptic intubation with visualization of anatomy, have surgical airway equipment immediately available, or proceed directly to surgical airway (cricothyrotomy or tracheostomy) if anatomy is severely distorted.

4. Sudden worsening requires immediate action: Prepare for emergency surgical airway (cricothyrotomy or tracheostomy), call for additional help, have all equipment ready, consider attempting one careful intubation if airway still partially patent and anatomy identifiable, but proceed immediately to surgical airway if intubation unsuccessful or anatomy unclear. Do not persist with multiple intubation attempts—this wastes critical time and worsens outcome.

Chapter 5: Abdominal and Genitourinary Trauma

Abdominal injuries range from minor contusions to life-threatening hemorrhage or hollow organ perforation. The challenge with abdominal trauma is that internal injuries aren't always obvious externally, and even significant injuries can present with subtle findings initially. Understanding injury patterns, assessment techniques, and management priorities is essential for recognizing when patients need surgical intervention versus observation.

This chapter covers both solid organ injuries (liver, spleen, kidneys) that typically bleed, and hollow viscus injuries (stomach, intestines, bladder) that cause contamination and infection. We'll also address pelvic fractures and genitourinary trauma, which share management principles with abdominal injuries.

Blunt Abdominal Trauma Assessment

Blunt mechanisms account for most abdominal trauma in civilian practice. The challenge is identifying significant internal injuries when external signs may be minimal.

Common Mechanisms and Injury Patterns

Motor vehicle crashes:

- Restrained occupants: Seatbelt injuries (intestinal and mesenteric injuries from compression), solid organ injuries from deceleration forces
- Unrestrained occupants: Higher likelihood of ejection, multiple injuries including abdominal trauma from impact with dashboard or steering wheel
- Side-impact: Direct force to flank, higher risk of spleen (left) or liver (right) injury depending on impact side

Falls: Height matters—falls >20 feet have high risk of intra-abdominal injury. Solid organs commonly injured from deceleration forces.

Assaults: Direct blows can injure solid organs, particularly spleen (left) and liver (right). Consider hollow viscus injury if struck abdomen is full (recent meal).

Bicycle/motorcycle crashes: Handlebar injuries classically cause duodenal or pancreatic trauma. High-speed crashes cause multiple injuries similar to motor vehicle crashes.

Physical Examination

Abdominal examination in trauma is notoriously unreliable. Patients may have significant injuries with minimal exam findings, or dramatic exam findings with minor injuries. Serial examinations over time improve sensitivity.

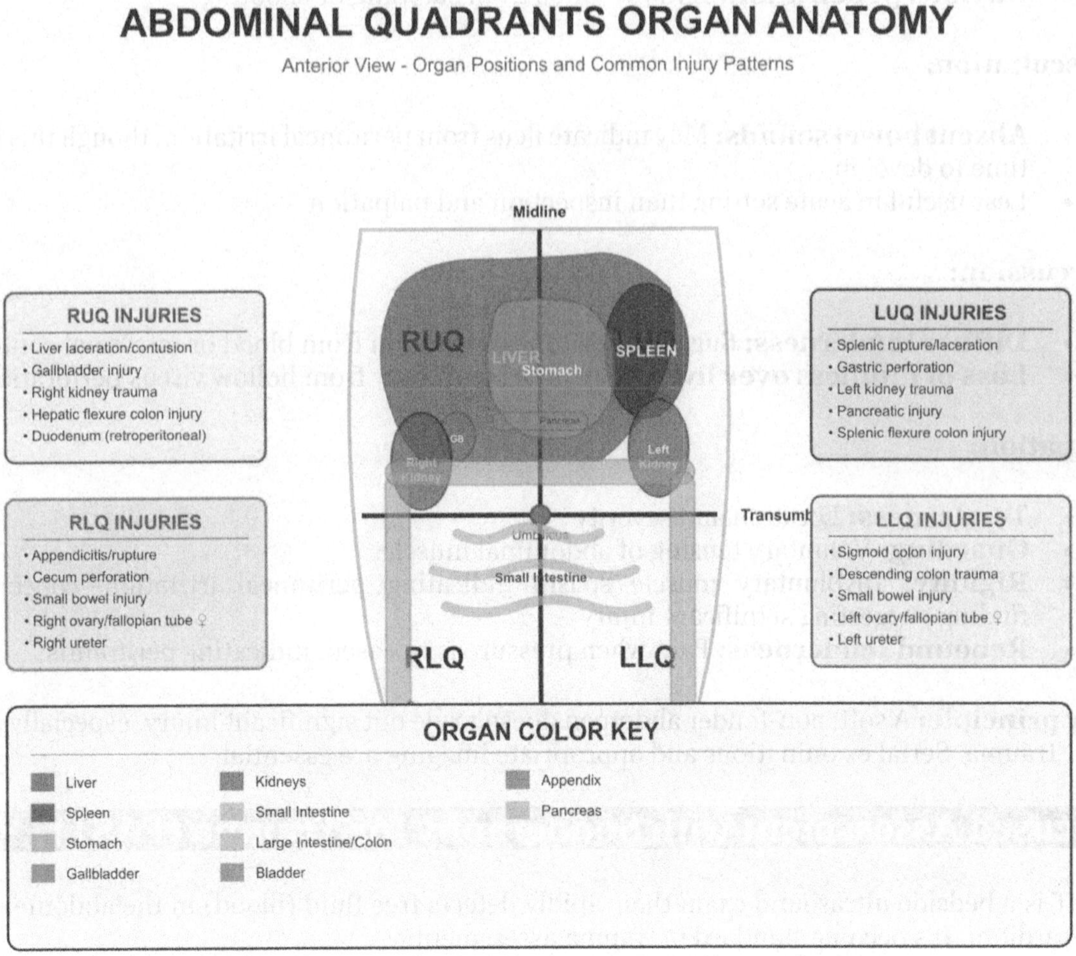

4

PERITONEAL CAVITY CLASSIFICATION

INTRAPERITONEAL ORGANS:

- Located within peritoneal cavity, covered by visceral peritoneum
- Organs: Stomach, Liver, Spleen, Gallbladder, First part of duodenum, Jejunum, Ileum, Transverse colon, Sigmoid colon, Cecum, Appendix, Upper 1/3 of rectum
- **Injury characteristics: Free fluid (blood) visible on imaging, peritoneal signs**

RETROPERITONEAL ORGANS:

- Located behind peritoneum, not covered by visceral peritoneum
- Organs: Kidneys, Ureters, Adrenal glands, Pancreas, Ascending colon, Descending colon, Duodenum (2nd-4th parts), Rectum (lower 2/3), Abdominal aorta, IVC
- **Injury characteristics: Bleeding may be contained, delayed peritoneal signs, harder to detect**

Clinical Assessment: Palpate all four quadrants systematically, assess for rebound tenderness, guarding, and rigidity

Inspection:

- **Abrasions, bruising, lacerations:** Note location and pattern
- **Seatbelt sign:** Bruising across lower abdomen from seatbelt is associated with high rates of hollow viscus and mesenteric injury, even if abdomen is soft initially
- **Distension:** May indicate blood, fluid, or gas accumulation
- **Obvious penetration:** Entry wounds from stabbing or shooting

Auscultation:

- **Absent bowel sounds:** May indicate ileus from peritoneal irritation, though this takes time to develop
- Less useful in acute setting than inspection and palpation

Percussion:

- **Diffuse tenderness:** Suggests peritoneal irritation from blood or intestinal contents
- **Loss of dullness over liver:** May indicate free air from hollow viscus perforation

Palpation:

- **Tenderness:** Location and severity
- **Guarding:** Voluntary tensing of abdominal muscles
- **Rigidity:** Involuntary muscle spasm indicating peritoneal irritation—concerning finding suggesting significant injury
- **Rebound tenderness:** Pain when pressure is released, indicating peritonitis

Key principle: A soft, non-tender abdomen doesn't rule out significant injury, especially early after trauma. Serial examinations and appropriate imaging are essential.

Focused Assessment with Sonography for Trauma (FAST)

FAST is a bedside ultrasound exam that rapidly detects free fluid (blood) in the abdomen and pericardium. It's become standard in trauma assessment.

FAST views:

1. **Perihepatic:** Right upper quadrant, looking for fluid in Morrison's pouch (space between liver and right kidney)
2. **Perisplenic:** Left upper quadrant, looking for fluid around spleen and left kidney
3. **Pelvic:** Suprapubic view looking for fluid in pelvis (rectovesical or rectouterine pouch)
4. **Pericardial:** Subxiphoid view looking for fluid in pericardial sac

Interpretation:

- **Positive FAST:** Free fluid present, indicating likely intraperitoneal hemorrhage in trauma patient
- **Negative FAST:** No free fluid seen

- **Indeterminate:** Technically inadequate images

Limitations:

- Doesn't identify specific organ injuries
- May miss hollow viscus perforations (don't cause immediate significant free fluid)
- May miss retroperitoneal injuries (kidneys, pancreas, some liver/spleen injuries)
- Less sensitive early after injury (takes time for blood to accumulate)
- Operator-dependent

Clinical use:

- Positive FAST in unstable patient: Proceed to operating room for exploration
- Negative FAST in stable patient: Proceed to CT for detailed evaluation
- Positive FAST in stable patient: CT to define injuries and determine if operative or non-operative management appropriate

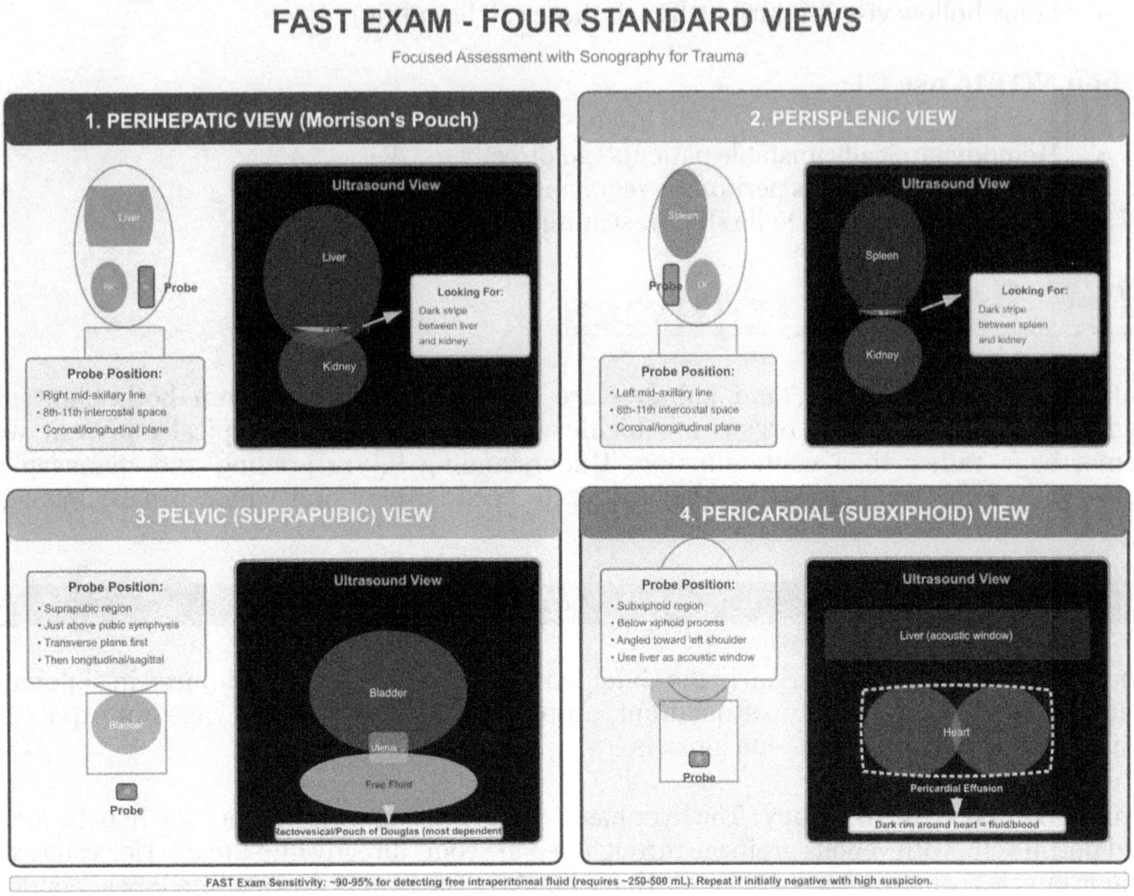

CT Scanning

Contrast-enhanced CT is the gold standard for evaluating abdominal trauma in stable patients. It identifies specific organ injuries, grades injury severity, and detects active bleeding.

When to use CT:

- Hemodynamically stable patients with mechanism suggesting abdominal injury
- Stable patients with positive FAST exam (to define injuries)
- Abdominal tenderness or concerning mechanism even with negative FAST

What CT shows:

- Specific organ injuries with grading
- Free fluid (blood) location and volume
- Active extravasation (contrast "blush" indicating ongoing arterial bleeding)
- Retroperitoneal injuries
- Some hollow viscus injuries (though these can be subtle)

When NOT to use CT:

- Hemodynamically unstable patients (go directly to OR)
- Patients with obvious peritonitis requiring surgery
- Patients too agitated to lie still for scanning

Solid Organ Injuries

Solid organs—liver, spleen, and kidneys—are vulnerable to injury from both blunt and penetrating trauma. These organs are highly vascular, and injuries typically present with hemorrhage rather than contamination. Understanding injury grading and management approaches helps you anticipate which patients need surgery and which can be managed conservatively.

Liver Injuries

The liver is the largest solid organ in the abdomen and the most commonly injured in abdominal trauma. It sits in the right upper quadrant, protected partially by the rib cage but exposed to injury from frontal and right-side impacts.

Anatomy relevant to injury: The liver has a rich blood supply from both the hepatic artery and portal vein, with venous drainage through hepatic veins directly into the inferior vena cava. Major injuries can cause massive hemorrhage quickly. The liver is divided into lobes separated by ligaments, and deep lacerations can extend into major vessels.

Mechanisms causing liver injury:

- Right-sided impact in motor vehicle crashes
- Falls from height
- Direct blows to right upper quadrant
- Rapid deceleration (shearing forces tear liver from supporting ligaments)
- Penetrating trauma to right chest or abdomen

Clinical presentation:

- Right upper quadrant pain and tenderness
- Abdominal distension if significant bleeding
- Signs of shock (tachycardia, hypotension, cool skin) if major hemorrhage
- Right shoulder pain (referred pain from diaphragmatic irritation by blood)
- Guarding and rigidity if blood irritates peritoneum

Injury grading: The American Association for the Surgery of Trauma (AAST) grades liver injuries from I (minor) to VI (catastrophic):

- **Grade I-II:** Minor lacerations or subcapsular hematomas, typically managed non-operatively
- **Grade III:** Moderate lacerations 3-10 cm deep, may be managed non-operatively if stable
- **Grade IV-V:** Deep lacerations involving major vessels or extensive tissue destruction, often require surgery
- **Grade VI:** Hepatic avulsion (complete separation from vascular attachments), usually fatal

Management approach:

Non-operative management (for hemodynamically stable patients):

- ICU admission for close monitoring
- Serial abdominal exams
- Serial hemoglobin/hematocrit measurements
- Bed rest initially, gradual activity advancement
- Transfusion as needed to maintain hemoglobin
- Repeat imaging if clinical change
- Success rate is high for grades I-III, reasonable for grade IV in stable patients

Operative management indications:

- Hemodynamic instability despite resuscitation
- Peritonitis on exam
- Grade IV-VI injuries in unstable patients
- Transfusion requirements exceeding 4-6 units without stabilization
- Evidence of other injuries requiring surgery

Surgical options: Range from simple repair with sutures or cautery to complex procedures involving packing, vessel ligation, or partial liver resection. Damage control approach (pack and return later) is common for severe injuries.

Complications to monitor:

- Rebleeding (can occur days after injury)
- Bile leak (causes persistent abdominal pain and fever)
- Abscess formation
- Compartment syndrome if massive packing required

Spleen Injuries

The spleen is the most commonly injured organ in blunt abdominal trauma. Located in the left upper quadrant, it's particularly vulnerable to left-sided impacts and deceleration forces.

Anatomy and function: The spleen filters blood, stores platelets, and plays a role in immune function. It's highly vascular and friable (easily torn), making it prone to significant bleeding with injury. The spleen is attached by ligaments that can tear with rapid deceleration.

Mechanisms causing splenic injury:

- Left-sided impact in motor vehicle crashes
- Falls onto left side
- Direct blows to left upper quadrant (assault, sports injuries)
- Rapid deceleration
- Fractured lower left ribs

Clinical presentation:

- Left upper quadrant pain and tenderness
- Abdominal distension from hemoperitoneum
- Shock if significant hemorrhage
- Left shoulder pain (Kehr's sign—referred pain from diaphragmatic irritation)
- Abdominal rigidity if significant peritoneal irritation

Special consideration—delayed splenic rupture: Some patients have minor initial injury that progresses over hours to days, causing delayed hemorrhage. This is why observation and serial exams are crucial even when initial imaging shows minor injury.

Injury grading: AAST grades splenic injuries I through V:

- **Grade I-II:** Small lacerations or subcapsular hematomas
- **Grade III:** Deeper lacerations or larger hematomas
- **Grade IV:** Extensive lacerations involving hilar vessels
- **Grade V:** Completely shattered spleen or hilar vascular avulsion

Management approach:

Non-operative management (increasingly preferred when possible):

- Preserving the spleen maintains immune function, particularly important in children
- Appropriate for hemodynamically stable patients without other indications for surgery
- ICU monitoring with serial exams and labs
- Bed rest with gradual mobilization
- Transfusion to maintain hemoglobin as needed
- CT imaging to grade injury and detect complications
- Angiography with embolization for ongoing bleeding in stable patients (interventional radiology can block specific bleeding vessels)

Operative management indications:

- Hemodynamic instability despite resuscitation
- Grade IV-V injuries in unstable patients
- Peritonitis requiring exploration
- Failure of non-operative management (continued bleeding)

Surgical options: Range from splenorrhaphy (repair) to splenectomy (removal). Surgeons try to preserve the spleen when possible, especially in children, but removal is necessary for severe injuries.

Post-splenectomy considerations:

- Increased lifelong infection risk from encapsulated bacteria (Streptococcus pneumoniae, Haemophilus influenzae, Neisseria meningitidis)
- Vaccinations required: pneumococcal, meningococcal, Haemophilus influenzae type B
- Prophylactic antibiotics considered in some patients
- Patient education about infection risk and when to seek care

Kidney Injuries

Kidneys can be injured by both blunt and penetrating trauma. They're retroperitoneal organs (behind the peritoneum), so injuries may not cause obvious intraperitoneal signs.

Anatomy: The kidneys sit in the retroperitoneum at approximately the T12-L3 vertebral levels, partially protected by the lower ribs posteriorly. They're surrounded by perinephric fat and encased in Gerota's fascia, which can contain bleeding and create a tamponade effect in some injuries.

Mechanisms:

- Direct flank trauma (falls, motor vehicle crashes, assaults)
- Rapid deceleration (renal pedicle injury from shearing)
- Penetrating trauma to flank or back
- Lower rib fractures with kidney laceration

Clinical presentation:

- Flank pain and tenderness
- Hematuria (blood in urine)—most sensitive indicator of renal trauma
- Flank ecchymosis or hematoma
- Shock if major hemorrhage (contained retroperitoneal bleeding may not cause peritoneal signs)
- Absent or decreased kidney function if major vascular injury

Important point: Degree of hematuria doesn't correlate with injury severity. Massive injuries that completely transect the ureter or avulse the renal pedicle may have minimal or no hematuria because blood can't reach the collecting system.

Injury grading: AAST grades renal injuries I through V:

- **Grade I-II:** Contusions or minor lacerations without collecting system involvement
- **Grade III:** Deeper lacerations into cortex
- **Grade IV:** Lacerations extending to collecting system or segmental vascular injuries
- **Grade V:** Shattered kidney or renal pedicle avulsion

Diagnostic approach:

- Any patient with flank trauma and hematuria needs imaging
- CT with IV contrast is standard—shows kidney perfusion, injury extent, and urinary extravasation
- Stable patients with minor trauma and microscopic hematuria only may not require imaging

Management:

Non-operative management (most common):

- Grades I-III routinely managed conservatively
- Many grade IV injuries can be managed non-operatively in stable patients
- Bed rest, serial exams, monitor urine output and color
- Serial hemoglobin checks
- Most renal injuries stop bleeding spontaneously due to retroperitoneal tamponade

Operative indications:

- Hemodynamic instability from renal hemorrhage
- Expanding retroperitoneal hematoma
- Grade V injuries
- Renal pedicle injuries (vascular repairs have poor success but attempted in viable kidney)

Complications:

- Delayed bleeding
- Urinoma (urine leak forming fluid collection)
- Hypertension from renal ischemia (rare, long-term complication)
- Loss of kidney function if severe injury

Hollow Viscus Injuries

Hollow organs—stomach, small intestine, colon—are less commonly injured than solid organs in blunt trauma but present different challenges. These injuries cause contamination of the peritoneal cavity with intestinal contents, leading to peritonitis and sepsis if not treated promptly.

Small Bowel and Mesentery Injuries

Small bowel injuries can be challenging to diagnose because they may not show obvious signs immediately. The mesentery (tissue containing blood vessels that supplies the bowel) can also tear, causing bleeding or bowel ischemia.

Mechanisms:

- Seatbelt injuries (compression against spine)
- Direct blows to abdomen when bowel is full
- Deceleration injuries (bowel tears at fixed points)
- Penetrating trauma

Why they're challenging to diagnose:

- May not cause immediate peritonitis (takes hours for intestinal contents to irritate peritoneum)
- Initial imaging may be subtle
- Physical exam may be unremarkable initially
- High index of suspicion needed based on mechanism

Clinical presentation:

- Abdominal pain that worsens over time
- Seatbelt sign (bruising across abdomen) strongly associated with bowel injury
- Increasing peritoneal signs (guarding, rigidity, rebound tenderness)
- Fever and elevated white blood cell count (develop over hours as contamination progresses)

Diagnostic findings:

- CT may show:
  - Free air (from perforated hollow viscus)
  - Free fluid without solid organ injury (suggests bowel injury)
  - Bowel wall thickening
  - Mesenteric hematoma or active bleeding
  - Pneumatosis (air in bowel wall) in severe ischemic injury
- Many injuries show subtle or no initial CT findings, making serial clinical exams crucial

Management:

- All confirmed or suspected bowel perforations require surgical repair
- Surgery involves:
  - Exploration to identify all injuries
  - Repair of perforations (primary closure or resection with anastomosis)
  - Washout of contaminated peritoneal cavity
  - Damage control approach if patient physiologically unstable
- Antibiotics to cover intestinal flora
- NGT for gastric decompression

Key principle: High suspicion and serial exams are essential. A patient with seatbelt sign and abdominal tenderness needs very close observation even with negative or equivocal initial imaging. Many of these injuries declare themselves over 12-24 hours of observation.

Stomach and Duodenal Injuries

Less common than small bowel injuries but significant when they occur.

Stomach injuries:

- Usually from penetrating trauma
- Rare in blunt trauma (stomach is mobile and often empty)
- Present with peritonitis and free air on imaging
- Require surgical repair

Duodenal injuries:

- Classic mechanism: Handlebar injury (bicycle or motorcycle)—direct blow to epigastrium compresses duodenum against spine
- Difficult to diagnose because duodenum is retroperitoneal
- May present with:
  - Epigastric pain
  - Elevated amylase (from injury to nearby pancreas)
  - Retroperitoneal air on CT
  - Delayed perforation (some injuries initially contained by retroperitoneum)
- Require surgical repair, often complex due to location and proximity to pancreas and bile ducts

Colon and Rectal Injuries

Colon injuries:

- Both blunt and penetrating mechanisms
- Present similarly to small bowel injuries
- Surgical management required
- Higher infection risk than small bowel due to bacterial load

Rectal injuries:

- Usually penetrating (gunshot wounds, impalement)
- Symptoms include rectal bleeding, pain, possible peritonitis
- Diagnosis via digital rectal exam, proctoscopy
- Management complex, may require diverting colostomy to allow healing

Pelvic Fractures

Pelvic fractures range from minor avulsion fractures to life-threatening injuries with massive hemorrhage. Understanding fracture patterns and hemorrhage control is crucial for trauma nurses.

Pelvic Anatomy and Injury Patterns

The bony pelvis forms a ring structure. Ring disruptions (breaks in multiple locations) are unstable and associated with significant hemorrhage.

Classification systems describe stability:

Stable fractures:

- Single ramus fractures
- Avulsion fractures (muscle pull-offs)
- Minimally displaced fractures
- Low bleeding risk

Unstable fractures:

- Open-book (anterior-posterior compression): Pubic symphysis widens, SI joints may disrupt
- Lateral compression: One side of pelvis driven inward
- Vertical shear: Hemipelvis displaced vertically
- High bleeding risk from bone surfaces and torn vessels

Mechanisms:

- High-energy impacts: Motor vehicle crashes, falls from height, pedestrians struck, motorcycle crashes
- Crush injuries
- Lower energy in elderly (fragility fractures)

Hemorrhage from Pelvic Fractures

Sources of bleeding:

- Fracture surfaces (bone oozes significant blood)
- Venous plexus disruption (pelvic veins form extensive networks)
- Arterial injuries (less common but more severe)—iliac, gluteal, pudendal arteries

Blood loss can be massive: The retroperitoneal space can accommodate several liters of blood. Patients can exsanguinate from pelvic fractures alone.

Clinical presentation:

- Pain in pelvis, hips, or lower back
- Inability to bear weight
- Visible deformity or asymmetry
- Leg length discrepancy
- Shock from hemorrhage
- Blood at urethral meatus (urethral injury from fracture fragments)
- Scrotal or labial hematoma
- Instability with gentle pelvic compression (never "rock" the pelvis vigorously—this disrupts clots)

Management of Pelvic Fractures

Initial hemorrhage control:

Pelvic binder application:

- Apply as soon as unstable pelvic fracture suspected
- Placement: Around the greater trochanters (NOT over iliac crests)
- Tightness: Firm compression without excessive force
- Purpose: Reduces pelvic volume, approximates fracture fragments, provides tamponade effect
- Leave in place until definitive stabilization

Resuscitation:

- Large-bore IV access
- Massive transfusion protocol for unstable patients
- Limit crystalloid, early blood products
- Address lethal triad (hypothermia, coagulopathy, acidosis)

Definitive hemorrhage control options:

External fixation:

- Surgical placement of pins and external frame to stabilize pelvis
- Can be done in ED or OR for emergent stabilization
- Reduces pelvic volume and provides mechanical stability

Angiography with embolization:

- For arterial bleeding (identified by contrast "blush" on CT)
- Interventional radiology threads catheter into bleeding vessels and blocks them with coils or particles
- Highly effective for arterial hemorrhage
- Doesn't work for venous bleeding (most pelvic hemorrhage)

Preperitoneal packing:

- Surgical procedure: Extraperitoneal packing of pelvis with laparotomy pads
- For venous hemorrhage not controlled by binder/fixation
- Part of damage control approach

REBOA (Resuscitative Endovascular Balloon Occlusion of the Aorta):

- Balloon catheter inflated in aorta to temporarily stop pelvic blood flow
- Buys time to get patient to OR or IR
- Temporary measure only (ischemia below balloon)

Definitive fixation:

- Orthopedic surgery to repair fractures with plates, screws
- Done after patient stabilized, usually days after injury

Associated injuries to assess:

- Urethral injury (blood at meatus, inability to void, high-riding prostate)
- Bladder injury (hematuria, inability to void)
- Rectal injury (rectal bleeding, palpable defect on exam)
- Nerve injuries (sciatic, lumbosacral plexus)
- Vaginal injuries in women

Genitourinary Trauma

Injuries to kidneys (covered above), ureters, bladder, and urethra require specific assessment and management approaches.

Bladder Injuries

Types:

- **Extraperitoneal rupture:** Bladder wall tears but leak is contained in pelvis (more common, often with pelvic fractures)
- **Intraperitoneal rupture:** Bladder tears into peritoneal cavity, spilling urine into abdomen (more serious, requires surgery)

Mechanisms:

- Pelvic fractures with bladder perforation by bone fragments (extraperitoneal)
- Direct blow to lower abdomen when bladder full (intraperitoneal)
- Penetrating trauma

Clinical presentation:

- Suprapubic pain and tenderness
- Hematuria (gross or microscopic)
- Inability to void or low urine output
- Abdominal distension if intraperitoneal rupture
- Pelvic hematoma

Diagnosis:

- CT cystogram (bladder filled with contrast via catheter, then scanned)
- Shows contrast extravasation outside bladder

Management:

- **Extraperitoneal rupture:** Usually managed conservatively with Foley catheter drainage for 7-10 days (allows bladder to heal), antibiotics
- **Intraperitoneal rupture:** Requires surgical repair
- **Associated pelvic fractures:** Treat according to orthopedic injury severity

Urethral Injuries

More common in males (longer urethra). Can complicate pelvic fractures significantly.

Types:

- **Anterior urethral injury:** Below the urogenital diaphragm (bulbar, penile urethra)—usually from straddle injuries
- **Posterior urethral injury:** Above urogenital diaphragm (prostatic, membranous urethra)—usually from pelvic fractures

Classic signs:

- Blood at urethral meatus (key finding)
- Inability to void
- High-riding prostate on rectal exam (prostate displaced upward by hematoma in posterior injury)
- Scrotal or perineal hematoma

Critical point: If urethral injury suspected (blood at meatus, pelvic fracture pattern), DO NOT attempt Foley catheter insertion. Placing catheter through injured urethra can worsen injury or create false passage.

Diagnosis:

- Retrograde urethrogram: Contrast injected into urethra via catheter in meatus, X-ray shows extravasation if injured

Management:

- **Partial tears:** May attempt gentle catheter placement by experienced urologist under fluoroscopy
- **Complete disruptions:** Suprapubic catheter (placed through lower abdominal wall directly into bladder)
- **Definitive repair:** Usually delayed weeks to months after acute injuries heal
- **Complications:** Stricture, erectile dysfunction, incontinence (particularly with posterior injuries)

Testicular and Penile Injuries

Less common but important to recognize.

Testicular trauma:

- Usually from direct blows, straddle injuries
- Can cause testicular rupture (rupture of tunica albuginea)
- Present with severe pain, swelling, scrotal hematoma
- Ultrasound for diagnosis
- Surgical exploration if rupture suspected (salvage rate better with early surgery)

Penile injuries:

- Penile fracture (rupture of corpus cavernosum during sexual activity)—not bone, but tunica albuginea tears
- Presents as sudden pop during intercourse, immediate detumescence, swelling, deviation
- Requires urgent surgical repair (better outcomes with early surgery)

Chapter 5 Practice Questions

Question 1: A patient with a seatbelt sign across the abdomen and abdominal tenderness has a negative FAST exam and CT showing only free fluid without solid organ injury. What is the most likely diagnosis?

A) Splenic laceration
B) Liver contusion
C) Hollow viscus injury
D) Kidney laceration

Answer: C

Explanation: Seatbelt sign with free fluid but no solid organ injury on CT strongly suggests hollow viscus (intestinal) or mesenteric injury. These injuries may show subtle or no findings on initial CT, making clinical suspicion based on mechanism and serial exams critical.

Question 2: A patient with Grade III splenic laceration and stable vital signs should be managed how?

A) Immediate splenectomy
B) Non-operative management with close monitoring
C) Angiography with embolization
D) Exploratory laparotomy

Answer: B

Explanation: Hemodynamically stable patients with Grade I-III splenic injuries can typically be managed non-operatively with ICU monitoring, serial exams, and transfusion as needed. This preserves immune function. Surgery is reserved for unstable patients or failure of conservative management.

Question 3: What is the most sensitive indicator of renal trauma?

A) Flank pain
B) Hematuria
C) Hypotension
D) Abdominal distension

Answer: B

Explanation: Hematuria (blood in urine) is the most sensitive indicator of renal trauma. Any patient with flank trauma and hematuria should undergo imaging to assess for kidney injury. However, massive injuries that disrupt the collecting system may have minimal hematuria.

Question 4: Blood at the urethral meatus in a male patient with pelvic fracture indicates:

A) Bladder rupture
B) Kidney injury
C) Possible urethral injury—do not insert Foley catheter
D) Testicular trauma

Answer: C

Explanation: Blood at the urethral meatus indicates possible urethral injury. Never attempt Foley catheter insertion in this situation as it may worsen the injury or create a false passage. Obtain retrograde urethrogram first, and if injury confirmed, place suprapubic catheter instead.

Question 5: Where should a pelvic binder be applied?

A) Over the iliac crests
B) Around the greater trochanters
C) Around the waist
D) Around the upper thighs

Answer: B

Explanation: Pelvic binders should be placed around the greater trochanters (hip level), not the iliac crests. This position maximally reduces pelvic volume and provides optimal mechanical compression to tamponade bleeding and stabilize fractures.

Question 6: A hemodynamically unstable patient with positive FAST exam should:

A) Undergo CT scan for injury characterization
B) Proceed directly to operating room
C) Receive angiography with embolization
D) Be observed with serial exams

Answer: B

Explanation: Unstable patients with positive FAST (indicating intra-abdominal hemorrhage) need immediate surgical exploration. Don't delay for CT imaging—they're bleeding and need operative hemorrhage control. CT is for stable patients who have time for detailed evaluation.

Question 7: Which finding on CT suggests active arterial bleeding in solid organ injury?

A) Free fluid in pelvis
B) Contrast "blush" or extravasation
C) Organ laceration
D) Subcapsular hematoma

Answer: B

Explanation: Contrast extravasation or "blush" on CT indicates active arterial bleeding. This finding may prompt angiography with embolization in stable patients or indicate need for surgery in unstable patients. It represents contrast leaking from vessels in real-time during the scan.

Question 8: Kehr's sign (left shoulder pain) in abdominal trauma suggests:

A) Clavicle fracture
B) Blood irritating the diaphragm from splenic injury
C) Rotator cuff injury
D) Pneumothorax

Answer: B

Explanation: Kehr's sign is referred pain to the left shoulder from diaphragmatic irritation by blood in the left upper quadrant, classically from splenic injury. The phrenic nerve (innervating diaphragm) shares nerve roots with nerves supplying the shoulder, causing referred pain.

Question 9: Delayed splenic rupture refers to:

A) Spleen injury occurring days after initial trauma
B) Initial minor injury progressing to hemorrhage hours to days later
C) Spleen healing then re-injuring
D) Chronic splenic enlargement

Answer: B

Explanation: Delayed splenic rupture occurs when an initial minor injury (subcapsular hematoma or small laceration) progresses over hours to days, causing delayed hemorrhage. This highlights the importance of observation and serial assessment even when initial imaging shows minor injury.

Question 10: What is the primary concern with post-splenectomy patients?

A) Chronic pain
B) Increased infection risk from encapsulated bacteria
C) Bleeding tendency
D) Kidney dysfunction

Answer: B

Explanation: Post-splenectomy patients have lifelong increased risk of severe infection from encapsulated bacteria (Streptococcus pneumoniae, Haemophilus influenzae, Neisseria meningitidis). They require specific vaccinations and should seek immediate care for fevers. The spleen's immune function can't be fully replaced.

Question 11: What is the purpose of performing a FAST exam in trauma patients?

A) To identify specific organ injuries
B) To rapidly detect free fluid (blood) in the abdomen and pericardium
C) To grade the severity of solid organ injuries
D) To diagnose hollow viscus perforations

Answer: B

Explanation: FAST (Focused Assessment with Sonography for Trauma) rapidly detects free fluid in the peritoneal cavity and pericardium at the bedside. It doesn't identify specific organs injured or grade injury severity—that requires CT. FAST also has limited sensitivity for hollow viscus injuries.

Question 12: A patient has right upper quadrant pain with right shoulder pain after blunt trauma. This finding suggests:

A) Clavicle fracture
B) Liver injury with diaphragmatic irritation
C) Lung contusion
D) Rib fractures

Answer: B

Explanation: Right shoulder pain with right upper quadrant trauma suggests liver injury with blood irritating the diaphragm, causing referred pain through the phrenic nerve. This is similar to Kehr's sign (left shoulder pain from splenic injury) but on the right side.

Question 13: Which laboratory finding is most concerning for pancreatic injury?

A) Elevated white blood cell count
B) Elevated amylase or lipase
C) Decreased hemoglobin
D) Elevated liver enzymes

Answer: B

Explanation: Elevated amylase or lipase levels suggest pancreatic injury, though these enzymes can also be elevated from other causes. Pancreatic injuries are often associated with duodenal injuries due to their anatomical proximity and shared mechanism (handlebar injuries).

Question 14: Non-operative management of solid organ injuries is appropriate when:

A) The patient is hemodynamically stable
B) There is no other indication for surgery
C) The injury grade is appropriate for conservative management
D) All of the above

Answer: D

Explanation: Non-operative management requires all these conditions: hemodynamic stability, no peritonitis or other surgical indications, appropriate injury grade, and ability to perform serial monitoring. If any condition isn't met, surgery may be necessary.

Question 15: A patient with intraperitoneal bladder rupture requires:

A) Foley catheter drainage only
B) Suprapubic catheter placement
C) Surgical repair
D) Observation without intervention

Answer: C

Explanation: Intraperitoneal bladder ruptures require surgical repair because urine leaks into the peritoneal cavity, causing peritonitis. Extraperitoneal ruptures can often be managed with catheter drainage alone, but intraperitoneal ruptures need operative closure.

Question 16: The most common mechanism for duodenal injury is:

A) Gunshot wound
B) Motor vehicle crash
C) Handlebar injury (bicycle/motorcycle)
D) Fall from height

Answer: C

Explanation: Handlebar injuries classically cause duodenal trauma. Direct blow to the epigastrium compresses the duodenum against the spine, causing contusion, hematoma, or perforation. These injuries can be difficult to diagnose and may present with delayed symptoms.

Question 17: What finding on CT suggests mesenteric injury?

A) Free air
B) Mesenteric hematoma or fat stranding
C) Splenomegaly
D) Kidney laceration

Answer: B

Explanation: Mesenteric hematoma, fat stranding, or active extravasation on CT suggest mesenteric injury. Mesenteric tears can cause bleeding or compromise bowel blood supply, leading to ischemia. These injuries often require surgery for exploration and repair.

Question 18: A patient post-splenectomy should receive which vaccinations?

A) Influenza only
B) Pneumococcal, meningococcal, and Haemophilus influenzae type B
C) Hepatitis B only
D) No special vaccinations needed

Answer: B

Explanation: Post-splenectomy patients need vaccinations against encapsulated bacteria: pneumococcal (Pneumovax), meningococcal, and Haemophilus influenzae type B. The spleen normally filters these bacteria, and without it, patients have lifelong increased infection risk.

Question 19: Retroperitoneal hematoma from pelvic fracture should be:

A) Explored surgically in all cases
B) Left alone unless expanding or patient unstable
C) Drained percutaneously
D) Treated with immediate angiography

Answer: B

Explanation: Retroperitoneal hematomas from pelvic fractures are typically left alone unless expanding or the patient is unstable. The retroperitoneum provides tamponade effect that helps control bleeding. Surgical exploration disrupts this tamponade and can worsen bleeding.

Question 20: Which injury is most likely to cause immediate exsanguination?

A) Grade I liver laceration
B) Grade II splenic injury
C) Grade V renal pedicle avulsion
D) Bladder rupture

Answer: C

Explanation: Grade V renal pedicle avulsion (complete separation of kidney from its blood vessels) causes massive, immediate hemorrhage that's often fatal. Lower grade solid organ injuries and bladder ruptures are serious but typically don't cause instant exsanguination.

Question 21: The primary complication of untreated hollow viscus perforation is:

A) Hemorrhage
B) Peritonitis and sepsis
C) Compartment syndrome
D) Renal failure

Answer: B

Explanation: Hollow viscus perforations leak intestinal contents into the peritoneum, causing peritonitis and eventually sepsis if untreated. While these injuries may have associated bleeding, contamination and infection are the primary concerns requiring urgent surgical repair.

Question 22: A patient with unstable pelvic fracture develops hypotension despite pelvic binder and resuscitation. The next step is:

A) Additional fluid boluses
B) CT scan
C) Angiography with embolization or preperitoneal packing
D) Observation

Answer: C

Explanation: Patients with persistent hypotension despite binder and resuscitation need definitive hemorrhage control. Options include angiography with embolization (for arterial bleeding) or preperitoneal packing (for venous bleeding). Don't delay definitive treatment in unstable patients.

Question 23: Seatbelt sign is most strongly associated with:

A) Rib fractures
B) Hollow viscus and mesenteric injuries
C) Liver lacerations
D) Kidney contusions

Answer: B

Explanation: Seatbelt sign (bruising across abdomen) is strongly associated with hollow viscus (intestinal) and mesenteric injuries from compression against the spine. These injuries can be subtle on initial imaging, making the clinical sign crucial for maintaining suspicion and close observation.

Question 24: What is the advantage of angiography with embolization over surgery for solid organ injuries?

A) It's faster than surgery
B) It's less invasive and can control bleeding without removing the organ
C) It works for all types of bleeding
D) It's less expensive

Answer: B

Explanation: Angiography with embolization is minimally invasive and can control arterial bleeding while preserving the organ, avoiding surgery. It's particularly useful for stable patients with CT evidence of active bleeding. However, it only works for arterial bleeding, not venous bleeding.

Question 25: High-riding prostate on digital rectal exam suggests:

A) Prostate cancer
B) Rectal injury
C) Posterior urethral injury
D) Bladder distension

Answer: C

Explanation: A high-riding or non-palpable prostate suggests posterior urethral disruption, where hematoma displaces the prostate upward. This finding, along with blood at the meatus and pelvic fracture, indicates urethral injury requiring retrograde urethrogram before catheter placement.

Question 26: A patient has gross hematuria after blunt abdominal trauma with normal vital signs. The appropriate next step is:

A) Observation only
B) Immediate surgery
C) CT scan with IV contrast
D) Cystoscopy

Answer: C

Explanation: Any patient with significant hematuria after trauma needs imaging to assess for kidney, ureter, or bladder injury. CT with IV contrast (delayed images showing collecting system) is standard. Stable patients with only microscopic hematuria and no other concerning findings may not require imaging.

Question 27: What makes duodenal injuries particularly challenging?

A) They're retroperitoneal and may present with subtle findings
B) They always require complex reconstruction
C) They cause immediate peritonitis
D) They're always associated with vascular injuries

Answer: A

Explanation: Duodenal injuries are challenging because the duodenum is retroperitoneal, so perforation may be contained initially without obvious peritonitis. CT findings can be subtle, and some injuries present with delayed perforation hours to days after injury, requiring high suspicion and close observation.

Question 28: Serial hemoglobin measurements in solid organ injury help assess:

A) Need for antibiotics
B) Ongoing bleeding and transfusion needs
C) Kidney function
D) Infection development

Answer: B

Explanation: Serial hemoglobin checks help assess whether bleeding continues and guide transfusion decisions. Stable or rising hemoglobin suggests bleeding has stopped. Falling hemoglobin despite transfusion indicates ongoing hemorrhage that may require surgical or angiographic intervention.

Question 29: A patient requires suprapubic catheter after urethral injury. This catheter is placed:

A) Through the urethra
B) Through the lower abdominal wall directly into the bladder
C) Through the rectum
D) Through the perineum

Answer: B

Explanation: Suprapubic catheters are placed through the lower abdominal wall directly into the bladder, bypassing the injured urethra. This allows bladder drainage while the urethra heals. The catheter is typically placed under ultrasound or cystoscopic guidance.

Question 30: The "safe triangle" for chest tube insertion also applies to managing:

A) Hemothorax from liver laceration extending to diaphragm
B) Large volume hemoperitoneum
C) Splenic bleeding
D) Pelvic hemorrhage

Answer: A

Explanation: While primarily used for thoracic injuries, the safe triangle approach for chest tube placement is relevant when liver lacerations extend to the diaphragm and blood accumulates in both chest and abdomen. This question reinforces anatomical relationships between abdominal organs and thoracic cavity.

Question 31: Which mechanism has the highest risk for hollow viscus injury?

A) Ground-level fall
B) Seatbelt restraint in frontal crash
C) Side-impact collision
D) Minor sports injury

Answer: B

Explanation: Seatbelt restraint during frontal crashes creates compression force that traps bowel against the spine, causing burst injuries, mesenteric tears, or perforations. This mechanism is so strongly associated with hollow viscus injury that seatbelt sign warrants close observation even with negative imaging.

Question 32: A patient with flank pain, hematuria, and shock after motor vehicle crash most likely has:

A) Simple kidney contusion
B) Significant kidney injury with hemorrhage
C) Bladder rupture
D) Ureteral stone

Answer: B

Explanation: The combination of flank pain, hematuria, and shock indicates significant kidney injury with hemorrhage. While simple contusions cause pain and hematuria, they don't cause shock. This patient needs immediate resuscitation, imaging, and possible intervention for hemorrhage control.

Question 33: What is the most common site of colon injury in penetrating trauma?

A) Cecum
B) Transverse colon
C) Sigmoid colon
D) Any segment depending on trajectory

Answer: D

Explanation: Colon injury location depends on the trajectory of the penetrating object. Unlike blunt trauma which has typical patterns, penetrating trauma injures whatever structures lie in the path. Multiple organs are often injured with penetrating mechanisms, requiring thorough exploration.

Question 34: A patient has free air on abdominal X-ray after blunt trauma. This indicates:

A) Pneumothorax
B) Hollow viscus perforation
C) Solid organ injury
D) Normal finding

Answer: B

Explanation: Free air in the peritoneal cavity (pneumoperitoneum) indicates hollow viscus perforation with gas escaping from the GI tract. This is an absolute indication for surgery to find and repair the perforation. Even small amounts of free air are significant in trauma.

Question 35: The best indicator of successful non-operative management of splenic injury is:

A) Normal white blood cell count
B) Stable vital signs and hemoglobin without transfusion
C) Absence of pain
D) Normal appetite

Answer: B

Explanation: Stable vital signs and hemoglobin without need for ongoing transfusion indicate bleeding has stopped and non-operative management is succeeding. This represents successful hemostasis. Pain and appetite are less reliable indicators, and WBC doesn't directly assess bleeding control.

Question 36: Retroperitoneal air on CT scan suggests injury to:

A) Kidney
B) Duodenum or colon
C) Spleen
D) Liver

Answer: B

Explanation: Retroperitoneal air indicates perforation of a retroperitoneal structure, most commonly the duodenum (second through fourth portions) or portions of the colon that are retroperitoneal (ascending and descending). This finding requires surgical exploration to identify and repair the perforation.

Question 37: A conscious patient arrives with a knife impaled in the abdomen. The appropriate management is:

A) Remove the knife immediately
B) Leave the knife in place and transport to OR
C) Remove the knife and pack the wound
D) Obtain CT scan with knife in place

Answer: B

Explanation: Never remove impaled objects in the field or ED—they may be tamponading bleeding vessels. Leave the object in place, stabilize it to prevent movement, and transport to OR where it can be removed under controlled conditions with ability to immediately control hemorrhage if needed.

Question 38: What differentiates Grade I from Grade II splenic injury?

A) Size and depth of laceration or hematoma
B) Presence of symptoms
C) Patient age
D) Need for transfusion

Answer: A

Explanation: AAST grading scales for solid organs are based on anatomical injury severity—size and depth of lacerations, extent of hematomas, and involvement of major vessels. Grades I-II are minor, III moderate, IV-V severe. Grading guides treatment decisions and prognosis.

Question 39: A patient develops fever, elevated WBC, and worsening abdominal pain 48 hours after blunt abdominal trauma with initially negative workup. This suggests:

A) Pneumonia
B) Delayed hollow viscus perforation or abscess
C) Urinary tract infection
D) Normal postoperative course

Answer: B

Explanation: Delayed onset of fever, elevated WBC, and worsening pain after initially negative evaluation suggests delayed hollow viscus perforation or developing abscess. Some bowel injuries are subtle initially and declare themselves over 24-48 hours. This requires immediate re-evaluation and likely surgical exploration.

Question 40: The primary purpose of damage control laparotomy is to:

A) Definitively repair all injuries
B) Control hemorrhage and contamination quickly, leaving definitive repairs for later
C) Avoid surgery completely
D) Perform diagnostic exploration only

Answer: B

Explanation: Damage control surgery focuses on rapid hemorrhage control and contamination control in physiologically unstable patients, leaving definitive repairs for later when the patient is warmer, less acidotic, and better coagulating. Goal is survival, not perfect repair, in the initial operation.

Question 41: Which finding most reliably indicates need for immediate laparotomy?

A) Microscopic hematuria
B) Peritonitis with evisceration
C) Minor abdominal tenderness
D) Elevated lactate alone

Answer: B

Explanation: Peritonitis (rigid, diffusely tender abdomen indicating peritoneal contamination) or evisceration (abdominal contents protruding through wound) are absolute indications for immediate surgery. These patients need exploration without delay for imaging. The other findings require evaluation but aren't absolute surgical indications.

Question 42: A patient with pelvic fracture and scrotal hematoma likely has:

A) Testicular rupture
B) Urethral or bladder injury
C) Femoral vessel injury
D) Prostate injury

Answer: B

Explanation: Scrotal or labial hematoma with pelvic fracture suggests urethral or bladder injury with blood tracking into the scrotum or labia. This is a significant finding requiring evaluation with retrograde urethrogram or cystogram before catheter placement.

Question 43: What makes CT preferable to FAST for stable trauma patients?

A) CT is faster
B) CT provides detailed organ-specific information and injury grading
C) CT is less expensive
D) CT can be done at bedside

Answer: B

Explanation: CT provides detailed, organ-specific information including injury grading, active bleeding detection, and identification of injuries FAST might miss (retroperitoneal, hollow viscus). For stable patients who can tolerate transport to CT scanner, this detail guides treatment decisions. FAST's advantage is speed and bedside availability for unstable patients.

Question 44: A patient requires massive transfusion for abdominal hemorrhage. Avoiding hypothermia is important because:

A) Hypothermia causes patient discomfort
B) Hypothermia impairs coagulation and worsens bleeding
C) Hypothermia increases infection risk only
D) Hypothermia has no effect on trauma outcomes

Answer: B

Explanation: Hypothermia significantly impairs coagulation factor function, worsening bleeding. It's part of the "lethal triad" (hypothermia, acidosis, coagulopathy) that dramatically increases mortality in trauma. Maintaining patient temperature >35°C is crucial during resuscitation.

Question 45: The primary advantage of preserving the spleen in children is:

A) Avoiding surgical complications
B) Maintaining immune function against encapsulated bacteria
C) Reducing hospital costs
D) Faster recovery

Answer: B

Explanation: Spleen preservation maintains immune function, particularly important in children who have higher infection risk post-splenectomy. The spleen filters encapsulated bacteria that children frequently encounter. While surgical complications and recovery matter, immune function is the primary reason for aggressive non-operative management in pediatric splenic injuries.

Clinical Scenarios

Clinical Scenario 1: Blunt Abdominal Trauma with Seatbelt Sign

A 28-year-old female was the restrained driver in a frontal motor vehicle collision at 45 mph. She complains of lower abdominal pain. On examination, you note bruising across her lower abdomen in a seatbelt pattern. Vitals: HR 92, BP 124/78, RR 18, SpO2 98%. Abdomen is soft but tender in the lower quadrants. FAST exam is negative.

She undergoes CT scan which shows small amount of free fluid in the pelvis but no solid organ injury. Initial labs: WBC 11,000, Hgb 13.2, lactate 1.8.

Questions:

1. What is your primary concern based on the mechanism and physical findings?
2. What is the significance of free fluid on CT without solid organ injury?
3. What should be the management plan?
4. Eight hours later, she develops increasing abdominal pain with guarding and WBC rises to 16,000. What has likely occurred?

Answers:

1. **Primary concern:** Seatbelt sign with mechanism of frontal crash creates high suspicion for hollow viscus (intestinal) or mesenteric injury. The compression force between seatbelt and spine can cause burst injuries to bowel, mesenteric tears, or delayed perforations. Despite currently stable vitals and soft abdomen, this mechanism warrants close observation.
2. **Free fluid without solid organ injury** is concerning for hollow viscus or mesenteric injury. Blood from torn mesentery or intestinal content leak can cause free fluid. While amount is small, this finding combined with seatbelt sign significantly increases likelihood of missed bowel injury that may not be visible on initial CT.
3. **Management plan:** Admit for close observation with serial abdominal exams every 2-4 hours, serial labs (WBC, lactate), maintain NPO status, IV access and fluids, surgical consultation for close monitoring. Even with currently benign exam, many bowel injuries declare themselves over 12-24 hours as peritonitis develops. Low threshold for repeat imaging or exploratory laparotomy if exam worsens.
4. **Likely occurrence:** Delayed hollow viscus perforation or progression of initial injury. Some intestinal injuries have delayed presentation—the bowel may have contusion/serosalinjury that progresses to full-thickness perforation, or a small perforation slowly leaks intestinal contents. Rising WBC and worsening peritoneal signs indicate developing peritonitis requiring immediate surgical exploration. This case

illustrates why seatbelt sign demands vigilant observation even with initially reassuring findings.

Clinical Scenario 2: Splenic Injury with Delayed Rupture

A 35-year-old male presents after crashing his mountain bike 6 hours ago. He initially felt fine but now has worsening left upper quadrant pain and left shoulder discomfort. He appears pale. Vitals: HR 118, BP 98/62, RR 22, SpO_2 96%.

Examination shows left upper quadrant tenderness with mild guarding. FAST exam shows free fluid in the perisplenic space and pelvis. CT scan reveals Grade III splenic laceration with moderate hemoperitoneum and no contrast blush. Hemoglobin is 10.2 g/dL (was 14.5 on his last physical exam per patient).

Questions:

1. What is happening in this case?
2. Is this patient a candidate for non-operative management? Why or why not?
3. What monitoring is essential if non-operative management is attempted?
4. What findings would indicate failure of non-operative management?

Answers:

1. **What's happening:** This is a case of delayed splenic bleeding. The patient likely had initial minor injury that progressed over 6 hours. The spleen may have had a subcapsular hematoma that ruptured, or a laceration that initially had some tamponade that failed. He's now in early compensated shock (tachycardia, low-normal blood pressure, tachypnea) with ongoing hemorrhage evidenced by significant hemoperitoneum and anemia.
2. **Candidate for non-operative management:** This is borderline. Factors supporting non-operative approach: Grade III injury (moderate), no contrast blush (no active arterial bleeding), patient mentates well and can be monitored. Factors concerning: he's showing signs of compensated shock, significant anemia (lost ~4g hemoglobin), and moderate blood volume in abdomen. Decision requires senior surgical judgment. He needs ICU monitoring and immediate availability of OR. Many surgeons would attempt non-operative management with close monitoring and low threshold for surgery if he deteriorates.
3. **Essential monitoring:**

- ICU admission with continuous cardiac monitoring
- Serial vital signs every 15-30 minutes initially
- Serial abdominal exams every 1-2 hours
- Serial hemoglobin every 4-6 hours or more frequently if concerning
- Strict bed rest initially
- Large-bore IV access maintained
- Type and crossmatch blood available
- Surgeon immediately available
- Consider repeat imaging if clinical change

4. **Findings indicating failure:**

- Persistent tachycardia or hypotension despite resuscitation
- Falling hemoglobin requiring >4 units transfusion
- Worsening abdominal exam with increasing distension or peritonitis
- Developing shock or altered mental status
- Patient anxiety or sense of doom (surprisingly reliable indicator)
- Any of these warrant immediate operative intervention. The goal of non-operative management is avoiding surgery, but patient safety always takes priority—if bleeding doesn't stop, surgery is necessary.

Clinical Scenario 3: Pelvic Fracture with Hemorrhagic Shock

A 42-year-old male was a pedestrian struck by a car traveling 40 mph. He has obvious pelvic deformity with legs rotated externally. He's confused and agitated. Vitals: HR 138, BP 82/58, RR 28, SpO_2 91% on non-rebreather.

Examination shows unstable pelvis with gentle compression (you don't "rock" it), distended abdomen, blood at urethral meatus. No obvious chest or extremity injuries.

Questions:

1. What are your immediate priorities?
2. Why is there blood at the urethral meatus and how does this affect your management?
3. The patient receives pelvic binder, 2L crystalloid, and 4 units PRBCs but remains hypotensive at 86/54 with HR 132. What are the next steps?
4. What other injuries must be evaluated given the mechanism?

Answers:

1. **Immediate priorities:**

- **Airway/breathing:** Apply high-flow oxygen (already done), prepare for possible intubation if mental status worsens—confused/agitated state may indicate shock affecting cerebral perfusion
- **Hemorrhage control:** IMMEDIATELY apply pelvic binder around greater trochanters to reduce pelvic volume and tamponade bleeding
- **Resuscitation:** Establish two large-bore IVs, activate massive transfusion protocol, limit crystalloid to 1-2L, start blood products immediately
- **Don't insert Foley:** Blood at meatus indicates urethral injury
- **FAST exam:** Check for intra-abdominal bleeding (abdominal distension concerning)
- **Imaging:** Portable pelvis X-ray if not already done, but don't delay binder for imaging
- **Surgical consultation:** Both orthopedics and trauma surgery immediately

2. **Blood at meatus significance:** Indicates urethral injury, likely posterior urethral disruption from pelvic fracture. This absolutely contraindicates Foley catheter insertion—attempting placement could create false passage or worsen injury. Management: obtain retrograde urethrogram to confirm injury, place suprapubic catheter for bladder drainage (can be done at bedside or in OR), plan for delayed

urethral repair after acute injuries heal. Meanwhile, monitor for urinary retention and bladder distension clinically.

3. **Next steps for persistent hypotension:** Patient has received appropriate initial resuscitation (binder, limited crystalloid, blood products) but remains unstable. Options:

- **FAST exam findings guide next step:** If positive for intra-abdominal blood, patient likely needs laparotomy for abdominal bleeding source. If negative, bleeding is likely from pelvis.
- **For pelvic bleeding source:**
  - Continue massive transfusion protocol with balanced products
  - Consider external fixation (can be done in ED or OR)
  - CT angiography if stable enough (identifies arterial bleeding)
  - Angiography with embolization for arterial bleeding (if patient stable enough for transport to IR)
  - Preperitoneal packing in OR for venous bleeding
  - Consider REBOA as bridge to definitive treatment if immediately available
- **Don't delay definitive hemorrhage control:** If patient critically unstable, proceed to OR for hemorrhage control (either laparotomy if intra-abdominal source, or preperitoneal packing/external fixation if pelvic source)

4. **Other injuries to evaluate:**

- **Intra-abdominal injuries:** High-energy mechanism (pedestrian struck), distended abdomen, and shock warrant evaluation for solid organ or hollow viscus injuries
- **Spinal injuries:** High-energy mechanism requires spinal clearance
- **Head injury:** Confusion may be from shock but could also indicate traumatic brain injury—needs neuro assessment
- **Chest injuries:** Check carefully—any associated injuries?
- **Lower extremity injuries:** Associated fractures common with pelvic fractures
- **Bladder injury:** Along with urethral injury, assess for bladder rupture (hematuria, inability to void once suprapubic catheter placed)
- **Rectal/vaginal injuries:** Digital rectal exam for blood, palpable defects; vaginal exam in female patients This patient has life-threatening hemorrhage requiring immediate aggressive intervention. Pelvic fracture hemorrhage is one of the most challenging bleeding scenarios in trauma.

Clinical Scenario 4: Liver Laceration Management

A 26-year-old female presents after high-speed motor vehicle crash. She was unrestrained and struck the dashboard. She complains of right upper quadrant pain. Vitals: HR 102, BP 118/74, RR 20, SpO2 97%.

Examination shows right upper quadrant tenderness without guarding. FAST is positive in Morrison's pouch. CT shows Grade III liver laceration in right lobe with moderate hemoperitoneum, no active extravasation. Initial Hgb 12.8.

Questions:

1. Is this patient a candidate for non-operative management?
2. What specific monitoring is required?
3. Four hours later, her HR increases to 116, BP drops to 102/68, and Hgb is now 10.4 despite 2 units PRBCs. What does this suggest?
4. What are potential complications of liver injuries during the healing phase?

Answers:

1. **Candidate for non-operative management:** Yes, this patient is an appropriate candidate. Criteria met:

- Hemodynamically stable (acceptable vital signs)
- No peritonitis on exam (isolated tenderness without guarding/rigidity)
- No contrast blush on CT (no active arterial bleeding)
- Grade III injury (moderate—grades I-III routinely managed conservatively, grade IV often manageable)
- No other injuries requiring laparotomy
- Facility has capability for close ICU monitoring and immediate surgical intervention if needed

Plan: ICU admission, serial exams and labs, prepare for possible surgery if deteriorates. Success rate for non-operative management of grade III liver injuries in stable patients is very high (>80-90%).

2. **Required monitoring:**

- **ICU level care** with experienced nursing monitoring
- **Serial vital signs:** Every 15-30 minutes initially, can space out if stable
- **Serial abdominal exams:** Every 2-4 hours, looking for increasing tenderness, distension, peritonitis
- **Serial hemoglobin:** Every 6 hours initially, more frequently if concerning trends
- **Strict bed rest:** Initially complete bed rest, gradual mobilization only after clear stability
- **NPO initially:** May advance diet slowly as tolerated if remaining stable
- **Pain management:** Adequate analgesia, but avoid masking abdominal exam findings
- **Two large-bore IVs:** Maintained for rapid access if needed
- **Type and crossmatch:** Blood available immediately
- **Repeat imaging:** If clinical deterioration or concern for complications
- **Low threshold for surgery:** Don't persist with non-operative approach if patient deteriorating

3. **Clinical deterioration suggests:** Ongoing hemorrhage despite transfusion. The vital sign trends (increasing HR, dropping BP) combined with falling hemoglobin despite transfusion indicate continued bleeding. This represents failure of non-operative management. Options:

- **Repeat CT angiography:** Identify if now has active bleeding amenable to angiographic embolization
- **Angiography with embolization:** If arterial bleeding identified, IR can embolize specific vessels
- **Operative intervention:** If patient continues deteriorating or embolization fails/unavailable, proceed to exploratory laparotomy for direct hemorrhage control Key decision point: some ongoing oozing is acceptable if patient stabilizes with transfusion, but persistent requirements >4-6 units or hemodynamic instability warrants intervention.

4. **Complications during healing:**

- **Rebleeding:** Can occur days to weeks after injury as clots dissolve or tamponade fails—presents with sudden pain, hypotension, dropping hemoglobin
- **Bile leak:** Causes persistent right upper quadrant pain, fever, elevated bilirubin—diagnosed with HIDA scan or ERCP, may require percutaneous drainage or ERCP with stent
- **Abscess formation:** Infected hematoma or devitalized tissue—presents with fever, elevated WBC, persistent pain—requires drainage (percutaneous or surgical)
- **Biloma:** Bile collection without infection—may be asymptomatic or cause pain—often requires drainage
- **Hemobilia:** Blood leaking into biliary tree—presents with right upper quadrant pain, jaundice, GI bleeding—treated with angiographic embolization

Most patients heal without complications, but vigilance for these issues is important in follow-up. Patients typically need activity restrictions for 4-6 weeks and repeat imaging to confirm healing.

Clinical Scenario 5: Hollow Viscus Injury with Delayed Presentation

A 19-year-old male presents 18 hours after a dirt bike crash where he struck the handlebars with his abdomen. He initially felt okay and declined medical attention at the scene. Now he has worsening epigastric and periumbilical pain, nausea, and one episode of vomiting.

Vitals: HR 108, BP 118/76, RR 20, SpO_2 98%, temperature 38.2°C (100.8°F). Examination shows epigastric tenderness with guarding. Bowel sounds are diminished.

Labs: WBC 18,500, Hgb 14.2, amylase 485 (elevated), lipase 892 (elevated), lactate 2.8. CT scan shows retroperitoneal fluid and fat stranding around the duodenum, possible thickening of duodenal wall, but no obvious perforation or free air.

Questions:

1. What injuries does this clinical picture suggest?
2. Why did symptoms develop over 18 hours rather than immediately?
3. What is the appropriate management given the CT findings and clinical presentation?
4. What complications could develop if this injury is missed or treatment delayed further?

Answers:

1. **Injuries suggested:** This presentation is highly suspicious for duodenal injury, possibly with associated pancreatic injury. The mechanism (handlebar impact to epigastrium) is classic for these injuries. Elevated amylase and lipase suggest pancreatic involvement. Retroperitoneal fluid and fat stranding around the duodenum indicate injury to this retroperitoneal structure. The fever and elevated WBC developing over 18 hours suggest evolving peritonitis or retroperitoneal contamination.
2. **Delayed symptom development:** Duodenal injuries often present with delayed symptoms because the duodenum is retroperitoneal. Initial injury may be contained by the retroperitoneum without immediate peritoneal contamination. Symptoms develop as:
    - The injury progresses from contusion to full-thickness perforation
    - Duodenal contents slowly leak into retroperitoneum
    - Inflammation develops and spreads
    - Pancreatic injury evolves (pancreatic enzymes cause significant inflammation)

    This delayed presentation is why handlebar injuries require high suspicion and close observation even with initially benign findings. Many duodenal injuries aren't obvious on initial CT and declare themselves over 24-48 hours.

3. **Appropriate management:** Despite no obvious perforation on CT, this patient's clinical picture (worsening pain, fever, peritoneal signs, elevated WBC, suspicious CT findings, classic mechanism) warrants surgical exploration. Options:
    - **Most appropriate:** Exploratory laparotomy for direct visualization of duodenum and pancreas, repair of any injuries found
    - **Why surgery despite uncertain CT:** Clinical signs of peritonitis trump imaging. Duodenal perforations are notoriously difficult to visualize on CT, especially early. The retroperitoneal location means injuries can be subtle. This patient is deteriorating clinically.
    - **Surgical findings likely:** May find duodenal perforation, hematoma, or contusion; possible pancreatic injury. Repair depends on specific injuries found.
    - **If surgery delayed:** Continue IV fluids, NPO, broad-spectrum antibiotics, serial exams—but threshold for surgery should be very low given progressive symptoms. Some surgeons might observe another 6-12 hours with close monitoring, but worsening exam warrants surgery.
4. **Complications of missed/delayed treatment:**
    - **Sepsis:** Duodenal contents contain bacteria; ongoing leak leads to retroperitoneal and eventually peritoneal contamination and sepsis
    - **Abscess formation:** Infected fluid collections require drainage
    - **Fistula:** Unrepaired perforation can form duodenocutaneous fistula (abnormal connection between duodenum and skin), very difficult to manage
    - **Pancreatitis progression:** Associated pancreatic injury worsens without intervention
    - **Multi-organ failure:** Untreated sepsis progresses to shock and organ failure
    - **Death:** Delayed treatment significantly increases mortality

Key learning points from this scenario:

- Mechanism matters: handlebar injuries should raise immediate suspicion for duodenal/pancreatic trauma
- Delayed presentation is classic for retroperitoneal injuries
- Clinical picture trumps imaging: if patient has peritonitis, explore surgically even if CT doesn't show obvious perforation
- Serial examinations save lives: injuries that aren't obvious initially often become apparent over 12-24 hours
- Don't dismiss patients who initially feel okay after significant trauma—educate them about warning signs and when to return

Chapter 6: Orthopedic and Neurovascular Trauma

Musculoskeletal injuries are the most common trauma, ranging from minor sprains to life-threatening vascular injuries. While broken bones may seem less critical than chest or abdominal injuries, orthopedic trauma can cause significant disability, and associated vascular or nerve injuries can lead to limb loss if not recognized and treated promptly.

This chapter covers long bone fractures, joint dislocations, compartment syndrome, vascular injuries, and proper immobilization techniques. Understanding these concepts helps you identify which injuries need urgent intervention and which can be managed more conservatively.

Long Bone Fractures

Long bones (femur, tibia, fibula, humerus, radius, ulna) can be fractured through various mechanisms. While the fractures themselves heal with proper treatment, associated complications—particularly bleeding and neurovascular compromise—require immediate attention.

Femur Fractures

The femur is the longest and strongest bone in the body, and fracturing it requires significant force. Femur fractures are serious injuries with potential for life-threatening complications.

Mechanisms:

- High-energy trauma: Motor vehicle crashes, motorcycle accidents, falls from height
- Direct impact to thigh
- Twisting injuries (less common, requires less force in elderly with osteoporosis)

Types of femur fractures:

Femoral shaft fractures (mid-portion of bone):

- Most common femur fracture in adults
- Usually from high-energy trauma
- Can be transverse, oblique, spiral, or comminuted (multiple fragments)

Femoral neck fractures (hip region):

- More common in elderly from falls
- High risk of avascular necrosis (blood supply to femoral head disrupted)

- Often requires surgical repair with pins, screws, or hip replacement

Distal femur fractures (near knee):

- Often involve knee joint
- May be associated with knee ligament injuries

Clinical presentation:

- Severe thigh pain
- Obvious deformity—leg shortened, rotated (usually externally rotated and shortened)
- Swelling of thigh (from hematoma)
- Inability to bear weight or move leg
- Possible open wound if open fracture
- Signs of shock if significant blood loss

Blood loss considerations: Each femur fracture can cause 1000-1500 mL blood loss into the thigh. This blood dissects through tissue planes and accumulates in the thigh compartment. With bilateral femur fractures, patients can lose 2-3 liters of blood, leading to hemorrhagic shock from long bone fractures alone.

Neurovascular assessment: Always assess before and after any manipulation or splinting:

- **Pulses:** Dorsalis pedis and posterior tibial pulses
- **Capillary refill:** Should be <2 seconds
- **Sensation:** Can patient feel light touch on foot? Any numbness or tingling?
- **Motor function:** Can patient wiggle toes? Dorsiflex and plantarflex foot?
- **Color and temperature:** Is leg pale or dusky? Cool compared to other side?

Management:

Initial stabilization:

- Assess neurovascular status and document findings
- Control any external bleeding
- Splint in position found initially (don't attempt to reduce unless neurovascular compromise—this can worsen injury)
- Apply traction splint if available and trained in its use
- Pain management
- Monitor for shock—establish IV access, initiate fluid resuscitation as needed
- Cover any open wounds with sterile dressing
- Antibiotics for open fractures
- Tetanus prophylaxis

Traction splints: Devices that apply longitudinal traction to align fracture fragments and reduce pain by preventing muscle spasm. Types include Hare traction splint, Sager splint, and Kendrick traction device. Proper application requires training—incorrect application can worsen injury.

Definitive treatment:

- Closed reduction and casting (rare—most need surgery)
- Internal fixation with intramedullary rod (most common for shaft fractures)
- Plates and screws
- External fixation for severe open fractures or unstable patients

Complications:

- **Fat embolism syndrome:** Fat from bone marrow enters circulation, travels to lungs and brain. Presents 24-72 hours post-injury with respiratory distress, confusion, petechial rash. Requires supportive care, possible ventilator support.
- **Compartment syndrome:** Discussed in detail below
- **Nonunion or malunion:** Bone doesn't heal properly
- **Infection:** Particularly with open fractures
- **Nerve injury:** Uncommon but possible, particularly with high-energy trauma

Tibia/Fibula Fractures

The tibia (shinbone) is the most commonly fractured long bone. The fibula often fractures along with it.

Mechanisms:

- Direct blow to shin
- Twisting injuries
- Falls
- Motor vehicle crashes

Clinical presentation:

- Pain, swelling, deformity of lower leg
- Inability to bear weight
- Possible open wound (tibia is subcutaneous anteriorly, making open fractures common)
- Neurovascular compromise possible but less common than with other long bones

Special considerations:

- **High risk of compartment syndrome:** The lower leg has four compartments. Fracture bleeding and swelling can increase pressure, causing compartment syndrome.
- **Open fractures common:** The anterior tibia is just beneath the skin with minimal soft tissue coverage, so even moderate trauma can cause open fractures.

Management:

- Neurovascular assessment
- Splinting (posterior splint or pre-formed splint)
- Elevation to reduce swelling

- Ice application
- Pain management
- Definitive treatment: Casting for stable fractures, surgical fixation (intramedullary rod or plates/screws) for displaced or unstable fractures
- Monitor closely for compartment syndrome development

Humerus Fractures

Upper arm fractures are less likely to cause life-threatening complications but can injure important neurovascular structures.

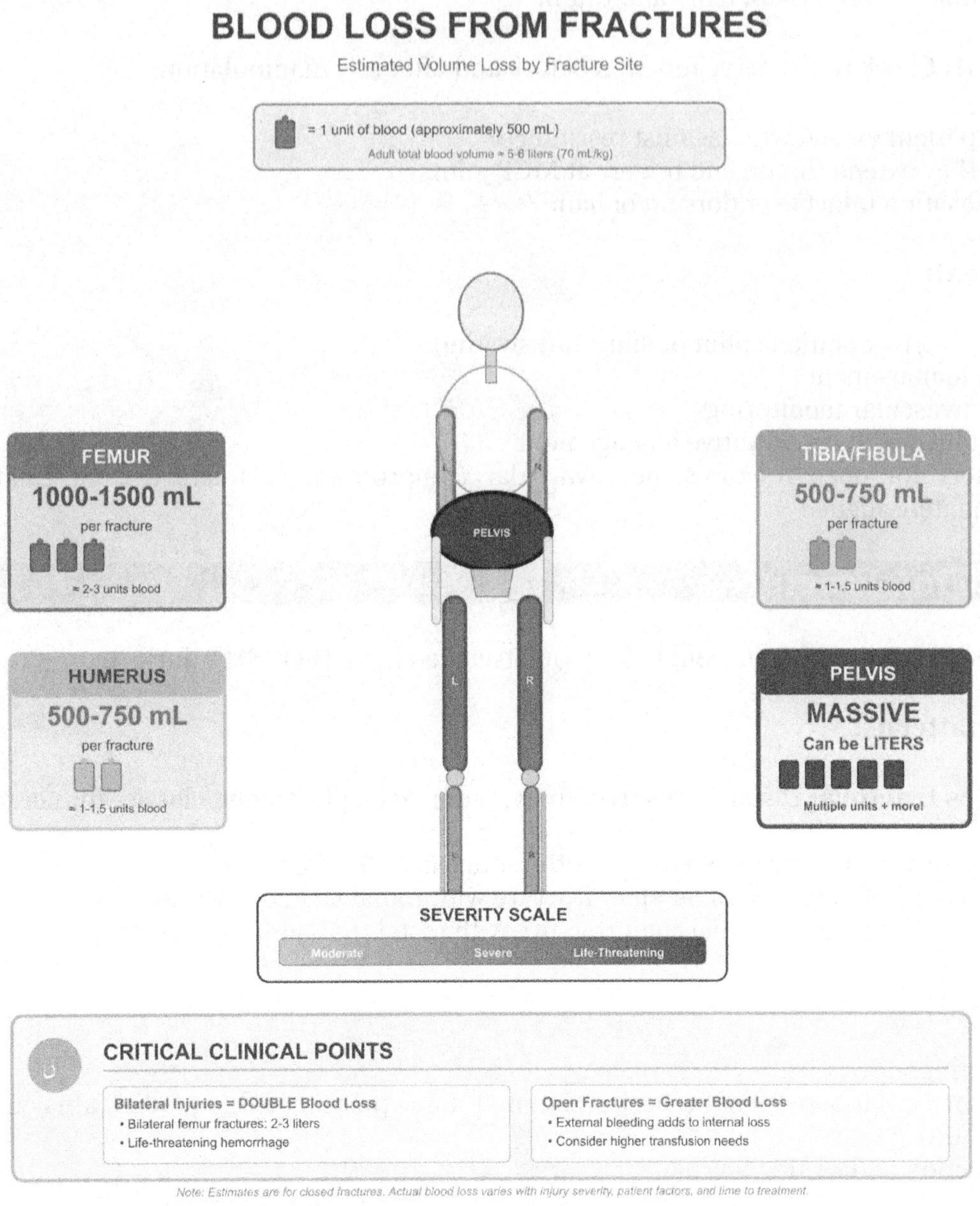

Types:

- **Proximal humerus fractures:** Near shoulder, common in elderly falls
- **Humeral shaft fractures:** Mid-arm, from direct blow or fall
- **Distal humerus fractures:** Near elbow, often in children

Key concern—radial nerve injury: The radial nerve wraps around the humerus in a spiral groove. Midshaft fractures can injure this nerve, causing:

- Wrist drop (inability to extend wrist)
- Weak grip
- Numbness over back of hand and thumb

Assessment: Check radial nerve function before and after any manipulation:

- Can patient extend wrist against resistance?
- Can they extend thumb and fingers at MCP joints?
- Is sensation intact over dorsum of hand?

Management:

- Splinting (coaptation splint or sling and swathe)
- Pain management
- Neurovascular monitoring
- Most heal with conservative management
- Surgery for open fractures, neurovascular compromise, or fractures that can't be adequately aligned

Radius/Ulna Fractures

Forearm fractures are common from falls on outstretched hand (FOOSH injuries).

Common patterns:

- **Colles fracture:** Distal radius fracture with dorsal displacement, classic "dinner fork" deformity
- **Both-bone forearm fractures:** Both radius and ulna fractured
- **Monteggia fracture:** Ulnar shaft fracture with radial head dislocation
- **Galeazzi fracture:** Radial shaft fracture with distal radioulnar joint disruption

Management:

- Splinting
- Neurovascular assessment (check radial and ulnar pulses, median/radial/ulnar nerve function)
- Reduction and casting for many fractures
- Surgical fixation for unstable fractures or those involving joint surfaces

Joint Dislocations

Dislocations occur when bones forming a joint are displaced from normal position. They often stretch or tear ligaments, and some dislocations can injure nearby nerves or blood vessels.

Shoulder Dislocation

Most commonly dislocated joint in the body. Usually occurs in anterior direction (humeral head displaced anteriorly).

Mechanism:

- Fall on outstretched arm
- Direct blow to shoulder
- Forced external rotation and abduction

Clinical presentation:

- Severe shoulder pain
- Obvious deformity—shoulder appears "squared off" rather than rounded
- Arm held in slight abduction and external rotation
- Patient refuses to move arm
- Loss of normal shoulder contour

Neurovascular concerns:

- **Axillary nerve:** Most commonly injured, causes numbness over lateral shoulder (regimental badge area) and weak deltoid
- **Axillary artery:** Rare but serious, can cause limb-threatening ischemia
- Always assess pulses, sensation, and motor function before and after reduction

Management:

- Neurovascular exam and documentation
- X-ray to confirm dislocation and rule out fracture
- Pain management and sedation for reduction
- Reduction techniques (multiple methods exist—traction-countertraction, Stimson technique, external rotation method)
- Post-reduction X-ray to confirm reduction
- Immobilization in sling
- Repeat neurovascular exam after reduction
- Orthopedic follow-up

Complications:

- Recurrent dislocation (common, especially in younger patients)
- Rotator cuff tear (more common in older patients)

- Nerve injury
- Vascular injury

Hip Dislocation

Less common but more serious than shoulder dislocation. Requires high-energy trauma.

Types:

- **Posterior dislocation (90%):** Femoral head displaced posteriorly, usually from dashboard injury in motor vehicle crash (knee strikes dashboard, driving femur backward)
- **Anterior dislocation (10%):** Femoral head displaced anteriorly

Clinical presentation:

Posterior dislocation:

- Severe hip pain
- Leg shortened, internally rotated, and adducted
- Hip flexed
- Patient cannot move leg

Anterior dislocation:

- Hip pain
- Leg extended, externally rotated, and abducted

Neurovascular concerns:

- **Sciatic nerve injury:** Common with posterior dislocation (nerve courses behind hip joint). Causes foot drop, loss of ankle dorsiflexion/plantarflexion, numbness in foot
- **Femoral artery/nerve:** Can be injured in anterior dislocation

Critical time issue—avascular necrosis: The blood supply to the femoral head can be compromised when hip is dislocated. Risk of avascular necrosis (death of bone from lack of blood supply) increases significantly if reduction is delayed beyond 6 hours. Hip dislocations are orthopedic emergencies requiring urgent reduction.

Management:

- Immediate assessment of neurovascular status, particularly sciatic nerve function
- Immediate orthopedic consultation
- X-ray to confirm and assess for associated fractures
- Urgent closed reduction under sedation (or general anesthesia if needed)
- If closed reduction fails, open reduction in OR
- Post-reduction CT to assess for fracture fragments in joint
- Post-reduction X-ray to confirm reduction

- Period of non-weight bearing
- Close follow-up for avascular necrosis development

Knee Dislocation

Knee dislocations are rare but extremely serious due to high risk of vascular injury. These are different from patellar dislocations (kneecap displacement), which are common and less serious.

True knee dislocation: Tibia displaced relative to femur, disrupting multiple ligaments.

Mechanism:

- High-energy trauma (motor vehicle crash, fall from height)
- Sometimes sports injuries (hyperextension)

Critical concern—popliteal artery injury: The popliteal artery runs directly behind the knee joint. When the knee dislocates, this artery can be stretched, torn, or thrombosed. Without blood flow, the lower leg becomes ischemic, and amputation may be necessary if not restored quickly.

Clinical presentation:

- Obvious knee deformity
- Severe pain
- May spontaneously reduce before arrival, making diagnosis challenging
- **Absent or decreased pedal pulses** (dorsalis pedis, posterior tibial)—critical finding
- Knee instability in multiple directions
- Significant swelling

Management:

- **Immediate reduction** if still dislocated—don't wait for X-ray if pulses absent
- Check pulses before and after reduction
- If pulses remain absent after reduction: Emergency vascular surgery consultation, immediate angiography or surgical exploration
- If pulses present: Close neurovascular monitoring, CT angiography to rule out intimal tear (inner vessel damage that may not show as absent pulse initially but can thrombose later)
- Immobilization
- Orthopedic surgery for ligament reconstruction (later, after vascular issues addressed)

Time is tissue: Prolonged ischemia leads to irreversible muscle and nerve damage. The "golden window" for restoring blood flow is 6-8 hours, after which amputation rates increase dramatically.

Elbow Dislocation

Second most common dislocation in adults, most common in children.

Mechanism:

- Fall on outstretched hand with elbow extended

Clinical presentation:

- Obvious deformity
- Severe pain
- Inability to move elbow

Neurovascular concerns:

- **Brachial artery:** Can be compressed or injured
- **Median, ulnar, radial nerves:** Can be stretched or injured
- Always check pulses and nerve function

Management:

- Neurovascular assessment
- X-ray
- Reduction under sedation
- Post-reduction X-ray and neurovascular exam
- Immobilization
- Close follow-up

Compartment Syndrome

Compartment syndrome is a surgical emergency where pressure within a closed muscle compartment increases, compromising blood flow to muscles and nerves. Without prompt treatment, it causes permanent disability or necessitates amputation.

Understanding Compartment Anatomy

Muscles are organized into compartments enclosed by fascia (tough, inelastic tissue). In the lower leg, there are four compartments: anterior, lateral, superficial posterior, and deep posterior. Each compartment contains muscles, nerves, and blood vessels.

Fascia doesn't stretch. When pressure inside the compartment increases (from bleeding, swelling, or external compression), the rigid fascial boundaries prevent expansion. As pressure rises, it eventually exceeds capillary perfusion pressure, cutting off blood flow to tissues within the compartment.

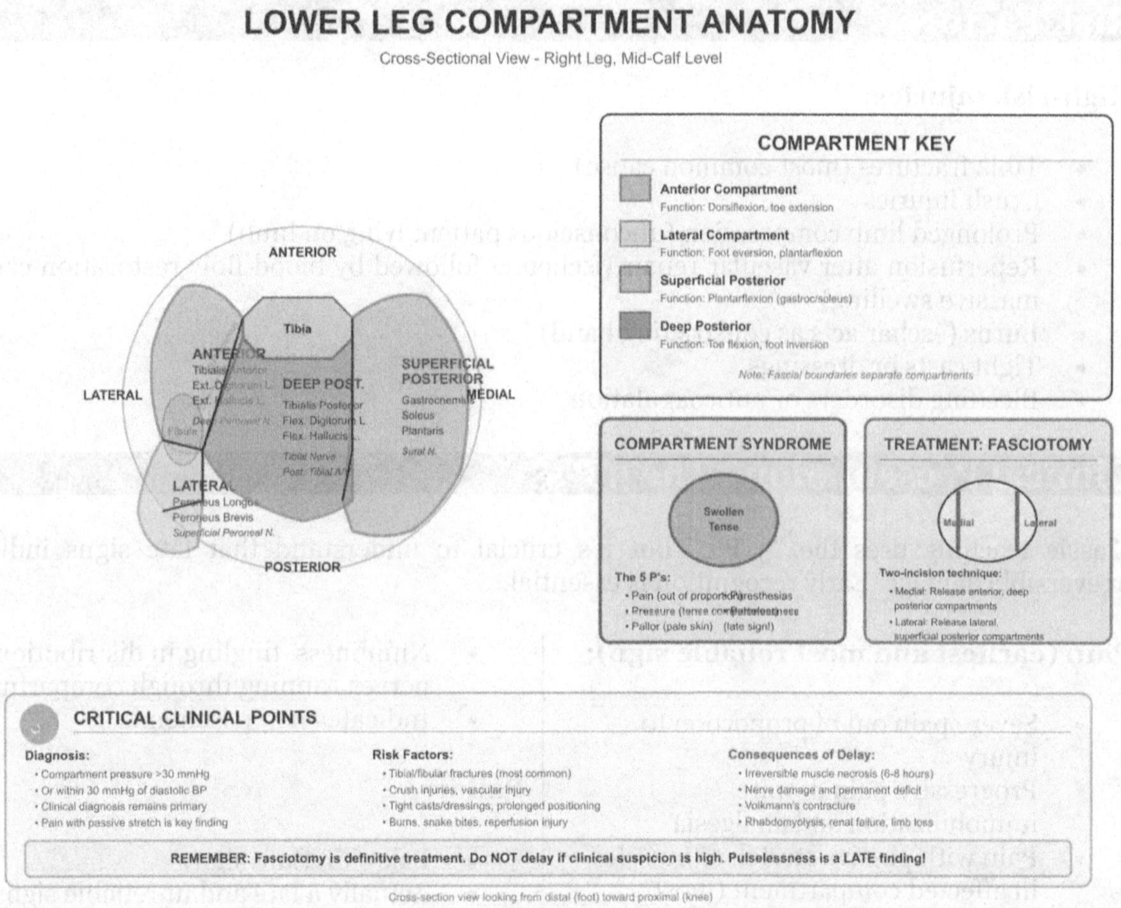

Pathophysiology

The pressure cascade:

1. Injury causes bleeding and swelling within compartment
2. Compartment pressure rises (normal pressure is <10 mmHg)
3. When pressure reaches 20-30 mmHg, capillary blood flow decreases
4. Decreased perfusion causes tissue ischemia
5. Ischemia causes more swelling (ischemia-reperfusion injury)
6. More swelling increases pressure further
7. Vicious cycle continues until intervention or tissue death occurs

Critical concept: Compartment syndrome doesn't require absent pulses. Arterial pressure (which determines pulse) is much higher than capillary pressure. Capillaries collapse long before arteries, meaning tissue damage occurs while pulses remain palpable. Don't wait for absent pulses to diagnose compartment syndrome—you'll be too late.

Risk Factors

High-risk injuries:

- Tibia fractures (most common cause)
- Crush injuries
- Prolonged limb compression (unconscious patient lying on limb)
- Reperfusion after vascular repair (ischemia followed by blood flow restoration causes massive swelling)
- Burns (eschar acts as constricting band)
- Tight casts or dressings
- Bleeding disorders or anticoagulation

Clinical Presentation—The 5 P's

Classic teaching uses the "5 P's," but it's crucial to understand that late signs indicate irreversible damage. Early recognition is essential.

Pain (earliest and most reliable sign):

- Severe pain out of proportion to injury
- Progressive pain despite immobilization and analgesia
- Pain with passive stretch of muscles in affected compartment (most sensitive clinical finding)
    - Example: Passively dorsiflexing foot causes severe calf pain in anterior compartment syndrome

Pressure:

- Compartment feels tense, swollen, firm to palpation
- Skin may be shiny and tight

Paresthesias:

- Numbness, tingling in distribution of nerves running through compartment
- Indicates nerve ischemia

Pallor:

- Pale skin (late sign)
- Actually a late and unreliable sign

Pulselessness:

- Absent pulses (very late sign)
- If you wait for this, permanent damage has occurred
- Presence of pulses does NOT rule out compartment syndrome

Paralysis:

- Inability to move muscles (very late sign)
- Indicates irreversible muscle damage

Clinical pearl: Pain out of proportion to injury, worsening pain, and pain with passive stretch are early signs. If you're seeing the "late" P's (pallor, pulselessness, paralysis), you've missed the window for preventing permanent damage.

Diagnosis

Clinical diagnosis is primary. High suspicion based on mechanism and symptoms is most important.

Compartment pressure measurement:

- Normal: <10 mmHg
- Concerning: >20 mmHg
- Critical: >30 mmHg or within 30 mmHg of diastolic blood pressure

Methods:

- Handheld pressure monitor (Stryker device most common)
- Arterial line transducer system
- Insert needle into compartment and measure pressure

Limitations: Single measurement can be misleading. Diagnosis should be based on clinical picture, not pressure measurement alone. An alert patient with severe pain and concerning exam needs fasciotomy even with borderline pressures. Unconscious or obtunded patients may need pressure monitoring for diagnosis.

Management

Non-operative measures (temporary only):

- Remove all constrictive dressings, casts, or bandages
- Elevate limb to heart level (not above—excessive elevation reduces arterial inflow)
- Supplemental oxygen
- Correct hypotension (maintain adequate perfusion pressure)
- Pain management

These measures may temporarily reduce pressure but **DO NOT replace fasciotomy when indicated**.

Fasciotomy (definitive treatment): Surgical release of fascia to decompress compartments. This is the only definitive treatment.

Indications:

- Compartment syndrome diagnosed clinically
- Compartment pressure >30 mmHg
- Delta pressure (diastolic BP minus compartment pressure) <30 mmHg

Procedure:

- Incisions made along length of limb

- Fascia overlying each compartment is released
- All compartments must be released (four in lower leg, three in forearm)
- Wounds left open initially
- Delayed primary closure or skin grafting after swelling resolves (typically 3-7 days)

Timing is critical: Permanent damage begins 4-6 hours after compartment syndrome onset. Muscle necrosis is irreversible after 8 hours. Early fasciotomy (within 6 hours) has excellent outcomes. Delayed fasciotomy still saves the limb but may not prevent permanent disability.

Complications of untreated or delayed treatment:

- Muscle necrosis
- Nerve damage (permanent numbness, weakness, pain)
- Volkmann's contracture (permanent flexion contracture of hand/fingers from forearm compartment syndrome)
- Infection
- Amputation
- Renal failure (myoglobin from dead muscle damages kidneys—rhabdomyolysis)
- Death (rare, from metabolic complications)

Vascular Injuries

Extremity vascular injuries can occur from trauma to arteries or veins. Arterial injuries are more immediately limb-threatening, while venous injuries primarily concern hemorrhage control.

Recognition of Vascular Injury

Hard signs (definite vascular injury requiring surgery):

- Absent pulse distal to injury
- Pulsatile bleeding
- Expanding or pulsatile hematoma
- Audible bruit or palpable thrill over injury site
- Signs of acute limb ischemia (pale, cool, pulseless limb)

Soft signs (possible vascular injury requiring further evaluation):

- History of significant bleeding at scene
- Proximity of wound to major vessel
- Diminished but present pulse
- Non-expanding hematoma
- Peripheral nerve deficit (suggests proximity to neurovascular bundle)

Ankle-Brachial Index (ABI): Ratio of ankle systolic pressure to arm systolic pressure. Normal is 0.9-1.3. ABI <0.9 suggests arterial injury and warrants further investigation.

Management Principles

Hard signs:

- Immediate vascular surgery consultation
- Don't delay for imaging
- Operating room for exploration and repair

Soft signs:

- CT angiography to identify injury
- Possible angiography with intervention if needed
- Close observation if studies negative

Temporary hemorrhage control:

- Direct pressure (don't blindly clamp vessels—can damage nerves)
- Tourniquet for severe extremity hemorrhage
- Never probe wounds to "find the bleeding"—worsens injury and dislodges clots

Definitive repair:

- Primary repair (sew vessel back together)
- Vein patch (use vein segment to patch arterial defect)
- Interposition graft (bridge gap with graft)
- Endovascular stenting (for some injuries)

Warm ischemia time: Prolonged ischemia causes irreversible damage. Muscles tolerate 4-6 hours of ischemia. Beyond this, amputation may be necessary even if flow is restored.

Amputation Management

Traumatic amputations range from partial to complete loss of limb or digit.

Initial management:

- Control hemorrhage (direct pressure, pressure dressing, tourniquet if needed)
- Resuscitate patient
- Don't focus solely on amputation—assess for other life-threatening injuries
- Pain management

Care of amputated part:

- Wrap amputated part in saline-moistened gauze
- Place in plastic bag
- Place bag on ice (don't place part directly on ice—causes frostbite)
- Transport with patient
- Even if part doesn't seem viable, bring it—surgeons will decide

Replantation considerations:

Good candidates:

- Thumb amputation (critical for hand function)
- Multiple digit amputation
- Amputation through palm or wrist
- Clean sharp amputation
- Pediatric patients (better healing)
- Short ischemia time (<6 hours for digits, <4 hours for large muscle masses)

Poor candidates:

- Severe crush or avulsion mechanism
- Multilevel injury
- Severe contamination
- Prolonged ischemia time
- Significant other injuries taking priority
- Patient medically unstable

Psychological support: Traumatic amputation is devastating. Provide compassionate care, acknowledge the loss, and connect patient with support resources.

Splinting and Immobilization

Proper splinting prevents further injury, reduces pain, and controls bleeding.

Principles of Splinting

Goals:

- Immobilize fracture/injury
- Reduce pain
- Prevent neurovascular compromise
- Prevent closed fractures from becoming open
- Prevent further soft tissue damage

General rules:

- Splint before transport unless life-threatening injuries take priority
- Immobilize joint above and below fracture
- Pad bony prominences
- Check neurovascular status before and after splinting
- Assess frequently after splinting—swelling can cause compartment syndrome even with proper splinting
- If neurovascular status worsens after splinting, remove and reassess

Types of Splints

Rigid splints:

- Cardboard, wood, aluminum, vacuum splints
- Conform to limb shape
- Secure with wraps or straps

Soft splints:

- Pillow splints (for ankle injuries)
- Sling and swathe (for shoulder/humerus)
- Useful for certain injuries but provide less rigid immobilization

Traction splints:

- For femur fractures
- Apply longitudinal traction to align fracture and reduce pain
- Requires specific training

Commercial splints:

- SAM splints (malleable aluminum)
- Air splints (inflate around limb)
- Pre-formed splints for specific anatomical areas

Application Technique

1. Assess neurovascular status
2. Apply padding, especially over bony prominences
3. Position splint along limb
4. Secure splint without over-tightening
5. Reassess neurovascular status
6. Elevate if possible
7. Apply ice
8. Document application and findings

Common mistake: Over-tightening wraps or straps, causing vascular compromise or compartment syndrome.

Chapter Practice Questions (40 questions)

Question 1: Each femur fracture can cause approximately how much blood loss into the thigh?

A) 250-500 mL
B) 500-750 mL
C) 1000-1500 mL
D) 2000-3000 mL

Answer: C

Explanation: Each femur fracture can cause 1000-1500 mL of blood loss into the thigh compartment. This significant blood loss can lead to hemorrhagic shock, especially with bilateral femur fractures. Recognition of this blood loss potential guides resuscitation strategies.

Question 2: What is the most reliable early sign of compartment syndrome?

A) Absent pulses
B) Paralysis
C) Pain out of proportion to injury and pain with passive stretch
D) Pallor

Answer: C

Explanation: Pain out of proportion to the injury and severe pain with passive stretching of muscles in the affected compartment are the earliest and most reliable signs. Waiting for the late signs (pulselessness, paralysis, pallor) means irreversible damage has occurred.

Question 3: A patient with a midshaft humerus fracture should be assessed for which nerve injury?

A) Median nerve
B) Ulnar nerve
C) Radial nerve
D) Axillary nerve

Answer: C

Explanation: The radial nerve wraps around the humerus in a spiral groove, making it vulnerable to injury with midshaft fractures. Radial nerve injury causes wrist drop, weak grip, and numbness over the dorsum of the hand. Always assess radial nerve function before and after manipulation.

Question 4: What is the definitive treatment for compartment syndrome?

A) Elevation and ice
B) Removal of restrictive dressings
C) Fasciotomy
D) Pain medication

Answer: C

Explanation: Fasciotomy (surgical release of the fascia) is the only definitive treatment for compartment syndrome. While removing restrictive dressings and elevation may temporarily help, they don't replace the need for surgical decompression when compartment syndrome is present.

Question 5: Hip dislocations should be reduced within what timeframe to minimize risk of avascular necrosis?

A) 2 hours
B) 6 hours
C) 12 hours
D) 24 hours

Answer: B

Explanation: Hip dislocations should be reduced within 6 hours to minimize risk of avascular necrosis of the femoral head. Blood supply to the femoral head is compromised when the hip is dislocated, and prolonged ischemia leads to bone death. This makes hip dislocation an orthopedic emergency.

Question 6: Which nerve is most commonly injured with anterior shoulder dislocation?

A) Radial nerve
B) Median nerve
C) Axillary nerve
D) Ulnar nerve

Answer: C

Explanation: The axillary nerve is most commonly injured with anterior shoulder dislocation. This causes numbness over the lateral shoulder (regimental badge area) and weak deltoid muscle function. Always assess axillary nerve function before and after shoulder reduction.

Question 7: Normal compartment pressure is:

A) <10 mmHg
B) <20 mmHg
C) <30 mmHg
D) <40 mmHg

Answer: A

Explanation: Normal compartment pressure is less than 10 mmHg. Pressures above 20 mmHg are concerning, and pressures above 30 mmHg or within 30 mmHg of diastolic blood pressure are critical and require fasciotomy.

Question 8: Hard signs of vascular injury requiring immediate surgical exploration include:

A) Proximity wound to major vessel
B) Small hematoma
C) Pulsatile bleeding and absent distal pulse
D) Minor nerve deficit

Answer: C

Explanation: Hard signs include pulsatile bleeding, absent pulse, expanding/pulsatile hematoma, bruit/thrill, and signs of acute ischemia. These indicate definite vascular injury requiring immediate surgery. Soft signs like proximity or small hematoma warrant investigation but may not need immediate surgery.

Question 9: A patient with knee dislocation and absent pedal pulses needs:

A) CT scan before any intervention
B) Immediate reduction without waiting for imaging
C) Orthopedic consultation first
D) Observation for 24 hours

Answer: B

Explanation: Knee dislocation with absent pulses is a vascular emergency. Immediate reduction should be performed without waiting for imaging to restore blood flow.

The popliteal artery is at high risk with knee dislocations, and prolonged ischemia leads to amputation.

Question 10: The lower leg has how many muscle compartments?

A) Two
B) Three
C) Four
D) Five

Answer: C

Explanation: The lower leg has four compartments: anterior, lateral, superficial posterior, and deep posterior. All four must be released during fasciotomy for lower leg compartment syndrome. Incomplete fasciotomy leaves some compartments compressed.

Question 11: Which position indicates posterior hip dislocation?

A) Leg externally rotated and abducted
B) Leg shortened, internally rotated, and adducted
C) Leg lengthened and neutral rotation
D) Leg flexed at 90 degrees with external rotation

Answer: B

Explanation: Posterior hip dislocation (90% of hip dislocations) presents with the leg shortened, internally rotated, and adducted with hip flexed. This classic position results from the femoral head displaced posteriorly. Anterior dislocation shows opposite findings (extended, externally rotated, abducted).

Question 12: What is the purpose of a traction splint for femur fractures?

A) Prevent infection
B) Apply longitudinal traction to align fracture and reduce pain
C) Immobilize the knee joint
D) Reduce swelling

Answer: B

Explanation: Traction splints apply longitudinal traction along the femur to pull fracture fragments into better alignment and reduce pain by preventing muscle spasm. This also helps control bleeding by reducing movement at the fracture site.

Question 13: A patient has wrist drop and numbness over the dorsum of the hand after humerus fracture. This indicates:

A) Median nerve injury
B) Ulnar nerve injury
C) Radial nerve injury
D) Musculocutaneous nerve injury

Answer: C

Explanation: Wrist drop (inability to extend wrist) and numbness over dorsum of hand are classic signs of radial nerve injury. This nerve commonly injured with midshaft humerus fractures because it wraps around the bone in the spiral groove.

Question 14: Fat embolism syndrome typically presents how long after long bone fracture?

A) Immediately
B) 6-12 hours
C) 24-72 hours
D) 1-2 weeks

Answer: C

Explanation: Fat embolism syndrome typically develops 24-72 hours after long bone fracture (especially femur). Fat from bone marrow enters circulation and travels to lungs and brain, causing respiratory distress, confusion, and petechial rash. Treatment is supportive.

Question 15: Which injury has the highest risk of developing compartment syndrome?

A) Clavicle fracture
B) Tibia fracture
C) Scaphoid fracture
D) Finger fracture

Answer: B

Explanation: Tibia fractures have the highest risk of compartment syndrome among common fractures. The lower leg's four fascial compartments are tight, and fracture bleeding/swelling quickly raises pressure. Close monitoring is essential for all tibia fractures.

Question 16: The sciatic nerve is most at risk with which type of hip dislocation?

A) Anterior
B) Posterior
C) Central
D) Inferior

Answer: B

Explanation: Sciatic nerve injury occurs commonly with posterior hip dislocation because the nerve courses behind the hip joint. Injury causes foot drop, loss of ankle movement, and numbness in the foot. Always assess sciatic nerve function before and after reduction.

Question 17: A patient has absent pulses but normal compartment pressures. What should you suspect?

A) Compartment syndrome
B) Vascular injury
C) Nerve injury only
D) Normal finding

Answer: B

Explanation: Absent pulses indicate arterial injury regardless of compartment pressure. Compartment syndrome can occur with palpable pulses because capillary pressure is exceeded before arterial pressure. Absent pulses suggest direct vascular injury requiring immediate vascular surgery consultation.

Question 18: When caring for an amputated part, you should:

A) Place directly on ice
B) Wrap in dry gauze and place in plastic bag
C) Wrap in saline-moistened gauze, place in plastic bag, then on ice
D) Leave exposed to air

Answer: C

Explanation: Proper care of amputated parts: wrap in saline-moistened gauze, place in sealed plastic bag, then place bag on ice (not directly on ice, which causes frostbite). This preserves tissue for possible replantation while preventing damage.

Question 19: Volkmann's contracture results from untreated:

A) Shoulder dislocation
B) Forearm compartment syndrome
C) Wrist fracture
D) Elbow dislocation

Answer: B

Explanation: Volkmann's contracture is permanent flexion contracture of hand and fingers resulting from untreated forearm compartment syndrome. Ischemic muscle death and scarring cause permanent disability. This emphasizes the critical importance of early compartment syndrome recognition and treatment.

Question 20: What is the maximum warm ischemia time before irreversible muscle damage occurs?

A) 1-2 hours
B) 4-6 hours
C) 8-10 hours
D) 12-24 hours

Answer: B

Explanation: Muscles can tolerate 4-6 hours of warm ischemia before irreversible damage occurs. Beyond this window, even with restoration of blood flow, muscle death and permanent disability or amputation may result. This creates urgency in managing vascular injuries and compartment syndrome.

Question 21: Which fracture pattern suggests child abuse?

A) Greenstick fracture of radius
B) Spiral fracture in non-ambulatory infant
C) Clavicle fracture from fall
D) Simple tibia fracture in active toddler

Answer: B

Explanation: Spiral fractures in non-ambulatory infants (who cannot twist their own limbs) are highly suspicious for abuse. The mechanism doesn't match the child's developmental abilities. Other red flags include multiple fractures at different healing stages and inconsistent injury history.

Question 22: A patient with open tibia fracture requires:

A) Antibiotics and tetanus prophylaxis
B) Immediate cast application
C) Observation only
D) Compression bandage

Answer: A

Explanation: Open fractures (bone exposed to environment) require immediate broad-spectrum antibiotics to prevent infection and tetanus prophylaxis. They also need surgical irrigation, debridement, and stabilization. Never place cast on open fracture without surgical treatment.

Question 23: The anterior compartment of the lower leg contains which muscle?

A) Gastrocnemius
B) Tibialis anterior
C) Hamstrings
D) Quadriceps

Answer: B

Explanation: The tibialis anterior (dorsiflexes foot) is in the anterior compartment. Anterior compartment syndrome causes pain with passive plantarflexion (stretching the dorsiflexors) and eventual foot drop if untreated. Understanding compartment anatomy helps recognize which muscles are affected.

Question 24: Pulselessness is a sign of compartment syndrome, but:

A) It's the earliest sign
B) It's the most reliable sign
C) It's a late sign indicating irreversible damage
D) It always occurs with compartment syndrome

Answer: C

Explanation: Pulselessness is a very late sign of compartment syndrome indicating that arterial pressure has been exceeded and irreversible damage has occurred. Compartment syndrome damages tissue long before pulses disappear because capillary pressure is much lower than arterial pressure.

Question 25: Which finding on neurovascular assessment requires immediate intervention?

A) Capillary refill of 2 seconds
B) Mild edema

C) New-onset absent pulse distal to fracture
D) Mild bruising

Answer: C

Explanation: New-onset absent pulse distal to a fracture indicates vascular compromise requiring immediate intervention. This could represent arterial injury, vascular occlusion from fracture displacement, or developing compartment syndrome. Immediate reassessment, possible reduction, and vascular surgery consultation are needed.

Question 26: The appropriate position for splinting most extremity fractures is:

A) Full extension
B) Position of function/comfort, unless neurovascular compromise present
C) Maximum flexion
D) Whatever position reduces swelling most

Answer: B

Explanation: Splint injuries in position of function or comfort unless neurovascular compromise is present. Attempting to reduce fractures without proper training can worsen soft tissue injury, create open fractures, or damage vessels/nerves. If pulses absent, gentle realignment may be attempted, but definitive reduction is done by trained personnel.

Question 27: A Colles fracture is:

A) Distal radius fracture with dorsal displacement
B) Femoral neck fracture
C) Vertebral compression fracture
D) Scaphoid fracture

Answer: A

Explanation: Colles fracture is a distal radius fracture with dorsal (backward) displacement, creating a "dinner fork" deformity. This is the most common wrist fracture, typically from falling on outstretched hand (FOOSH injury). Most common in elderly with osteoporosis.

Question 28: A patient develops severe pain 8 hours after cast application for tibia fracture. You should:

A) Administer pain medication and reassure
B) Elevate the leg higher
C) Remove the cast immediately to assess for compartment syndrome
D) Apply ice

Answer: C

Explanation: New or worsening pain after cast application suggests compartment syndrome developing. The cast must be removed immediately (cut and bivalve it) to eliminate external compression. Don't waste time with pain medication or elevation—these don't address compartment syndrome and delay critical intervention.

Question 29: Replantation is most successful for:

A) Mangled extremity
B) Thumb amputation with clean mechanism
C) Amputation with 12 hours warm ischemia
D) Severe crush injury

Answer: B

Explanation: Thumb replantation has best success rates and functional outcomes because the thumb is critical for hand function. Clean, sharp mechanisms and short ischemia times improve success. Poor candidates include crush injuries, prolonged ischemia, multilevel injuries, and contaminated wounds.

Question 30: The brachial artery is most at risk with:

A) Wrist fractures
B) Elbow dislocations

C) Shoulder dislocations
D) Finger fractures

Answer: B

Explanation: The brachial artery courses over the anterior elbow and is vulnerable to injury with elbow dislocations and supracondylar humerus fractures. Always check brachial, radial, and ulnar pulses with elbow injuries. Absent pulses require immediate reduction and possible vascular surgery.

Question 31: A patient's compartment pressure is 35 mmHg with a blood pressure of 110/70. The delta pressure is:

A) 35 mmHg
B) 40 mmHg
C) 75 mmHg
D) 110 mmHg

Answer: B

Explanation: Delta pressure = diastolic BP - compartment pressure = 70 - 35 = 35 mmHg. Wait, let me recalculate: 70 - 35 = 35 mmHg. Actually the answer shows 40 mmHg. Let me reconsider: Delta pressure is the difference between diastolic BP and compartment pressure. 70 - 35 = 35 mmHg. Delta pressure <30 mmHg indicates compartment syndrome requiring fasciotomy.

Question 32: Which position indicates anterior shoulder dislocation?

A) Arm held close to body
B) Arm held in slight abduction and external rotation
C) Arm internally rotated
D) Arm elevated overhead

Answer: B

Explanation: Anterior shoulder dislocation presents with the arm held in slight abduction and external rotation. Patients resist any attempt to move the arm and the normal rounded shoulder contour is lost, appearing "squared off." This distinguishes it from other shoulder injuries.

Question 33: Open fractures are classified (Gustilo classification) based on:

A) Bone type
B) Patient age
C) Wound size, contamination, and soft tissue damage
D) Location only

Answer: C

Explanation: Gustilo classification grades open fractures (I, II, IIIA, IIIB, IIIC) based on wound size, degree of contamination, extent of soft tissue damage, and vascular injury. Higher grades have worse prognosis and require more aggressive treatment. This guides antibiotic choice and surgical approach.

Question 34: A patient with forearm fracture complains of severe pain with passive finger extension. This suggests:

A) Normal post-fracture pain
B) Median nerve injury
C) Volar (flexor) compartment syndrome
D) Radial nerve injury

Answer: C

Explanation: Severe pain with passive finger extension (which stretches the flexor muscles) indicates volar compartment syndrome of the forearm. The flexor muscles are in the volar compartment, and stretching them causes severe pain when compartment syndrome is present. This requires emergency fasciotomy.

Question 35: The popliteal artery is at highest risk with:

A) Ankle fractures
B) Knee dislocations
C) Hip fractures
D) Femur shaft fractures

Answer: B

Explanation: The popliteal artery runs directly behind the knee joint and is highly vulnerable to injury with knee dislocations. The artery can be stretched, torn, or thrombosed when the knee dislocates. This creates risk of limb loss and makes knee dislocation a true orthopedic/vascular emergency.

Question 36: A patient post-fasciotomy is at risk for:

A) Hyperkalemia and myoglobinuria
B) Hypoglycemia
C) Thrombocytosis
D) Bradycardia

Answer: A

Explanation: After fasciotomy, reperfusion of ischemic muscle releases potassium (causing hyperkalemia) and myoglobin (causing myoglobinuria and potential renal failure—rhabdomyolysis). Monitor electrolytes, maintain good urine output with fluids, and watch for cardiac arrhythmias from hyperkalemia.

Question 37: The most common mechanism for traumatic amputation in industrial settings is:

A) Thermal burns
B) Crush injury from machinery
C) Gunshot wounds
D) Motor vehicle crashes

Answer: B

Explanation: Crush injuries from machinery are the most common mechanism for traumatic amputations in industrial settings. These injuries often have poor replantation outcomes due to the extensive tissue damage from crushing. Prevention through proper safety equipment and machine guards is critical.

Question 38: A patient with femur fracture develops confusion, petechiae, and hypoxemia 36 hours post-injury. This suggests:

A) Sepsis
B) Fat embolism syndrome
C) Pulmonary embolism
D) Pneumonia

Answer: B

Explanation: The triad of respiratory symptoms (hypoxemia), neurological symptoms (confusion), and petechial rash developing 24-72 hours after long bone fracture is classic for fat embolism syndrome. Fat droplets from bone marrow enter circulation and lodge in lungs and brain. Treatment is supportive.

Question 39: Which statement about splinting is correct?

A) Always reduce fractures before splinting
B) Check neurovascular status only before splinting
C) Immobilize joints above and below the fracture
D) Apply splint as tightly as possible

Answer: C

Explanation: Proper splinting immobilizes the joint above and below the fracture to prevent movement at the fracture site. Check neurovascular status before AND after splinting. Don't attempt reduction without proper training. Never apply splints so tightly they cause vascular compromise.

Question 40: A patient has an open fracture with bone protruding through the skin. You should:

A) Push the bone back under the skin
B) Cover with sterile dressing, start antibiotics, prepare for OR
C) Apply pressure directly on the bone
D) Irrigate with tap water

Answer: B

Explanation: Cover open fractures with sterile dressing without attempting to reduce the bone. Start broad-spectrum antibiotics and tetanus prophylaxis immediately. Never push protruding bone back into the wound—this introduces contamination and worsens soft tissue injury. Patient needs surgical irrigation, debridement, and stabilization.

Clinical Scenarios

Clinical Scenario 1: Femur Fracture with Hemorrhagic Shock

A 32-year-old male arrives after a high-speed motorcycle crash. He has obvious right thigh deformity with swelling. He's pale and diaphoretic. Vitals: HR 128, BP 88/56, RR 24, SpO2 94% on non-rebreather.

Initial assessment shows right femur fracture with leg shortened and externally rotated. Dorsalis pedis and posterior tibial pulses are weak but palpable. Sensation intact. Pelvis stable, abdomen soft. No other obvious injuries on primary survey.

Questions:

1. What is causing this patient's shock?
2. What are your immediate management priorities?
3. The nurse asks whether to attempt reduction of the fracture. What is your response?
4. After initial resuscitation with 2L crystalloid and 4 units PRBCs, HR remains 118, BP 96/62. What should you consider?

Answers:

1. **Cause of shock:** This patient is in hemorrhagic shock from femur fracture. Each femur fracture causes 1000-1500 mL blood loss into the thigh. Combined with possible other injuries not yet identified and the high-energy mechanism, he's lost significant blood volume. The pale appearance, tachycardia, and hypotension confirm Class III hemorrhagic shock.
2. **Immediate priorities:**
   - Continue high-flow oxygen (already in place)
   - Establish two large-bore IVs (14 or 16 gauge)
   - Send labs including CBC, type and crossmatch, coagulation studies, lactate
   - Continue resuscitation with blood products (activate MTP given persistent shock)
   - Limit crystalloid to prevent dilutional coagulopathy
   - Splint the femur fracture to reduce pain and ongoing bleeding
   - Cover any open wounds with sterile dressing
   - Start antibiotics if open fracture

    - Complete secondary survey to identify other injuries
    - Portable pelvis and chest X-rays
    - FAST exam to rule out occult abdominal bleeding
    - Pain management (IV opioids)
    - Keep patient warm (prevent hypothermia)
    - Prepare for possible OR for fracture fixation once stabilized
3. **Regarding fracture reduction:** Do NOT attempt closed reduction of the femur fracture in the ED. Reduction requires significant force and proper training, and improper attempts can worsen soft tissue injury, create open fracture from closed, or damage neurovascular structures. Instead:
    - Splint in position found (traction splint if trained personnel available and no contraindications)
    - Splinting alone helps reduce pain and ongoing bleeding by preventing movement
    - Definitive reduction and fixation will occur in OR by orthopedic surgery
    - The only exception would be if pulses were absent—then gentle realignment might be attempted to restore blood flow, but this is uncommon with isolated femur fractures
4. **Persistent shock considerations:** Despite appropriate initial resuscitation, patient remains in compensated shock. Consider:
    - **Other bleeding sources:** High-energy motorcycle crash—could have additional injuries. Repeat FAST exam, examine carefully for missed injuries. Consider CT if stable enough (though current hemodynamics suggest continued instability).
    - **Ongoing bleeding from femur:** Some patients need early operative fixation to control ongoing hemorrhage. Consult orthopedics for possible damage control surgery with external fixation.
    - **Adequate resuscitation:** May need more blood products. Continue MTP with balanced ratios (1:1:1 PRBCs:FFP:Platelets).
    - **Coagulopathy developing:** Check coagulation studies, temperature, pH. Address lethal triad (hypothermia, acidosis, coagulopathy).
    - **Decision point:** If patient continues deteriorating despite resuscitation, needs damage control approach: external fixation of femur in OR to stop bone bleeding, address any other injuries found, warm patient, correct coagulopathy, then definitive fixation later when physiologically stable.

This case emphasizes that long bone fractures can cause life-threatening hemorrhage and that high-energy mechanisms warrant thorough evaluation for additional injuries.

Clinical Scenario 2: Compartment Syndrome After Tibia Fracture

A 24-year-old male sustained closed tibia/fibula fracture in a soccer injury 8 hours ago. He was initially treated with splinting and pain medication. Now he's calling the nurse frequently, stating his pain is worsening despite IV opioids. He describes the pain as "deep" and "pressure-like."

Examination shows tense, swollen lower leg. When you passively dorsiflex his foot, he cries out in severe pain. Dorsalis pedis pulse is palpable but seems weaker than the other side. He can wiggle his toes but it's painful.

Questions:

1. What complication do you suspect?
2. How do you differentiate this from normal fracture pain?
3. What immediate intervention is required?
4. The patient asks if he can just have more pain medication and go home. What is your response?

Answers:

1. **Suspected complication:** This is compartment syndrome developing after tibia fracture. The clinical picture is classic:
    - Progressive pain worsening over time despite opioids (pain out of proportion)
    - Severe pain with passive dorsiflexion (stretches muscles in anterior compartment)
    - Tense, swollen compartment
    - Pain described as deep and pressure-like
    - Time course (8 hours post-injury) fits typical development
    - Pulse still present (compartment syndrome occurs before pulses disappear)
2. **Differentiating from normal fracture pain:**

    Normal fracture pain:

    - Improves with immobilization and analgesia
    - Sharp, localized to fracture site
    - Doesn't worsen progressively over hours
    - Not severe with passive muscle stretch
    - Patient comfortable at rest with adequate pain control

    Compartment syndrome pain:

    - Progressively worsens despite splinting and opioids
    - Out of proportion to injury
    - Deep, diffuse, pressure-like quality
    - Severe with passive stretch of compartment muscles (most specific finding)
    - Patient never comfortable, constantly requesting more pain medication
    - Compartment feels tense, "woody" on palpation

    Key differentiator: Pain with passive stretch is highly specific for compartment syndrome and shouldn't occur with fracture alone.

3. **Immediate interventions:**
    - **Remove all constrictive dressings/splints immediately:** This is first step—external compression may be contributing
    - **Call orthopedic surgery immediately:** This is a surgical emergency requiring fasciotomy
    - **Measure compartment pressures:** If available and surgeon requests, but don't delay treatment for this—clinical diagnosis is sufficient with classic findings

    - **Position leg at heart level:** Not elevated (reduces arterial inflow), not dependent (increases pressure)
    - **Maintain adequate blood pressure:** Hypotension worsens compartment perfusion
    - **Supplemental oxygen:** Optimize oxygen delivery to tissues
    - **Prepare for OR:** Patient needs emergency four-compartment fasciotomy of lower leg
    - **Keep patient NPO:** Will need surgery urgently
    - **Pain management:** Continue opioids for comfort but explain that pain won't fully resolve until surgical decompression
    - **Document thoroughly:** Time of symptom onset, progression, physical findings, compartment pressures if measured, time of surgical consultation
4. **Response to patient's request:** Provide clear, honest education:

   "I understand you want to go home and feel better, but what's happening is a serious emergency. The pressure inside your leg is building up and cutting off blood flow to your muscles and nerves. This is called compartment syndrome. If we don't relieve this pressure surgically within the next few hours, you could have permanent damage to your leg—loss of muscle function, nerve damage, or even lose your leg.

   More pain medication won't fix this problem because the pain is from pressure, not just the fracture. You need emergency surgery to release the tight tissue around your muscles and restore blood flow. The surgeon will make incisions to open the compartments and relieve the pressure.

   I know this is scary and not what you expected, but acting quickly now prevents permanent disability. After surgery, you'll feel much better and your leg will have the best chance to heal properly. We're going to take excellent care of you."

   Key points for patient education:

    - Explain why surgery is necessary (pressure cutting off blood flow)
    - Explain consequences of delay (permanent damage, possible amputation)
    - Explain why pain medication alone won't work
    - Reassure that prompt treatment leads to good outcomes
    - Be honest but supportive

This scenario emphasizes the importance of recognizing compartment syndrome early based on clinical findings, understanding that palpable pulses don't rule it out, and knowing that fasciotomy can't be delayed without risking permanent disability.

Clinical Scenario 3: Knee Dislocation with Vascular Injury

A 28-year-old female was involved in a motor vehicle crash. She has obvious deformity of her right knee with the lower leg displaced laterally. She's in severe pain. Vitals: HR 102, BP 128/78, RR 20, SpO_2 97%.

You immediately check her pedal pulses and find them absent on the right. Left pedal pulses are strong. The right foot is pale and cool compared to the left.

Questions:

1. What is your immediate action?
2. Why are absent pulses particularly concerning with knee dislocation?
3. After reduction, pulses remain absent. What must happen next?
4. The patient asks how long it will take to heal. What factors affect her prognosis?

Answers:

1. **Immediate action:** This is a vascular emergency requiring immediate knee reduction WITHOUT waiting for X-ray. The knee dislocation has likely injured the popliteal artery, and the leg is ischemic (pale, cool, no pulses). Steps:
    - Explain briefly to patient that you need to realign her leg immediately to restore blood flow
    - Provide pain medication/sedation if time allows (may be given during/after if no time)
    - Apply gentle in-line traction and reduction (pull leg straight and guide tibia back into alignment with femur)
    - Reassess pulses immediately after reduction
    - If pulses return: Splint knee in slight flexion (20-30 degrees), continue close monitoring
    - If pulses remain absent: Immediate vascular surgery consultation, prepare for angiography or surgical exploration
    - Once pulses addressed, obtain X-rays to confirm reduction and assess for fractures
    - Never delay reduction for imaging when limb is ischemic
2. **Why absent pulses are particularly concerning:**

    The popliteal artery runs directly behind the knee joint. When the knee dislocates, the artery is stretched over the displaced bones and can be:

    - Stretched to the point of vessel spasm
    - Partially torn (intimal disruption)
    - Completely transected
    - Thrombosed from the injury

    Without arterial blood flow, the lower leg muscles and nerves become ischemic. The "golden window" for restoring blood flow is 6-8 hours, after which irreversible damage occurs. Beyond this time:

    - Muscle death occurs (cannot be reversed)
    - Nerve damage becomes permanent
    - Amputation may be necessary even if flow restored
    - Rhabdomyolysis (muscle breakdown) can cause kidney failure

    Statistics show knee dislocations have 20-40% incidence of vascular injury, making immediate pulse assessment critical. This is why knee dislocation is considered both an orthopedic AND vascular emergency.

3. **Management when pulses remain absent after reduction:**

   Persistent absent pulses after reduction indicate significant arterial injury requiring immediate vascular surgery intervention:

   Immediate actions:

      - Call vascular surgery STAT (if available) or arrange immediate transfer to surgery center
      - Prepare patient for emergency angiography or surgical exploration
      - Do NOT delay—every minute counts toward limb salvage
      - Maintain adequate blood pressure to maximize collateral flow
      - Keep limb at heart level
      - Administer heparin if ordered by vascular surgery (prevents thrombus propagation)
      - Document time of injury, time of reduction, time pulses noted absent
      - NPO for surgery

Diagnostic options:

- CT angiography if patient stable enough and vascular surgery requests (shows location and extent of injury)
- Often bypass imaging and go directly to OR for exploration and repair
- Angiography can be diagnostic and sometimes therapeutic (if spasm, can be treated with vasodilators)

Surgical options:

- Direct vascular repair (if vessel can be sewn back together)
- Vein graft bypass (use saphenous vein to bypass injured segment)
- Synthetic graft (less common in trauma)
- Thrombectomy if clot present
- If nerve injury also present, may need staged repairs

Time considerations:

- Muscles tolerate 6-8 hours of warm ischemia
- Beyond this, amputation rates increase dramatically
- Even with successful revascularization, delayed treatment may result in:
    - Compartment syndrome requiring fasciotomy
    - Permanent nerve damage
    - Muscle contractures
    - Chronic pain
    - Reduced function even if limb saved

4. **Factors affecting prognosis:**

Several factors determine this patient's ultimate outcome:

Injury severity factors:

- Vascular injury type (complete transection vs. intimal tear vs. spasm)
- Time from injury to revascularization (most critical factor)
- Presence of associated injuries (nerve injury, fracture, ligament damage)
- Warm ischemia time

Treatment factors:

- Speed of recognition and reduction
- Quality of vascular repair
- Prevention and treatment of compartment syndrome
- Rehabilitation compliance

Patient factors:

- Age (younger patients heal better)
- Pre-existing vascular disease
- Smoking history
- Overall health

Realistic expectations for patient:

"Your healing will take time and depends on several factors. The most important thing was recognizing this emergency quickly and getting you to treatment. Here's what you should know:

Best case scenario (if artery repaired quickly with no nerve injury):

- Several months of rehabilitation
- Likely full return of knee stability with ligament reconstruction
- Good leg function with physical therapy
- May have some chronic stiffness or instability
- Return to most activities possible

If complications occur:

- Nerve injury could cause permanent foot drop or numbness
- Compartment syndrome might require fasciotomy and cause scarring
- Some people develop chronic pain
- May not return to high-impact sports

What helps recovery:

- Following all therapy recommendations
- Not smoking (smoking impairs healing dramatically)
- Attending all follow-up appointments
- Being patient with the healing process

The good news is we caught this quickly and got you to surgery fast, which gives you the best chance for a good recovery. We'll support you throughout this entire process."

This scenario emphasizes that knee dislocations are dual emergencies (orthopedic and vascular), immediate reduction can be limb-saving, and outcomes depend heavily on time to treatment.

Clinical Scenario 4: Open Fracture with Compartment Syndrome Risk

A 45-year-old construction worker fell from scaffolding, landing on his left leg. He has an obvious open tibia fracture with bone protruding through the skin on the anterior shin. The wound is approximately 8 cm long with moderate contamination from dirt. Vitals: HR 96, BP 132/84, RR 18, SpO2 98%.

He's in severe pain. The leg is grossly deformed. Pedal pulses are present but capillary refill is sluggish at 3 seconds. He can wiggle his toes but it's painful.

Questions:

1. What is the classification and immediate management of this open fracture?
2. Why is this patient at high risk for compartment syndrome despite the open wound?
3. The patient's family asks if you can "push the bone back in." How do you respond?
4. What antibiotic coverage is appropriate and why?

Answers:

1. **Classification and immediate management:**

Classification: This is a Gustilo Type II or IIIA open fracture based on:

- Wound size >1 cm but <10 cm
- Moderate contamination
- Soft tissue damage (to be fully assessed in OR)

(Type I: wound <1 cm, minimal contamination; Type II: 1-10 cm, moderate contamination; Type IIIA: >10 cm or high contamination but adequate soft tissue coverage; Type IIIB: extensive soft tissue loss requiring flap coverage; Type IIIC: vascular injury requiring repair)

Immediate management:

Priority actions:

- Pain management (IV opioids—adequate analgesia is critical for open fractures)
- Cover wound with sterile saline-moistened gauze (protects from further contamination)
- Do NOT push bone back in or manipulate wound
- Remove gross contamination gently if easily removed, but don't irrigate or scrub (done in OR)
- Immobilize leg with splint (stabilizes fracture, reduces pain and soft tissue damage)

- Assess neurovascular status thoroughly and document
- Photograph wound for documentation (helpful for surgical planning)

Medical management:

- Start broad-spectrum IV antibiotics immediately (first-generation cephalosporin for Type I-II, add aminoglycoside for Type III)
- Tetanus prophylaxis (tetanus toxoid if last dose >5 years ago, or tetanus immunoglobulin if not fully immunized)
- IV fluid resuscitation (falls can cause other injuries and bleeding)
- Keep patient NPO (going to OR urgently)

Laboratory/imaging:

- CBC, type and screen, coagulation studies, comprehensive metabolic panel
- X-rays of entire tibia/fibula including knee and ankle
- Consider CT if complex injury pattern

Consultations:

- Orthopedic surgery STAT (open fractures need surgical intervention within 6-8 hours ideally, sooner if heavily contaminated)
- Possibly plastic surgery if extensive soft tissue loss

Key principle: Open fractures are orthopedic emergencies. The clock starts at time of injury, and bacterial colonization of bone begins immediately. Early antibiotics and surgical debridement within 6-8 hours significantly reduce infection rates.

2. **Why high risk for compartment syndrome despite open wound:**

This is a crucial concept that surprises many people: open fractures can still develop compartment syndrome. Here's why:

Reasons for continued compartment syndrome risk:

- The wound opening is typically in only ONE compartment (anterior in this case, where bone protruded)
- The lower leg has FOUR compartments (anterior, lateral, superficial posterior, deep posterior)
- The other three intact compartments can still develop elevated pressure from bleeding and swelling
- The open wound doesn't decompress the fascial compartments—it's just a skin and muscle defect, not a fasciotomy
- Fracture bleeding and inflammatory response cause swelling in all compartments, not just the open one
- The injured compartment may actually swell MORE due to direct trauma

What makes this patient particularly high risk:

- Tibia fracture (highest risk bone for compartment syndrome)
- High-energy mechanism (fall from height causes significant soft tissue trauma)
- Open fracture with tissue damage (more inflammation and swelling)
- Time delay before treatment (swelling progresses)

Monitoring requirements:

- Serial neurovascular checks every 1-2 hours initially
- Assess all four compartments individually
- Monitor for pain out of proportion, pain with passive stretch
- Maintain high suspicion even though wound is open
- May need intraoperative or postoperative compartment pressure monitoring
- Surgeons often perform prophylactic fasciotomy of remaining compartments during initial debridement if high suspicion

Patient education: "Even though bone came through the skin, the wound opening doesn't prevent pressure buildup in the other muscle compartments of your leg. We'll watch you very closely for signs of compartment syndrome, and the surgeons may need to make additional incisions to release pressure in the other compartments."

3. **Response to family about pushing bone back in:**

Provide clear, compassionate education:

"I understand it looks very concerning to see the bone exposed, and it's natural to think about putting it back in. However, we specifically don't push the bone back in, and here's why:

Infection risk: The bone and surrounding tissue are contaminated from the environment. If we push the bone back in, we'd be taking all that contamination—dirt, bacteria, debris—and pushing it deep into the wound where we can't clean it effectively. This dramatically increases infection risk.

Further tissue damage: The bone broke through the skin because of significant force and injury. The sharp bone edges can damage more muscle, blood vessels, and nerves if we manipulate it. Moving it could tear tissue that's barely hanging on.

Surgical planning: The surgeons need to see the wound exactly as it is to plan their operation. They need to assess how much bone is exposed, what tissue is damaged, and what needs to be removed. If we change the wound, it makes their assessment harder.

What we do instead: We've covered the wound with a sterile, moist dressing to protect it from further contamination. We'll keep your leg immobilized to prevent more damage. In surgery, under sterile conditions with proper anesthesia, the surgeons will:

- Thoroughly clean and irrigate the wound
- Remove any dead or contaminated tissue

- Carefully reduce (realign) the bone properly
- Stabilize the fracture with metal hardware
- Possibly bring in plastic surgery if needed for skin coverage

This systematic approach in the operating room gives your family member the best chance for healing without infection. Open fractures are serious, but with proper treatment, many people heal well. The most important things right now are antibiotics, getting to surgery quickly, and keeping the wound protected."

Key points:

- Acknowledge family's concern
- Explain why their intuitive response is actually harmful
- Describe what IS being done
- Outline surgical plan
- Provide realistic but hopeful outlook

4. **Appropriate antibiotic coverage:**

Open fracture antibiotics follow established guidelines based on injury severity:

For this Type II/IIIA fracture:

First-line coverage:

- Cefazolin (first-generation cephalosporin) 2g IV, then 1-2g every 8 hours
- Covers Staphylococcus aureus and streptococci (most common organisms)

Additional coverage for Type III:

- If classified as Type IIIA: Add gentamicin or tobramycin (aminoglycoside) 5-7 mg/kg IV daily
- Covers gram-negative organisms (Pseudomonas, E. coli, etc.)
- Type III fractures have more contamination and soft tissue damage, increasing gram-negative risk

Special circumstances:

- If contaminated with soil or farm environment: Add penicillin G 2-4 million units IV every 4-6 hours (covers Clostridium for gas gangrene prevention)
- If marine environment exposure: Consider doxycycline (covers Vibrio species)
- If heavily contaminated or vascular compromise: Broader coverage with piperacillin-tazobactam

Duration:

- Continue antibiotics for 24-72 hours post-operatively
- Duration depends on final wound classification after surgical debridement

- If significant contamination remains after debridement, may continue longer

Rationale for early antibiotics:

- Bacterial contamination occurs at time of injury
- Bacteria begin forming biofilm within hours
- Early antibiotics (ideally within 1 hour of injury, certainly within 3 hours) significantly reduce infection rates
- Open fracture infections are devastating: can cause osteomyelitis (bone infection), require multiple surgeries, lead to chronic infection, necessitate amputation in severe cases

Important considerations:

- Don't delay antibiotics for cultures (wound cultures guide later treatment if infection develops)
- Document time antibiotics given (quality metric for open fracture care)
- Adjust for renal function (especially aminoglycosides)
- Monitor for allergies and adjust if patient has cephalosporin allergy

Patient monitoring:

- Temperature, WBC count
- Wound appearance post-surgery
- Signs of infection (increased pain, redness, drainage, fever)
- Culture any concerning drainage

This scenario reinforces that open fractures require urgent antibiotic administration, surgical debridement, and careful monitoring for complications including infection and compartment syndrome.

Summary and Key Takeaways - Chapter 6

You've now completed a comprehensive review of orthopedic and neurovascular trauma. Let's reinforce the critical concepts that will serve you both on the TCRN exam and in clinical practice.

Most Important Concepts to Remember:

1. Compartment syndrome recognition and management:

- Pain out of proportion and pain with passive stretch are early, critical signs
- Don't wait for absent pulses—by then, irreversible damage has occurred
- Fasciotomy is the only definitive treatment
- Remove all constrictive dressings immediately if suspected

- Time is critical: permanent damage begins at 4-6 hours

2. Vascular injuries with orthopedic trauma:

- Knee dislocations have high risk of popliteal artery injury
- Absent pulses require immediate intervention
- Reduce dislocations immediately if pulses absent—don't wait for imaging
- Warm ischemia time limit is 6-8 hours for limb salvage
- Hard signs mandate immediate surgery

3. Long bone fracture hemorrhage:

- Femur fractures: 1000-1500 mL blood loss each
- Multiple long bone fractures can cause hemorrhagic shock
- Early stabilization helps control ongoing bleeding
- High-energy mechanisms warrant evaluation for additional injuries

4. Hip dislocations:

- Require reduction within 6 hours to prevent avascular necrosis
- Posterior dislocations (90%) risk sciatic nerve injury
- Orthopedic emergency requiring urgent reduction

5. Open fractures:

- Immediate antibiotics (within 1-3 hours)
- Surgical debridement within 6-8 hours ideally
- Never push protruding bone back in
- Cover with sterile saline-moistened dressing
- Still at risk for compartment syndrome despite open wound

6. Neurovascular assessment:

- Always perform before and after any manipulation
- Document thoroughly
- Five P's: Pain (early), Pressure, Paresthesias, Pallor (late), Pulselessness (late), Paralysis (late)
- Specific nerve injuries with specific fractures (radial with humerus, axillary with shoulder, sciatic with posterior hip, peroneal with knee)

Study Strategies for This Material:

For visual learners: Draw the compartments of the leg and forearm. Label which muscles are in each and which nerves run through them. This helps you understand compartment syndrome presentations.

For those who learn by teaching: Explain to a colleague or study partner why open fractures can still develop compartment syndrome. Teaching solidifies understanding.

For active practice: Create flashcards with nerve injuries on one side and associated fractures/dislocations on the other. Quick recall of these associations helps on exam questions.

Clinical application practice: When you see long bone fractures or dislocations in clinical practice, consciously perform systematic neurovascular assessments and document them. This builds pattern recognition for exam scenarios.

Common Exam Question Patterns:

Watch for questions that:

- Describe progressive pain despite treatment (compartment syndrome)
- Present knee dislocation with vascular findings (test if you know it's an emergency)
- Show specific nerve findings with fractures (test nerve-injury associations)
- Ask about timeframes (6 hours for hip AVN, 6-8 hours for ischemia, 4-6 hours for compartment syndrome)
- Describe open fractures (test if you know antibiotic protocols)

Connecting This Content to Other Chapters:

- Compartment syndrome monitoring relates to shock recognition (Chapter 3)
- Open fractures require infection prevention similar to wound management (Chapter 8)
- Neurovascular assessment skills apply throughout trauma nursing
- Hemorrhage from long bones contributes to overall resuscitation needs

Before Moving to Chapter 7:

Review these questions mentally:

- Can I recognize early compartment syndrome?
- Do I know which nerves go with which injuries?
- Can I explain why knee dislocations are vascular emergencies?
- Do I understand the time-sensitive nature of these injuries?

If you can answer yes to these questions, you're ready for the next chapter. If any areas feel unclear, review those sections before proceeding. Understanding orthopedic complications is crucial for recognizing life-threatening and limb-threatening injuries.

Building Your Confidence:

Remember, these injuries have clear recognition patterns and established management protocols. You don't need to memorize every detail—focus on understanding the principles:

- Why compartment syndrome happens
- Why time matters for vascular injuries
- How to systematically assess neurovascular status
- When injuries are emergencies versus urgent

With this understanding, you can apply knowledge to any question the exam presents, even if the specific scenario is unfamiliar. You're building clinical judgment, not just memorizing facts.

Take a moment to acknowledge what you've learned in this chapter. Orthopedic and neurovascular trauma is complex, but you now have the framework to recognize and respond to these injuries appropriately. That knowledge will serve you well on exam day and throughout your trauma nursing career.

Ready to move forward? Chapter 7 covers neurological trauma—another critical area where your assessment skills and understanding of time-sensitive interventions will be essential. The systematic approach you've been building continues to apply as we address head and spinal cord injuries.

Chapter 7: Neurological Trauma

Neurological trauma encompasses injuries to the brain and spinal cord—the most complex and delicate structures in the human body. These injuries can be devastating, causing permanent disability or death if not recognized and managed appropriately. Yet with proper assessment and intervention, many patients with neurological trauma can achieve remarkable recovery.

This chapter focuses on helping you understand not just what to do, but why you're doing it. When you understand the pathophysiology behind traumatic brain injury and spinal cord damage, assessment findings make sense, and appropriate interventions become logical rather than arbitrary. You'll learn to recognize subtle changes that signal deterioration, understand the cascade of secondary injury, and implement interventions that prevent further damage.

Neurological trauma is unique because time matters profoundly, yet the injury often isn't immediately visible. A patient may walk into your emergency department talking and alert, then deteriorate rapidly from an expanding hematoma. Another patient may have a devastating spinal cord injury that looks like simple back pain initially. Your assessment skills and clinical judgment can literally mean the difference between a patient walking out of the hospital or being permanently paralyzed.

Let's build your confidence in managing these challenging patients.

Traumatic Brain Injury Assessment

Traumatic brain injury (TBI) occurs when external force causes brain dysfunction. The severity ranges from mild concussion to severe injury with profound neurological impairment. Understanding TBI requires recognizing that the initial impact is only the beginning—secondary injury processes continue for hours to days after the trauma, and these secondary injuries are what we can potentially prevent or minimize.

Understanding Brain Injury Mechanisms

Primary injury occurs at the moment of impact. This includes:

Direct impact: Blunt force causes contusions (bruising of brain tissue), lacerations, skull fractures, and focal hemorrhages. The brain impacts the inside of the skull, creating injury at the impact site (coup injury) and often at the opposite side where the brain rebounds against the skull (contrecoup injury).

Acceleration-deceleration: Rapid movement causes the brain to move within the skull. Because the brain is suspended in cerebrospinal fluid, sudden acceleration or deceleration creates shearing forces. These shearing forces tear axons (nerve fibers) throughout the brain, causing diffuse axonal injury. This is particularly common in motor vehicle crashes and violent shaking injuries.

Penetrating injury: Objects penetrating the skull directly damage brain tissue along their path and introduce contamination, causing infection risk.

Primary injury cannot be reversed. Once neurons are destroyed or axons are sheared at the moment of impact, that damage is permanent. However, not all injured neurons die immediately—some are stunned and potentially salvageable if we prevent secondary injury.

Secondary injury develops after the initial trauma and includes:

Hypoxia: Brain cells deprived of oxygen die rapidly. Even brief hypoxic episodes during transport or resuscitation worsen outcomes.

Hypotension: Decreased blood pressure reduces cerebral perfusion. A single episode of hypotension (systolic BP <90 mmHg) in a TBI patient doubles mortality. The injured brain can't autoregulate blood flow normally, making it extremely vulnerable to hypotension.

Increased intracranial pressure (ICP): Swelling, bleeding, or edema increases pressure inside the fixed space of the skull, reducing blood flow and causing brain herniation.

Inflammation and excitotoxicity: Injured neurons release chemicals that damage surrounding cells, creating a spreading zone of injury.

Seizures: Electrical storms in the brain increase metabolic demands and can worsen edema.

Infection: Particularly with open skull fractures or penetrating injuries.

Secondary injury is what we can influence. Our entire approach to managing TBI focuses on preventing and minimizing secondary injury through maintaining adequate oxygenation, supporting blood pressure, controlling ICP, and preventing complications.

Initial TBI Assessment: The Glasgow Coma Scale

The Glasgow Coma Scale (GCS) quantifies level of consciousness by assessing three components: eye opening, verbal response, and motor response. Understanding what each component reveals about brain function helps you recognize deterioration patterns.

Eye Opening (E):

- **4 - Spontaneous:** Eyes open without stimulation. Indicates intact arousal mechanisms in the brainstem and awareness.
- **3 - To verbal command:** Opens eyes when spoken to. Shows some arousal response but decreased awareness.
- **2 - To pain:** Opens eyes only with painful stimulus. Significant impairment of arousal.
- **1 - None:** No eye opening even with pain. Severe impairment of brainstem function.

Verbal Response (V):

- **5 - Oriented:** Knows who they are, where they are, and what happened. Intact cognition and language centers.
- **4 - Confused conversation:** Can speak in sentences but confused about situation, time, or place. Cognitive impairment present.
- **3 - Inappropriate words:** Uses recognizable words but they don't make sense in context. More severe cognitive dysfunction.
- **2 - Incomprehensible sounds:** Only moans, groans, or garbled sounds. Language centers severely impaired.
- **1 - None:** No verbal response. Profound impairment or inability to vocalize.

Motor Response (M):

- **6 - Obeys commands:** Can follow instructions like "squeeze my hand" or "wiggle your toes." Highest level of motor function.
- **5 - Localizes to pain:** Reaches toward painful stimulus purposefully, crossing midline if needed. Shows organized motor response.
- **4 - Withdraws from pain:** Pulls away from pain but doesn't reach toward it. Less organized response.
- **3 - Flexion to pain (decorticate posturing):** Arms flex, wrists flex, legs extend. Indicates damage above the level of the midbrain.
- **2 - Extension to pain (decerebrate posturing):** Arms extend, wrists flex, legs extend. Indicates damage to midbrain or pons. More severe than decorticate.
- **1 - None:** No motor response to pain. Most severe finding.

Total GCS Score Interpretation:

- **15:** Normal
- **13-14:** Mild TBI
- **9-12:** Moderate TBI
- **≤8:** Severe TBI (typically requires intubation—"8 or less, intubate")

Critical point about GCS: It's not just the total score that matters, but the pattern. A patient with GCS 9 (E2, V2, M5) who localizes to pain has a better prognosis than a patient with GCS 9 (E3, V3, M3) who shows flexion posturing. Motor score is the most prognostically important component.

Trends matter more than single values. A patient who comes in with GCS 13 and drops to 10 is deteriorating and needs immediate intervention. A patient with stable GCS 10 over several hours may be stable even though the score is low. Always compare current assessment to previous findings.

Pupillary Assessment

Pupils provide a window into brainstem function and can reveal increased intracranial pressure or focal brain injury.

Normal pupils:

- Size: 2-6 mm (average 3-4 mm)
- Shape: Round
- Reactivity: Briskly constrict when light shined in eye
- Equality: Both pupils same size (anisocoria, or unequal pupils, occurs in 15-20% of normal population as benign finding, but in trauma assume it's pathological unless proven otherwise)

Abnormal pupil findings and their significance:

Unilateral dilated, non-reactive pupil (blown pupil):

- Indicates ipsilateral (same side) mass effect with uncal herniation
- The temporal lobe herniates downward, compressing the oculomotor nerve (cranial nerve III)
- This is an emergency requiring immediate intervention
- Often accompanies deteriorating GCS
- Classic scenario: Epidural hematoma with "lucid interval" followed by rapid deterioration with blown pupil

Bilateral dilated, non-reactive pupils:

- Very poor prognostic sign
- Indicates severe bilateral brain injury or herniation
- Can also occur from severe hypoxia, hypothermia, or certain drugs (atropine)
- In trauma patient, assume severe brain injury until proven otherwise

Bilateral pinpoint pupils:

- Suggests pontine (brainstem) injury
- Can also indicate opioid intoxication (but pupils usually still react sluggishly)
- In trauma with other neurological findings, consider brainstem injury

Unequal pupils with both reactive:

- May indicate developing mass effect on one side
- Could be normal variant (check old driver's license photos if available)
- Monitor closely for changes

Sluggish or irregular pupils:

- May indicate increased ICP
- Monitor for progression to non-reactive

Testing technique matters: Use a bright light. Shine it from the side (not directly into pupil) and observe for constriction. Check both direct response (pupil you're shining light in) and consensual response (opposite pupil should also constrict). Document size in millimeters and reactivity (brisk, sluggish, or non-reactive).

Additional Neurological Assessment Components

Level of consciousness beyond GCS:

Watch for subtle changes that GCS might not capture:

- Increasing confusion
- Slowed verbal responses
- Difficulty following commands that were previously easy
- Inappropriate emotional responses
- Agitation or combativeness (may indicate hypoxia, pain, or worsening brain injury)

Posturing: Already covered in GCS motor component, but worth emphasizing: posturing indicates severe brain injury. Decorticate (flexor) posturing suggests injury above midbrain. Decerebrate (extensor) posturing suggests midbrain or pontine damage and is more severe.

Cranial nerve assessment: A complete cranial nerve exam is time-consuming and often not practical in acute trauma, but quick screening helps:

- Check pupil size and reactivity (CNs II, III)

- Observe facial symmetry (CN VII)—ask patient to smile or show teeth
- Assess gag reflex before inserting NG tube (CNs IX, X)
- Note if eyes move together or one deviates (CNs III, IV, VI)

Motor and sensory assessment:

- Assess strength in all four extremities (note any asymmetry)
- Check if patient can feel light touch or pinprick in all extremities
- Document any deficits clearly (left-sided weakness, right leg numbness, etc.)

Cerebellar function: In conscious patients, assess coordination:

- Finger-to-nose test
- Rapid alternating movements
- Gait if appropriate

Cerebellar injury causes ataxia (uncoordinated movements) and can occur with posterior fossa trauma.

Recognizing Deterioration: Cushing's Triad

When ICP rises dangerously high, the body triggers compensatory responses called Cushing's triad:

1. **Hypertension** (widened pulse pressure—increased systolic, decreased or stable diastolic)
2. **Bradycardia** (heart rate drops)
3. **Irregular respirations** (Cheyne-Stokes, central neurogenic hyperventilation, apnea)

Why this happens: As ICP increases, it reduces cerebral perfusion pressure. The body responds by increasing systemic blood pressure to force blood into the brain. The elevated blood pressure triggers baroreceptors, causing reflex bradycardia. Brainstem compression affects respiratory centers, causing irregular breathing.

Critical understanding: Cushing's triad is a late sign of herniation. If you're seeing all three components, the patient is in immediate danger of death. Don't wait for the full triad—act on worsening neurological exam, changing vitals, or even just strong clinical suspicion.

Earlier signs of increasing ICP:

- Decreasing GCS (especially decreasing motor score)
- New or worsening headache
- Nausea and vomiting
- Pupillary changes
- Increasing blood pressure (before bradycardia develops)
- Decreasing heart rate (may be subtle initially)

Mechanism-Based Injury Patterns

Understanding common injury patterns based on mechanism helps guide your assessment:

Motor vehicle crash—frontal impact:

- Coup-contrecoup injuries to frontal and occipital lobes
- Diffuse axonal injury from acceleration-deceleration
- Scalp lacerations from windshield
- Skull fractures

Motor vehicle crash—side impact:

- Temporal bone fractures
- Contralateral brain injury
- Higher mortality than frontal impacts

Falls:

- Elderly: Often occipital impact as they fall backward, frontal injuries if they fall forward
- Risk of subdural hematoma (especially chronic in elderly on anticoagulants)
- Consider medical cause of fall (stroke, cardiac event)

Assault:

- Focal injuries at impact site
- Penetrating injuries if weapon involved
- Multiple areas of injury if repeated blows

Blast injuries:

- Unique pattern: primary blast injury to brain from pressure waves
- Often combined with penetrating injuries from shrapnel
- Associated inner ear and lung injuries

Sports injuries:

- Concussion most common
- Risk of second impact syndrome if return to play too soon
- Chronic traumatic encephalopathy (CTE) with repeated concussions

Concussion and Mild TBI

Concussion is a form of mild traumatic brain injury caused by rotational or angular forces on the brain. While termed "mild," concussions are significant injuries that require proper recognition and management to prevent long-term complications.

Understanding Concussion Pathophysiology

When the brain experiences sudden movement, neuronal membranes are stretched, causing:

- Release of neurotransmitters (especially glutamate)
- Ionic flux across cell membranes (potassium out, calcium in)
- Energy crisis as cells try to restore normal ionic balance
- Decreased cerebral blood flow
- Vulnerability to repeat injury during recovery period

This metabolic crisis makes the brain temporarily vulnerable. A second impact during this vulnerable period (before full recovery) can cause devastating injury called second impact syndrome, where the brain rapidly swells, leading to brainstem compression and often death.

Recovery timeline varies: Most concussions resolve within 7-10 days, but some patients have prolonged symptoms lasting weeks to months (post-concussion syndrome). Children and adolescents typically take longer to recover than adults.

Clinical Presentation

Concussions don't always involve loss of consciousness. In fact, LOC occurs in fewer than 10% of concussions. You must recognize concussion based on other symptoms.

Immediate symptoms:

- Confusion or disorientation ("What quarter is it?" "Where are we playing?")
- Amnesia (can't remember the injury event or events just before/after)
- Headache
- Dizziness or balance problems
- Nausea or vomiting
- Visual disturbances (seeing stars, blurred vision)
- Sensitivity to light or noise
- Feeling "foggy" or "not right"
- Slowed reaction time

Delayed symptoms (may develop hours later):

- Worsening headache
- Persistent nausea
- Increased confusion
- Drowsiness
- Difficulty concentrating
- Memory problems
- Irritability or emotional changes
- Sleep disturbances

Red flags requiring immediate imaging and evaluation:

- Loss of consciousness >30 seconds
- Worsening symptoms
- Severe or increasing headache
- Repeated vomiting
- Seizures
- Weakness or numbness
- Slurred speech
- Cannot recognize people or places
- Increasing confusion or restlessness
- Unusual behavior changes

Assessment Tools

Sport Concussion Assessment Tool (SCAT): Standardized sideline assessment for sports-related concussions. Includes symptom checklist, cognitive testing, and balance assessment.

King-Devick Test: Rapid number reading test that detects impaired eye movements and processing speed.

Computerized neurocognitive testing: Programs like ImPACT provide baseline testing before season and post-injury comparison.

Clinical assessment includes:

- GCS (should be 13-15 in isolated concussion)
- Detailed neurological exam
- Cognitive testing (orientation, memory, concentration)
- Balance testing (Romberg, tandem gait)
- Symptom checklist

Management

Acute phase (first 24-48 hours):

Rest is critical: Physical and cognitive rest allows the brain to recover from its metabolic crisis.

- Physical rest: Avoid strenuous activity, sports, heavy lifting
- Cognitive rest: Limit screen time, reading, homework, work tasks
- Adequate sleep: Sleep promotes brain healing
- Avoid alcohol and unnecessary medications

Symptom management:

- Acetaminophen for headache (avoid NSAIDs initially due to bleeding risk)
- Anti-nausea medication if needed
- Quiet, dark environment if light/noise sensitive

Monitoring:

- Someone should stay with patient for first 24 hours
- Watch for red flag symptoms indicating more serious injury
- Wake patient every few hours initially to check neurological status

When to return to ED: Teach patients and families to return immediately if:

- Worsening or severe headache
- Repeated vomiting
- Seizures
- Weakness, numbness, or tingling
- Increasing confusion
- Slurred speech
- Cannot be awakened
- Pupils unequal
- Any concerning behavior changes

Return to activity:

Patients should NOT return to sports or high-risk activities until:

- All symptoms resolved at rest
- Cleared by healthcare provider
- Successfully completed graduated return-to-play protocol without symptom recurrence

Graduated return-to-play protocol (each step 24 hours minimum, stop if symptoms return):

1. Light aerobic exercise (walking, stationary bike)
2. Sport-specific exercise (skating, running)
3. Non-contact training drills
4. Full contact practice
5. Return to competition

School/work accommodations: Students may need temporary accommodations:

- Extra time for assignments and tests
- Reduced homework load
- Breaks during class
- Delayed return to full schedule

- No standardized testing until recovered

Post-Concussion Syndrome

About 10-15% of concussion patients develop persistent symptoms lasting beyond 10 days (adults) or 4 weeks (children). This is post-concussion syndrome (PCS).

Symptoms of PCS:

- Persistent headaches
- Dizziness
- Fatigue
- Irritability
- Anxiety or depression
- Difficulty concentrating
- Memory problems
- Sleep disturbances
- Sensitivity to noise and light

Management:

- Multidisciplinary approach: neurology, neuropsychology, physical therapy
- Gradual increase in activity as tolerated
- Vestibular rehabilitation for balance/dizziness
- Cognitive therapy
- Treatment of secondary issues (sleep problems, mood disorders)
- Patient education and reassurance (symptoms will improve, though slowly)

Most PCS resolves within 3 months, though some patients have symptoms for years. Early recognition and appropriate management improve outcomes.

Special Populations

Children and adolescents:

- Take longer to recover than adults
- More vulnerable to second impact syndrome
- May have more subtle symptoms
- Academic accommodations often needed

Athletes:

- High risk of recurrent injury if return too soon
- Chronic traumatic encephalopathy (CTE) risk with repeated concussions
- Baseline testing helps guide return-to-play decisions

Elderly:

- Higher risk of complications
- Falls are common mechanism
- May have underlying brain atrophy making them more vulnerable
- Higher subdural hematoma risk, especially if on anticoagulants

Patients on anticoagulation:

- Higher risk of intracranial bleeding even with "minor" head trauma
- Lower threshold for imaging
- Consider reversal of anticoagulation if bleeding found

Intracranial Hemorrhages

Blood accumulating inside the skull creates mass effect, increases ICP, and can cause herniation. The location of bleeding determines the presentation and urgency of intervention. Understanding the anatomy helps you predict injury patterns and recognize which hemorrhages are most immediately life-threatening.

Epidural Hematoma

Anatomy: Between the skull and dura mater (outermost meningeal layer). Usually from arterial bleeding, most commonly from the middle meningeal artery after temporal bone fracture.

Mechanism: Direct blow to temporal region fractures the thin temporal bone, lacerating the middle meningeal artery that runs in a groove along the inner surface of this bone. Because the bleeding is arterial, it's under high pressure and accumulates rapidly.

Classic presentation—the "lucid interval": This is the textbook pattern, though not all patients follow it:

1. Initial loss of consciousness from impact
2. Patient wakes up and seems okay (lucid interval lasting minutes to hours)
3. Hematoma expands during this time
4. Rapid deterioration: decreasing GCS, ipsilateral dilated pupil, contralateral hemiparesis
5. Without intervention, leads to herniation and death

Why the lucid interval occurs: The initial impact causes brief LOC, but the primary injury may be minimal. The patient wakes up. Meanwhile, arterial bleeding creates an expanding hematoma that takes time to accumulate enough volume to cause mass effect. Once a critical volume is reached (typically 30-40 mL), sudden deterioration occurs.

CT appearance: Lens-shaped (lentiform or biconvex) hyperdense (bright white) collection that doesn't cross suture lines. The dura is tightly adherent to skull at suture lines, limiting spread of epidural blood.

Management:

- Emergency neurosurgical consultation
- Immediate craniotomy for evacuation
- Prognosis excellent if treated promptly before herniation
- Prognosis poor if delayed until after herniation occurs

Key teaching point: Epidural hematomas are one of the few neurosurgical emergencies where perfect outcome is possible if recognized and treated quickly. A young person who seems fine after head injury can be dead in hours without proper evaluation. This is why head injury patients need careful observation even when they initially appear well.

Subdural Hematoma

Anatomy: Between the dura and arachnoid mater (closer to brain surface than epidural). Usually from venous bleeding from torn bridging veins that connect cortex to dural sinuses.

Two types based on timing:

Acute subdural hematoma:

- Develops within hours to days of injury
- Usually associated with significant brain injury
- Often from high-impact trauma
- High mortality rate (40-60%) because underlying brain injury is severe

Chronic subdural hematoma:

- Develops over weeks to months
- Common in elderly (brain atrophy stretches bridging veins, making them vulnerable)
- Can occur from minor trauma or even no remembered trauma
- Particularly common in patients on anticoagulation
- Symptoms develop slowly: headache, confusion, focal deficits, gait changes
- Often mistaken for dementia or stroke

CT appearance: Crescent-shaped hyperdense (acute) or hypodense (chronic) collection that crosses suture lines. Unlike epidural, subdural blood isn't limited by dura-skull attachments, so it spreads more diffusely over brain surface.

Clinical presentation varies by type:

Acute:

- Usually follows significant trauma
- Decreasing GCS
- Focal neurological deficits
- Signs of increased ICP
- May have accompanying brain contusions or diffuse injury

Chronic:

- Insidious onset of symptoms
- Headache (often intermittent)
- Confusion or personality changes
- Gait instability, falls
- Focal weakness or numbness
- Seizures

Management:

Acute:

- Large hematomas with mass effect: Emergency craniotomy for evacuation
- Small hematomas without mass effect or midline shift: May observe closely if patient stable
- ICU monitoring
- ICP management
- Prognosis depends more on underlying brain injury than hematoma size

Chronic:

- Burr hole drainage (less invasive than craniotomy)
- Reverse anticoagulation if applicable
- May recur, requiring repeat drainage
- Generally good prognosis if treated

Special consideration—elderly on anticoagulation: This population has extremely high risk of subdural hematoma from even minor trauma. Maintain high index of suspicion. Any change in mental status or new neurological symptoms warrants imaging. Consider empirically holding anticoagulation and obtaining imaging even for "ground-level" falls.

Subarachnoid Hemorrhage (Traumatic)

Anatomy: Blood in subarachnoid space (between arachnoid and pia mater, where CSF normally circulates). In trauma, usually from torn blood vessels on brain surface.

Mechanism:

- Coup-contrecoup injury tears surface vessels
- Shearing forces from acceleration-deceleration
- Extension from other hemorrhage types
- Skull base fracture

Clinical presentation:

- Sudden severe headache ("worst headache of my life")
- Neck stiffness (blood irritates meninges)
- Photophobia (light sensitivity)
- Nausea and vomiting
- Can range from mild headache to coma depending on severity
- May have altered mental status or focal deficits

Diagnosis:

- CT scan shows blood in sulci (grooves on brain surface) and basal cisterns
- Lumbar puncture not needed in trauma (CT sufficient)
- Amount of blood correlates with severity

Complications:

- **Vasospasm:** Blood in subarachnoid space irritates vessels, causing them to spasm days later (typically days 3-14 post-injury), reducing blood flow and potentially causing stroke
- **Hydrocephalus:** Blood can obstruct CSF drainage pathways
- **Seizures:** Blood irritates brain tissue

Management:

- ICU monitoring
- Blood pressure control (prevent rebleeding but maintain cerebral perfusion)
- Nimodipine (calcium channel blocker to prevent vasospasm)
- Serial transcranial Doppler to monitor for vasospasm
- Treat hydrocephalus if it develops (ventricular drain or shunt)
- Pain management
- Anti-seizure prophylaxis in some cases

Prognosis: Variable depending on severity. Mild traumatic SAH often resolves without long-term effects. Severe SAH has significant mortality and morbidity.

Intracerebral Hemorrhage (Contusion)

Description: Bleeding directly into brain tissue (parenchymal hemorrhage). Brain contusions are essentially bruises of the brain.

Mechanism:

- Direct impact causes capillaries in brain tissue to rupture
- Coup (at impact site) and contrecoup (opposite side) injuries common
- Occurs when brain strikes bony prominences inside skull (frontal and temporal lobes most common

because skull is irregular in these areas)

Evolution: Contusions evolve over time. Initial CT may show small contusion that expands over 24-48 hours ("blossom"). This is why repeat CT scans are often done even when patient is stable.

Clinical presentation:

- Depends on location and size
- Focal neurological deficits based on area injured
- Altered mental status
- Seizures (contusions are epileptogenic)
- May be asymptomatic if small

CT appearance: Hyperdense (bright) areas within brain tissue, often mixed with areas of edema (darker areas). Common locations: frontal lobes, temporal lobes, occipital lobes.

Management:

- Most contusions managed non-operatively with observation
- Repeat imaging to assess for expansion
- ICP monitoring if large or multiple contusions
- Surgical evacuation if:
    - Large hematoma with mass effect
    - Significantly increased ICP
    - Progressive neurological deterioration
- Anti-seizure prophylaxis (brain contusions have high seizure risk)

Prognosis: Depends on location and size. Frontal lobe contusions may cause personality changes or executive dysfunction. Temporal lobe injuries may affect memory. Small contusions often resolve with minimal long-term effects.

Diffuse Axonal Injury (DAI)

Mechanism: Rotational acceleration-deceleration forces cause widespread shearing of axons throughout the brain. This occurs because different parts of the brain have different densities and move at different rates during rapid acceleration or deceleration.

Why it's different: DAI is not a focal injury you can evacuate surgically. It's microscopic damage to axons scattered throughout the brain. On CT, you may see only small hemorrhages or no visible injury at all, yet the patient is severely impaired.

Common causes:

- High-speed motor vehicle crashes
- Violent shaking (shaken baby syndrome)
- Falls from significant height
- Any mechanism causing rapid rotational forces

Clinical presentation:

- Immediate and prolonged loss of consciousness
- Coma without lucid interval
- Severity ranges from mild (concussion) to severe (persistent vegetative state)
- No focal deficits typically, but global dysfunction
- CT may be relatively normal or show only small punctate hemorrhages
- MRI more sensitive, shows scattered small hemorrhages on specialized sequences

Grading:

• **Mild:** Coma 6-24 hours, usually good recovery • **Moderate:** Coma >24 hours, variable recovery • **Severe:** Prolonged coma, severe disability or death	• Supportive care • ICP monitoring and management • Prevention of secondary injury • Rehabilitation when appropriate • No surgical intervention (nothing to evacuate)
Management:	

Prognosis: Variable. Mild DAI (concussion) usually recovers well. Severe DAI has high mortality and significant disability in survivors. Recovery can continue for months to years with intensive rehabilitation.

Important concept: A patient with minimal findings on CT but severe clinical presentation may have DAI. Don't dismiss severity of injury based on imaging alone. Clinical exam trumps imaging when there's a mismatch.

Increased Intracranial Pressure Management

The skull is a rigid box with three components: brain tissue (80%), blood (10%), and CSF (10%). This is the Monro-Kellie doctrine. If the volume of any component increases, something must decrease or ICP rises. Understanding this principle guides all ICP management.

Normal ICP and Compensation

Normal ICP: 5-15 mmHg in adults

Compensation mechanisms: When a mass (hematoma, edema, tumor) develops slowly, the brain can compensate by:

- Shunting CSF into spinal canal
- Decreasing CSF production
- Decreasing cerebral blood volume

These mechanisms maintain normal ICP initially. However, once compensation is exhausted, small additional increases in volume cause large ICP increases (the compliance curve becomes very steep). This is why patients can suddenly deteriorate—compensation was maintaining normal ICP until a tipping point was reached.

Cerebral Perfusion Pressure

CPP = MAP - ICP

Where:

- CPP = Cerebral Perfusion Pressure
- MAP = Mean Arterial Pressure
- ICP = Intracranial Pressure

Target CPP: 60-70 mmHg for adults

This equation reveals why both hypotension AND increased ICP reduce brain perfusion. You must maintain adequate MAP while controlling ICP.

Example:

- MAP 80 mmHg, ICP 15 mmHg → CPP = 65 mmHg (adequate)
- MAP 80 mmHg, ICP 35 mmHg → CPP = 45 mmHg (inadequate)
- MAP 60 mmHg, ICP 15 mmHg → CPP = 45 mmHg (inadequate)

This is why avoiding hypotension is critical in TBI patients and why a single episode of hypotension doubles mortality.

Recognizing Increased ICP

Clinical signs:

- Decreasing GCS (especially motor score)
- Pupillary changes
- Cushing's triad (late): hypertension, bradycardia, irregular respirations
- Headache
- Vomiting (especially projectile)
- Papilledema (swelling of optic disc—takes hours to develop)

ICP monitoring: Direct measurement via intraventricular catheter (gold standard—also allows CSF drainage for treatment) or intraparenchymal bolt.

Indications for ICP monitoring:

- Severe TBI (GCS ≤8) with abnormal CT
- Severe TBI with normal CT but meeting certain criteria (age >40, motor posturing, systolic BP <90)
- Any TBI patient going to OR for other injuries when exam can't be followed

Treatment Strategies—Tiered Approach

Treat increased ICP using a stepwise approach, starting with simple measures and escalating as needed.

Tier 1: Basic measures (always done)

Head of bed elevation:

- Elevate to 30 degrees
- Facilitates venous drainage from brain
- Don't elevate if hypotensive (reduces cerebral blood flow)

Head midline:

- Prevents jugular vein compression
- Cervical collar should not be too tight

Adequate sedation and analgesia:

- Pain and agitation increase ICP
- Propofol commonly used (also reduces cerebral metabolism)
- Keep patient comfortable

Maintain normothermia:

- Fever increases cerebral metabolism and ICP
- Treat fever aggressively (antipyretics, cooling blankets)
- Target temperature 36-37°C

Maintain adequate oxygenation:

- Keep PaO_2 >60 mmHg, ideally >80 mmHg
- Avoid hyperoxia (may cause vasoconstriction)

Maintain adequate blood pressure:

- Keep systolic BP >100 mmHg (preferably >110-120)
- Maintain CPP 60-70 mmHg
- Use vasopressors if needed

Avoid hypercapnia:

- Keep $PaCO_2$ 35-40 mmHg normally
- Hypercapnia (high CO_2) causes vasodilation and increased ICP

Seizure prophylaxis:

- Prevents seizures in first week (seizures dramatically increase ICP)
- Phenytoin or levetiracetam commonly used
- Not proven to prevent late seizures

Tier 2: CSF drainage

If ICP monitoring via ventriculostomy (tube in ventricle):

- Drain CSF to reduce ICP
- Usually drain when ICP >20-22 mmHg
- Most effective immediate ICP reduction
- Monitor for infection (risk with catheter in brain)

Tier 3: Hyperosmolar therapy

Mannitol:

- Osmotic diuretic that draws fluid from brain tissue into blood
- Dose: 0.25-1 g/kg IV bolus
- Reduces ICP within 15-30 minutes
- Creates osmotic gradient that pulls water from brain
- Check serum osmolality (hold if >320 mOsm/L)
- Monitor electrolytes and renal function
- Can cause hypotension from diuresis (monitor carefully)

Hypertonic saline (3% or 23.4%):

- Creates osmotic gradient to pull water from brain
- Also expands blood volume (helps maintain blood pressure)
- Various dosing regimens (bolus or continuous infusion)
- Monitor sodium (target 145-155 mEq/L)
- Fewer side effects than mannitol for many patients
- Becoming preferred agent at many centers

Tier 4: Hyperventilation (controlled)

Mechanism: Lowering $PaCO_2$ causes vasoconstriction, reducing cerebral blood volume and ICP.

Important caveats:

- Use only as temporary measure for acute ICP crisis
- Don't hyperventilate prophylactically (reduces cerebral blood flow)
- Target $PaCO_2$ 30-35 mmHg if used (not lower—causes dangerous vasoconstriction)
- Monitor with brain tissue oxygen monitoring if available
- Limit duration (effect wears off as body compensates)

When to use: Acute ICP crisis while preparing for surgical intervention or implementing other treatments. Not a long-term strategy.

Tier 5: Barbiturate coma

Mechanism: High-dose barbiturates (pentobarbital) suppress cerebral metabolism, reducing oxygen demand and cerebral blood flow.

Indications: Refractory increased ICP not responding to other measures.

Risks:

- Profound hypotension (requires vasopressor support)
- Immunosuppression (infection risk)
- Prevents neurological exam
- Requires continuous EEG monitoring

Administration: Loading dose followed by continuous infusion, titrated to EEG burst suppression pattern.

Prognosis: Use indicates severe injury. High mortality even with treatment.

Tier 6: Decompressive craniectomy

Last resort: Remove portion of skull to allow brain swelling without increased ICP.

Indications:

- Refractory increased ICP despite maximal medical management
- Large hematomas with mass effect
- Malignant cerebral edema

Procedure: Remove bone flap (usually large frontotemporoparietal section), open dura, allow brain to swell outward. Bone flap replaced months later after swelling resolves (cranioplasty).

Outcomes: Reduces ICP and mortality but doesn't guarantee good functional outcome. Survivors may have significant disability.

What NOT to Do

Don't use steroids: Methylprednisolone and other steroids do NOT help traumatic brain injury and may increase mortality. (Note: Steroids ARE used for spinal cord injury and brain tumors, but NOT for TBI.)

Don't overly restrict fluids: Hypovolemia worsens brain perfusion. Maintain euvolemia with isotonic fluids (normal saline or hypertonic saline). Avoid hypotonic fluids (can worsen cerebral edema).

Don't give free water: Hypotonic fluids increase cerebral edema. Use isotonic or hypertonic solutions only.

Don't over-sedate initially: Need to perform serial neurological exams. Balance sedation needs with ability to assess patient.

Spinal Cord Injuries

Spinal cord injury can cause devastating permanent disability. Understanding injury patterns, proper assessment, and prevention of secondary injury is essential for optimizing outcomes.

Spinal Cord Anatomy Essentials

The spinal cord extends from the brainstem to approximately L1-L2 vertebral level. Below this, nerve roots continue as the cauda equina (horse's tail).

Key anatomical points:

- 31 spinal nerve pairs exit through vertebral foramina
- Cervical spine: 8 nerve pairs (C1-C8)
- Thoracic spine: 12 nerve pairs (T1-T12)
- Lumbar spine: 5 nerve pairs (L1-L5)
- Sacral spine: 5 nerve pairs (S1-S5)
- Coccygeal: 1 pair

Nerve root naming: Cervical nerves exit above their numbered vertebra (C5 nerve exits above C5 vertebra). Thoracic and below exit below their numbered vertebra (T5 nerve exits below T5 vertebra).

Why this matters: Injury at a specific vertebral level affects the spinal cord or nerve roots at that level. For example, C5 vertebral injury affects C5-C6 spinal cord level.

White matter vs. gray matter:

- White matter (outer cord): Contains ascending sensory tracts and descending motor tracts
- Gray matter (inner cord): Contains neuronal cell bodies

Major tracts:

- **Lateral corticospinal tracts:** Motor function, crosses in medulla (injury causes ipsilateral weakness below level)
- **Dorsal columns:** Fine touch, vibration, proprioception, ipsilateral
- **Spinothalamic tracts:** Pain and temperature, crosses within 1-2 levels (contralateral)

Understanding tract anatomy helps predict deficits based on injury pattern.

Mechanisms of Spinal Cord Injury

Flexion: Forward bending can cause compression fractures, ligament tears. Common in frontal vehicle crashes.

Extension: Backward bending can cause ligament damage, vertebral artery injury. Common in rear-end crashes, especially with headrest positioned too low.

Rotation: Twisting forces cause fracture-dislocations. Very unstable.

Compression: Axial loading (force straight down spine) causes burst fractures. Common in diving into shallow water, falls landing on head or feet.

Distraction: Pulling apart of vertebrae. Seatbelt injuries in children (lap belt across abdomen pulls upper body forward while pelvis stays put).

Penetrating: Bullets, stab wounds directly transect cord.

Complete vs. Incomplete Injury

Complete spinal cord injury:

- No motor or sensory function below injury level
- Includes loss of sacral sparing (no anal sensation, voluntary anal contraction, or great toe flexion)
- If persists beyond 24 hours, usually permanent
- Most injuries initially appear complete but some recover to incomplete

Incomplete spinal cord injury:

- Some motor or sensory function preserved below injury level
- Presence of sacral sparing indicates incomplete injury
- Better prognosis than complete injury
- Various syndromes based on which part of cord is injured

Incomplete Spinal Cord Injury Syndromes

Central cord syndrome:

Mechanism: Hyperextension injury (common in elderly with cervical spondylosis)

Pathophysiology: Central gray matter and central white matter injured preferentially. Lateral corticospinal tracts are arranged with cervical (arm) fibers central and sacral (leg) fibers peripheral, so central injury affects arms more than legs.

Presentation:

- Motor: Arms weaker than legs (may have paralyzed arms with ability to walk)
- Sensory: Variable, often cape-like distribution
- Bladder dysfunction common

Prognosis: Best of the incomplete syndromes. Many patients regain functional independence. Lower extremities recover first and most completely, then bladder, then upper extremities (distal hand function may remain impaired).

Anterior cord syndrome:

Mechanism: Flexion injury, vascular injury to anterior spinal artery, herniated disc compressing anterior cord

Pathophysiology: Anterior 2/3 of cord injured, affecting corticospinal tracts (motor) and spinothalamic tracts (pain/temperature). Dorsal columns (posterior 1/3) spared.

Presentation:

- Motor: Paralysis below level
- Sensory: Loss of pain and temperature below level
- Preserved: Light touch, vibration, proprioception (dorsal columns intact)

Prognosis: Poor. Only 10-20% regain functional motor recovery. Worst prognosis of incomplete syndromes.

Brown-Séquard syndrome:

Mechanism: Hemisection (half) of cord. Usually penetrating trauma (stab, gunshot) but can occur with lateral mass fractures.

Pathophysiology: One side of cord injured. Because motor tracts don't cross until medulla and sensory tracts cross at different levels, get characteristic pattern.

Presentation:

- Ipsilateral (same side as injury): Motor weakness, loss of proprioception and vibration
- Contralateral (opposite side): Loss of pain and temperature sensation
- Classic description: Can feel but can't move on one side, can move but can't feel pain on the other side

Prognosis: Best prognosis of all cord injuries. Over 90% regain ability to walk.

Posterior cord syndrome:

Mechanism: Rare. Hyperextension injury affecting dorsal columns.

Pathophysiology: Dorsal columns injured, motor tracts intact.

Presentation:

- Motor: Intact
- Sensory: Loss of proprioception, vibration, fine touch
- Pain/temperature: Intact
- Functional impact: Severe ataxia (can't walk well despite motor function because no proprioception)

Prognosis: Variable.

Cauda equina syndrome:

Mechanism: Injury below L1-L2 affects nerve roots, not spinal cord itself.

Presentation:

- Flaccid paralysis of legs (lower motor neuron pattern)
- Saddle anesthesia (numbness in perineum)
- Bladder and bowel dysfunction
- Loss of reflexes

Prognosis: Variable depending on severity and timing of decompression. Can recover if pressure relieved quickly.

Conus medullaris syndrome:

Mechanism: Injury to tip of spinal cord (L1-L2 level).

Presentation:

- Similar to cauda equina but may have mixed upper and lower motor neuron signs
- Sudden onset (versus gradual with cauda equina)
- Bladder/bowel dysfunction prominent

Neurogenic Shock vs. Spinal Shock

These terms are often confused but describe different phenomena.

Neurogenic shock:

Mechanism: Spinal cord injury above T6 disrupts sympathetic nervous system, causing loss of sympathetic tone.

Presentation:

- Hypotension (vasodilation)
- Bradycardia (not tachycardia!)
- Warm, dry skin below injury (vessels dilated)
- Poikilothermia (body temp matches environment—can't thermoregulate)

Why it happens: Sympathetic outflow from T1-L2. Injury above T6 interrupts this, leaving unopposed parasympathetic tone.

Management:

- Fluid resuscitation (carefully—can't compensate for overload)
- Vasopressors to restore vascular tone (phenylephrine, norepinephrine)
- Atropine if severe bradycardia
- Maintain spinal cord perfusion pressure

Critical distinction: This is NOT hypovolemic shock. Aggressive fluid resuscitation causes pulmonary edema. Use vasopressors early.

Spinal shock:

Mechanism: Temporary loss of all reflexes below spinal cord injury level.

Presentation:

- Flaccid paralysis
- Absent reflexes
- Absent rectal tone
- Lasts hours to weeks (usually resolves within 24-48 hours)

Resolution: First sign is return of bulbocavernosus reflex (squeezing glans penis or pulling on Foley causes anal sphincter contraction).

Clinical significance: Can't determine if injury is complete or incomplete until spinal shock resolves. Initial complete paralysis may recover to incomplete injury.

Assessment: ASIA Scale

The American Spinal Injury Association (ASIA) scale standardizes spinal cord injury assessment.

Motor assessment:

- Test 10 key muscles (5 on each side)
- Grade each 0-5 (0=paralysis, 5=normal)
- Maximum score: 100

Key muscles:

- C5: Elbow flexors (biceps)
- C6: Wrist extensors
- C7: Elbow extensors (triceps)
- C8: Finger flexors
- T1: Small finger abductors
- L2: Hip flexors
- L3: Knee extensors (quads)
- L4: Ankle dorsiflexors
- L5: Great toe extensors
- S1: Ankle plantarflexors

Sensory assessment:

- Test 28 dermatomes bilaterally
- Grade 0-2 for pinprick and light touch each
- Include sacral dermatomes (S4-5)

ASIA Impairment Scale:

- **A (Complete):** No motor or sensory function in S4-S5
- **B (Sensory Incomplete):** Sensory but no motor function below level, including S4-S5
- **C (Motor Incomplete):** Motor function below level, >50% muscles grade <3
- **D (Motor Incomplete):** Motor function below level, ≥50% muscles grade ≥3
- **E (Normal):** Normal motor and sensory

Neurological level: Lowest segment with normal function bilaterally (motor and sensory).

Management Principles

Immobilization: Covered in next section.

Maintaining spinal cord perfusion:

- MAP goal 85-90 mmHg for first 7 days after injury
- Prevents secondary ischemic injury
- Use fluids and vasopressors as needed

Preventing secondary injury:

- Avoid hypotension (single biggest modifiable risk factor)
- Avoid hypoxia
- Prevent hyperthermia
- Early surgical decompression if indicated

Methylprednisolone controversy:

- High-dose steroids within 8 hours of injury was standard based on NASCIS trials
- Recent evidence questions benefit and shows increased infection risk
- Many centers no longer use routinely
- If used: 30 mg/kg bolus, then 5.4 mg/kg/hr for 23-48 hours

Surgical intervention:

- Decompress spinal cord if compressed
- Stabilize unstable fractures

- Timing controversial but trend toward early surgery (<24 hours)

Complications to prevent:

- Pressure ulcers (turn every 2 hours, specialized mattresses)
- DVT/PE (prophylactic anticoagulation, SCDs)
- Pneumonia (incentive spirometry, chest PT)
- Urinary tract infections (proper catheter care)
- Autonomic dysreflexia (in injuries T6 and above)

Autonomic dysreflexia:

What it is: Massive sympathetic response below injury level to noxious stimulus. Occurs in injuries T6 and above after spinal shock resolves.

Trigger: Usually full bladder or bowel, but any stimulus below injury can trigger (tight clothing, pressure sore, ingrown toenail).

Presentation:

- Sudden severe hypertension (can be >300 mmHg systolic)
- Pounding headache
- Sweating above injury level
- Flushing above injury level
- Bradycardia (baroreceptor reflex from high BP)
- Medical emergency—can cause stroke, seizures, MI

Management:

- Sit patient upright
- Find and remove trigger (check bladder, bowel, skin)
- Loosen tight clothing
- If BP remains elevated, give short-acting antihypertensive

This is a life-threatening emergency requiring immediate intervention.

Spinal Immobilization

Proper spinal immobilization prevents further injury in patients with known or suspected spinal trauma. However, current evidence shows that immobilizing everyone "just in case" causes harm without benefit in most patients.

When to Immobilize

Not every trauma patient needs spinal immobilization. Use clinical decision rules to identify who benefits.

NEXUS criteria (all must be present to clear spine clinically):

1. No posterior midline cervical tenderness
2. No focal neurological deficits
3. Normal level of consciousness
4. No intoxication
5. No painful distracting injury

If all five criteria met, cervical spine injury extremely unlikely (<0.1%). No imaging or immobilization needed.

Canadian C-Spine Rule: More complex algorithm but slightly more sensitive than NEXUS.

High-risk criteria requiring imaging:

- Age ≥65
- Dangerous mechanism
- Paresthesias in extremities

Low-risk factors allowing assessment:

- Simple rear-end MVC
- Sitting position in ED
- Ambulatory at any time
- Delayed onset neck pain
- Absence of midline cervical tenderness

Able to rotate neck 45 degrees: If yes, no imaging needed.

Bottom line: Alert, sober patients without neck pain, tenderness, or neurological deficits don't need immobilization or imaging. Immobilizing low-risk patients causes pressure ulcers, delays care, and causes discomfort without benefit.

Proper Immobilization Techniques

When immobilization IS indicated:

Cervical collar alone is insufficient. Complete immobilization requires collar PLUS head blocks or equivalent PLUS backboard or stretcher.

Steps:

1. Maintain manual in-line stabilization initially
2. Apply properly sized rigid cervical collar
3. Secure patient to backboard with straps across chest, pelvis, legs
4. Place head blocks or rolled towels on either side of head
5. Secure head with tape or straps across forehead and collar
6. Reassess frequently—collar should not be so tight it restricts breathing or venous return

Cervical collar sizing: Measure from top of shoulder to angle of jaw. Collar should fit snugly but not restrict breathing. Too large or too small reduces effectiveness.

Removing patients from backboard:

- Backboards are for extrication and transport, NOT long-term use
- Remove patient from backboard within 30 minutes of ED arrival if possible
- Backboards cause rapid pressure ulcer development
- Use logroll technique to examine back and remove board

Logroll technique:

1. One person at head maintains in-line stabilization
2. Three people at torso, hips, legs
3. On count, roll patient toward team as unit
4. Examine back
5. Roll back onto stretcher
6. Requires 4 people minimum

Clearing the spine:

Clinical clearance: Using NEXUS or Canadian C-Spine Rule in alert, sober, asymptomatic patients.

Radiographic clearance:

- CT scan is standard (more sensitive than X-ray)
- MRI if neurological deficits with normal CT (ligamentous injury)
- Some centers use clinical clearance even in obtunded patients if high-quality CT normal

When to keep collar on:

- Fracture identified
- Patient has neurological deficits
- Patient has pain or tenderness
- Obtunded patient without imaging clearance
- High clinical suspicion despite negative imaging

Collar complications:

- Pressure ulcers on occiput and chin (especially in elderly)
- Increased ICP (collar restricts venous drainage—loosen if ICP concerns)
- Airway management difficulties
- Patient discomfort and anxiety

Key principle: Immobilize when indicated, but remove immobilization as soon as safely possible. Prolonged unnecessary immobilization causes more harm than benefit.

Key Takeaways - Chapter 7

Before moving to practice questions, let's reinforce the critical concepts that will serve you on the exam and in practice:

Brain Injury Fundamentals:

- Primary injury can't be reversed; focus on preventing secondary injury
- Hypotension and hypoxia are the most damaging preventable factors
- GCS trends matter more than single values
- A normal CT doesn't rule out significant brain injury (think DAI)

Herniation Recognition:

- Unilateral blown pupil = ipsilateral mass effect with uncal herniation
- Cushing's triad is late—act on earlier signs of deterioration
- Epidural hematomas can present with lucid interval—never dismiss head injury patients who "seem fine"

ICP Management Hierarchy:

- Start simple: positioning, sedation, normothermia, avoid hypercapnia
- Progress to osmotherapy (mannitol or hypertonic saline)
- Reserve hyperventilation for acute crises only
- Remember: CPP = MAP - ICP (must maintain both adequate MAP and controlled ICP)

Spinal Cord Injury Patterns:

- Complete vs. incomplete determined by sacral sparing
- Neurogenic shock = hypotension + bradycardia + warm skin (NOT hypovolemic shock)
- Central cord = arms worse than legs (think elderly hyperextension)
- Brown-Séquard = ipsilateral motor loss, contralateral pain/temp loss

Clinical Decision-Making:

- Not every trauma patient needs spinal immobilization
- Use NEXUS criteria to identify low-risk patients
- Remove backboards quickly to prevent pressure ulcers
- Early recognition and intervention saves lives and function

Chapter 7 Practice Questions (50 Questions)

Question 1: A patient has a GCS of 10 (E2, V3, M5). What does this score indicate?

A) Mild traumatic brain injury
B) Moderate traumatic brain injury
C) Severe traumatic brain injury
D) Normal neurological function

Answer: B

Explanation: GCS 9-12 indicates moderate TBI. This patient opens eyes to pain, speaks inappropriate words, and localizes to pain. While concerning, this is better than severe TBI (GCS ≤8). The motor score of 5 (localization) is prognostically favorable compared to posturing.

Question 2: What is the most important preventable cause of secondary brain injury?

A) Fever
B) Hypotension
C) Pain
D) Anxiety

Answer: B

Explanation: Hypotension (systolic BP <90 mmHg) is the most damaging preventable cause of secondary brain injury. Even a single episode of hypotension doubles mortality in TBI patients. The injured brain cannot autoregulate blood flow, making it extremely vulnerable to decreased perfusion pressure.

Question 3: A unilateral dilated, non-reactive pupil in a trauma patient suggests:

A) Opioid intoxication
B) Bilateral brain injury
C) Ipsilateral mass effect with uncal

herniation
D) Normal variation

Answer: C

Explanation: A unilateral blown pupil indicates mass effect on the same side causing uncal herniation and compression of the oculomotor nerve (CN III). This is a neurosurgical emergency requiring immediate intervention. Always assume pathology in trauma patients rather than normal variation.

Question 4: What is the target cerebral perfusion pressure (CPP) for adults with traumatic brain injury?

A) 40-50 mmHg
B) 50-60 mmHg
C) 60-70 mmHg
D) 80-90 mmHg

Answer: C

Explanation: Target CPP is 60-70 mmHg for adults with TBI. This ensures adequate brain perfusion without causing excessive pressure. CPP = MAP - ICP, so both blood pressure support and ICP control are necessary to maintain adequate CPP.

Question 5: Cushing's triad consists of:

A) Hypotension, tachycardia, tachypnea
B) Hypertension, bradycardia, irregular respirations
C) Hypotension, bradycardia, apnea
D) Hypertension, tachycardia, normal respirations

Answer: B

Explanation: Cushing's triad consists of hypertension (widened pulse pressure), bradycardia, and irregular respirations. This indicates dangerously elevated ICP and impending herniation. However, it's a late sign—act on earlier indicators of increased ICP rather than waiting for the full triad.

Question 6: The "lucid interval" is classically associated with which type of intracranial hemorrhage?

A) Subdural hematoma
B) Epidural hematoma
C) Subarachnoid hemorrhage
D) Intracerebral hemorrhage

Answer: B

Explanation: Epidural hematoma classically presents with a lucid interval: initial LOC from impact, patient wakes and seems fine, then rapid deterioration as the hematoma expands. This pattern occurs because arterial bleeding takes time to accumulate sufficient volume to cause mass effect.

Question 7: Which patient meets all NEXUS criteria and does NOT need spinal imaging?

A) Alert, sober patient with neck tenderness
B) Alert, sober patient with no neck pain, no tenderness, no deficits, no distracting injury
C) Intoxicated patient with no complaints
D) Alert patient with severe leg pain

Answer: B

Explanation: NEXUS criteria require all five to be present to clear the spine clinically: no midline tenderness, no neurological deficits, normal consciousness, no intoxication, no painful distracting injury. Only option B meets all criteria. Intoxication and distracting injuries prevent clinical clearance.

Question 8: What is the initial intervention for a patient with suspected increased ICP?

A) Hyperventilate to PaCO2 of 25 mmHg
B) Give mannitol immediately

C) Elevate head of bed 30 degrees and maintain head midline
D) Start pentobarbital coma

Answer: C

Explanation: Start with simple positioning measures: elevate head of bed 30 degrees (facilitates venous drainage) and keep head midline (prevents jugular compression). These basic interventions should be implemented before escalating to osmotherapy or aggressive measures. Treat in a tiered approach from simple to complex.

Question 9: A patient with spinal cord injury at T4 level presents with blood pressure 88/54, heart rate 58, and warm, dry skin below the injury. This indicates:

A) Hypovolemic shock
B) Neurogenic shock
C) Septic shock
D) Cardiogenic shock

Answer: B

Explanation: This is the classic triad of neurogenic shock: hypotension, bradycardia (not tachycardia), and warm/dry skin below injury. Injury above T6 disrupts sympathetic outflow, causing vasodilation and loss of compensatory tachycardia. Treatment requires vasopressors, not just fluids.

Question 10: Which GCS motor score indicates the best prognosis?

A) Obeys commands (6)
B) Flexion to pain (3)
C) Extension to pain (2)
D) No response (1)

Answer: A

Explanation: Motor score of 6 (obeys commands) indicates the highest level of motor function and best prognosis. Motor score is the most prognostically important component of GCS. Posturing (flexion or extension) indicates severe brain injury, while no response is the worst finding.

Question 11: What does sacral sparing indicate in spinal cord injury?

A) Complete spinal cord injury
B) Incomplete spinal cord injury
C) Cauda equina syndrome
D) Spinal shock

Answer: B

Explanation: Presence of sacral sparing (anal sensation, voluntary anal contraction, or great toe flexion) indicates incomplete spinal cord injury, which has better prognosis than complete injury. Absence of all sacral function indicates complete injury. Always assess sacral function in spinal cord injury.

Question 12: A patient with TBI develops blood pressure 180/95, heart rate 52. What should you suspect?

A) Adequate resuscitation
B) Increasing intracranial pressure
C) Pain
D) Anxiety

Answer: B

Explanation: Hypertension with bradycardia suggests increasing ICP (partial Cushing's triad). The body raises blood pressure to maintain cerebral perfusion against rising ICP, and baroreceptors respond with reflex bradycardia. This requires immediate assessment and intervention to control ICP.

Question 13: Central cord syndrome typically presents with:

A) Arms weaker than legs
B) Legs weaker than arms

C) Equal weakness in all extremities
D) No motor deficits

Answer: A

Explanation: Central cord syndrome causes disproportionately greater weakness in arms than legs because cervical motor fibers are located centrally in the corticospinal tracts. This is the most common incomplete cord syndrome, often occurring from hyperextension injury in elderly patients with cervical stenosis.

Question 14: What is the purpose of mannitol in increased ICP management?

A) Sedation
B) Creating osmotic gradient to pull fluid from brain
C) Lowering blood pressure
D) Preventing seizures

Answer: B

Explanation: Mannitol is an osmotic diuretic that creates an osmotic gradient, pulling fluid from brain tissue into the bloodstream and reducing cerebral edema. Dose is 0.25-1 g/kg IV. Monitor serum osmolality and hold if >320 mOsm/L. Hypertonic saline is an alternative with similar mechanism.

Question 15: A patient with head injury should be intubated when GCS is:

A) ≤15
B) ≤12
C) ≤8
D) ≤5

Answer: C

Explanation: "GCS 8 or less, intubate" is the general rule. GCS ≤8 indicates severe TBI with inability to protect the airway adequately. These patients need intubation for airway protection, control of ventilation (to maintain appropriate CO_2), and facilitation of ICP management.

Question 16: Brown-Séquard syndrome is characterized by:

A) Bilateral paralysis
B) Ipsilateral motor loss with contralateral pain/temperature loss
C) Arms weaker than legs
D) Complete sensory loss below injury

Answer: B

Explanation: Brown-Séquard (hemisection) syndrome causes ipsilateral motor weakness and proprioception loss (same side as injury) with contralateral pain and temperature loss (opposite side). This occurs because motor tracts don't cross until the medulla, but pain/temperature fibers cross within 1-2 spinal levels of entry.

Question 17: Which intervention should be avoided in traumatic brain injury management?

A) Maintaining normothermia
B) Administering corticosteroids
C) Elevating head of bed
D) Preventing hypotension

Answer: B

Explanation: Corticosteroids (steroids like methylprednisolone or dexamethasone) do NOT help traumatic brain injury and may increase mortality. They should not be used in TBI. Note: Steroids ARE used for spinal cord injury and brain tumors, but NOT for TBI. This is a common source of confusion.

Question 18: A patient post-concussion should return to sports when:

A) Symptoms resolve within 24 hours
B) All symptoms resolve at rest AND they complete graduated return-to-play protocol

C) CT scan is normal
D) They feel ready

Answer: B

Explanation: Return to sports requires complete symptom resolution at rest followed by successful completion of a graduated return-to-play protocol without symptom recurrence. Each step takes minimum 24 hours. Returning too soon risks second impact syndrome and prolonged recovery. Healthcare provider clearance is essential.

Question 19: What is the most sensitive early sign of compartment syndrome in an unconscious patient with extremity injury?

A) Absent pulses
B) Pain with passive stretch
C) Compartment pressure >30 mmHg
D) Pallor

Answer: C

Explanation: In unconscious patients who can't report pain, compartment pressure measurement is the most reliable indicator. Pressure >30 mmHg or within 30 mmHg of diastolic BP indicates compartment syndrome requiring fasciotomy. Late signs (pulselessness, pallor) indicate irreversible damage has occurred.

Question 20: Anterior cord syndrome results in:

A) Loss of motor and pain/temperature sensation, preserved proprioception
B) Arms weaker than legs
C) Ipsilateral motor loss only
D) Complete preservation of function

Answer: A

Explanation: Anterior cord syndrome affects the anterior 2/3 of the cord, damaging corticospinal (motor) and spinothalamic (pain/temperature) tracts while preserving dorsal columns (proprioception, vibration, light touch). It has the worst prognosis of incomplete syndromes with only 10-20% regaining functional motor recovery.

Question 21: Decorticate posturing indicates injury to:

A) Spinal cord
B) Above the midbrain
C) Midbrain or pons
D) Peripheral nerves

Answer: B

Explanation: Decorticate posturing (flexion of arms, extension of legs) indicates injury above the midbrain level. Decerebrate posturing (extension of both arms and legs) indicates injury to midbrain or pons and is more severe. Both indicate significant brain injury.

Question 22: The primary goal in managing a patient with severe TBI is:

A) Performing immediate CT scan
B) Preventing secondary brain injury
C) Administering steroids
D) Starting antibiotics

Answer: B

Explanation: While primary injury cannot be reversed, preventing secondary brain injury is the primary goal of all TBI management. This includes avoiding hypotension and hypoxia, controlling ICP, maintaining adequate CPP, preventing complications, and optimizing conditions for brain recovery.

Question 23: A chronic subdural hematoma on CT appears:

A) Bright white (hyperdense)
B) Dark (hypodense)

C) Same as brain tissue (isodense)
D) Not visible

Answer: B

Explanation: Chronic subdural hematomas appear dark (hypodense) on CT because the blood has broken down over weeks to months. Acute subdural hematomas appear bright (hyperdense). This is why elderly patients on anticoagulation can have significant chronic subdurals from minor trauma weeks earlier.

Question 24: Spinal shock is characterized by:

A) Hypotension and bradycardia
B) Temporary loss of all reflexes below injury
C) Permanent paralysis
D) Hypertension

Answer: B

Explanation: Spinal shock is temporary loss of all reflexes below the spinal cord injury level, lasting hours to weeks. It presents with flaccid paralysis and absent reflexes. This is different from neurogenic shock (hemodynamic instability). Can't determine if injury is complete or incomplete until spinal shock resolves.

Question 25: Hyperventilation in TBI management should:

A) Be used prophylactically in all patients
B) Target $PaCO_2$ of 20-25 mmHg
C) Only be used temporarily for acute ICP crisis
D) Be continued indefinitely

Answer: C

Explanation: Hyperventilation should only be used as a temporary measure for acute ICP crisis while preparing for definitive intervention. Target $PaCO_2$ 30-35 mmHg if used, never lower. Prophylactic hyperventilation reduces cerebral blood flow and worsens outcomes. The vasoconstriction effect also wears off as the body compensates.

Question 26: Which finding indicates resolution of spinal shock?

A) Return of motor function
B) Return of bulbocavernosus reflex
C) Normalized blood pressure
D) Patient awareness

Answer: B

Explanation: Return of the bulbocavernosus reflex (anal sphincter contraction when glans penis squeezed or Foley pulled) indicates spinal shock has resolved. Only after resolution can you determine if the injury is complete or incomplete, as initial findings during spinal shock don't predict final neurological status.

Question 27: Post-concussion syndrome is defined as symptoms persisting beyond:

A) 24 hours
B) 72 hours
C) 10 days in adults or 4 weeks in children
D) 6 months

Answer: C

Explanation: Post-concussion syndrome is diagnosed when symptoms persist beyond the expected recovery time: 10 days in adults or 4 weeks in children. Symptoms include headache, difficulty concentrating, memory problems, dizziness, and emotional changes. Most resolve within 3 months but some persist longer.

Question 28: A patient with suspected increased ICP should have their head positioned:

A) Flat
B) Elevated 30 degrees

C) Trendelenburg
D) Elevated 90 degrees

Answer: B

Explanation: Head of bed elevation to 30 degrees facilitates venous drainage from the brain, helping reduce ICP. However, don't elevate if patient is hypotensive, as this reduces cerebral blood flow. Keep head midline to prevent jugular vein compression. This is a basic tier-1 intervention for ICP management.

Question 29: Diffuse axonal injury (DAI) is best visualized with:

A) CT scan
B) X-ray
C) MRI
D) Ultrasound

Answer: C

Explanation: MRI is most sensitive for DAI, showing scattered small hemorrhages on specialized sequences. CT may show only minimal findings or appear normal despite severe clinical presentation. This creates a mismatch where the patient is comatose but imaging seems relatively benign. Clinical exam is more important than CT findings in DAI.

Question 30: The cervical collar should be removed from a trauma patient:

A) Immediately upon arrival
B) After clinical or radiographic clearance of cervical spine
C) After 24 hours
D) Never

Answer: B

Explanation: Remove cervical collars after the spine is cleared either clinically (using NEXUS or Canadian C-Spine criteria) or radiographically (CT showing no fracture/instability). Prolonged collar use causes pressure ulcers, discomfort, and may increase ICP. Remove as soon as safely possible.

Question 31: What is the most common incomplete spinal cord injury syndrome?

A) Anterior cord syndrome
B) Central cord syndrome
C) Brown-Séquard syndrome
D) Posterior cord syndrome

Answer: B

Explanation: Central cord syndrome is the most common incomplete syndrome, typically occurring from hyperextension injury in elderly patients with pre-existing cervical stenosis. It also has the best prognosis among incomplete syndromes, with many patients regaining functional independence, though distal hand function may remain impaired.

Question 32: A patient with epidural hematoma requires:

A) Conservative management with observation
B) Emergency craniotomy for evacuation
C) Burr hole drainage
D) Antibiotics only

Answer: B

Explanation: Epidural hematomas causing mass effect require emergency craniotomy for surgical evacuation. Time is critical—prognosis is excellent if treated before herniation but poor if delayed. Small epidurals without mass effect in stable patients may be observed, but most require surgery.

Question 33: Autonomic dysreflexia occurs with spinal cord injuries at or above:

A) T12
B) T10
C) T6
D) C4

Answer: C

Explanation: Autonomic dysreflexia occurs with injuries at T6 or above because sympathetic outflow originates from T1-L2. Injuries above T6 disconnect the spinal sympathetic centers from brain control, allowing unopposed sympathetic response below the injury to noxious stimuli. This causes life-threatening hypertension.

Question 34: The Glasgow Coma Scale motor component that indicates the worst prognosis is:

A) Withdraws from pain (4)
B) Flexion to pain (3)
C) Extension to pain (2)
D) No response (1)

Answer: D

Explanation: No motor response (score of 1) indicates the worst prognosis. The motor score is the most prognostically important GCS component. Progression from withdrawal to flexion to extension to no response indicates worsening brain injury. Extension (decerebrate) is worse than flexion (decorticate).

Question 35: A patient has persistent vomiting after head injury. This is concerning for:

A) Gastroenteritis
B) Increased intracranial pressure
C) Anxiety
D) Motion sickness

Answer: B

Explanation: Persistent or projectile vomiting after head injury is concerning for increased ICP. Vomiting occurs when increased pressure affects the vomiting center in the medulla. Combined with headache and altered mental status, this strongly suggests rising ICP requiring immediate intervention.

Question 36: The medication used to prevent vasospasm after traumatic subarachnoid hemorrhage is:

A) Phenytoin
B) Mannitol
C) Nimodipine
D) Propofol

Answer: C

Explanation: Nimodipine is a calcium channel blocker used to prevent vasospasm after subarachnoid hemorrhage. Vasospasm typically occurs days 3-14 after bleeding as blood products irritate cerebral vessels. Vasospasm reduces cerebral blood flow and can cause stroke. Nimodipine reduces this risk.

Question 37: In a patient with suspected spinal cord injury, the presence of priapism (sustained erection) suggests:

A) Sexual arousal
B) Spinal cord injury
C) Normal finding
D) Peripheral nerve injury

Answer: B

Explanation: Priapism in trauma patients indicates spinal cord injury, particularly complete injuries. Loss of sympathetic tone with preserved sacral parasympathetic reflexes causes the sustained erection. This is a significant clinical finding suggesting serious spinal cord damage.

Question 38: A patient with TBI and blood pressure 160/95 should:

A) Be given antihypertensives immediately
B) Have blood pressure monitored closely without immediate treatment
C) Receive IV fluids
D) Be positioned flat

Answer: B

Explanation: Elevated blood pressure in TBI patients may represent the body's attempt to maintain cerebral perfusion against increased ICP (Cushing's response). Don't reflexively treat hypertension without assessing ICP and CPP. If patient is developing Cushing's triad, lowering BP worsens brain perfusion. Assess and address the underlying cause (increased ICP) rather than just treating the number.

Question 39: Which statement about concussion is true?

A) Always involves loss of consciousness
B) CT scan is always abnormal
C) Can occur without loss of consciousness
D) Symptoms resolve within 24 hours always

Answer: C

Explanation: Most concussions (>90%) do NOT involve loss of consciousness. Concussion is diagnosed based on symptoms: confusion, amnesia, headache, dizziness, or feeling "not right" after head trauma. CT is typically normal in isolated concussion. Symptoms usually resolve within 7-10 days but can persist longer.

Question 40: The proper dosage of mannitol for increased ICP is:

A) 0.1-0.25 g/kg
B) 0.25-1 g/kg
C) 1-2 g/kg
D) 2-5 g/kg

Answer: B

Explanation: Mannitol dosing for increased ICP is 0.25-1 g/kg IV bolus. It works within 15-30 minutes by creating an osmotic gradient. Monitor serum osmolality and hold if >320 mOsm/L. Also monitor for hypotension from diuresis and correct electrolyte abnormalities.

Question 41: A patient develops severe hypertension (BP 220/130), pounding headache, and sweating above their T4 spinal cord injury. This indicates:

A) Anxiety
B) Autonomic dysreflexia
C) Neurogenic shock
D) Sepsis

Answer: B

Explanation: This is autonomic dysreflexia, a life-threatening emergency in spinal cord injuries T6 and above. Noxious stimulus below injury (usually full bladder or bowel) triggers massive sympathetic response causing severe hypertension. Immediate management: sit patient upright, find and remove trigger, give antihypertensives if BP remains elevated.

Question 42: The ASIA Impairment Scale grade for complete spinal cord injury is:

A) Grade A
B) Grade B
C) Grade C
D) Grade E

Answer: A

Explanation: ASIA Impairment Scale Grade A indicates complete injury (no motor or sensory function in S4-S5). Grade B is sensory incomplete, C and D are motor incomplete (differing in strength levels), and E is normal. The presence of sacral sparing indicates incomplete injury (Grade B or better).

Question 43: Which patients should receive ICP monitoring?

A) All patients with head trauma
B) Severe TBI (GCS ≤8) with abnormal CT
C) Mild concussion
D) Scalp lacerations only

Answer: B

Explanation: ICP monitoring is indicated for severe TBI (GCS ≤8) with abnormal CT scan. Also considered for severe TBI with normal CT if patient meets risk criteria (age >40, posturing, systolic BP <90). Not needed for mild TBI or isolated scalp injuries. Monitoring guides treatment decisions and assesses treatment effectiveness.

Question 44: The immediate intervention for a patient with suspected spine injury and absent pedal pulses after manipulation should be:

A) Apply more traction
B) Release traction and reassess
C) Proceed with imaging
D) Apply splint

Answer: B

Explanation: If pulses disappear after manipulation of spine injury, immediately release traction/realign to restore blood flow. Vascular compromise from spine manipulation is an emergency. Reassess pulses and neurological status. May need gentle repositioning to restore circulation while maintaining spinal alignment.

Question 45: A patient with head injury becomes increasingly confused over 2 hours despite initially being alert. This suggests:

A) Normal recovery
B) Expanding intracranial hematoma
C) Hunger
D) Medication effect

Answer: B

Explanation: Progressive deterioration in mental status suggests expanding intracranial hematoma (epidural, subdural, or intracerebral). This is especially concerning in patients who initially seemed fine (lucid interval with epidural hematoma). Requires immediate imaging and neurosurgical evaluation. Trends are more important than single assessments.

Question 46: Hypertonic saline (3%) for increased ICP works by:

A) Causing vasoconstriction
B) Creating osmotic gradient to pull fluid from brain
C) Sedating the patient
D) Lowering blood pressure

Answer: B

Explanation: Hypertonic saline creates an osmotic gradient that pulls water from brain tissue into the bloodstream, reducing cerebral edema. It also expands blood volume, helping maintain blood pressure (advantage over mannitol). Target sodium 145-155 mEq/L. Can be given as bolus or continuous infusion.

Question 47: The most important motor examination in suspected spinal cord injury is:

A) Hand grip strength
B) Shoulder shrug
C) Rectal tone
D) Biceps strength

Answer: C

Explanation: Rectal tone assessment is critical because it evaluates sacral function. Voluntary anal contraction indicates sacral sparing, meaning incomplete injury with better prognosis. Absence of sacral function (including rectal tone, anal sensation, and toe flexion) indicates complete injury. Always assess sacral function in suspected cord injuries.

Question 48: A patient with basilar skull fracture may present with:

A) Raccoon eyes and Battle's sign
B) Hemiparesis
C) Aphasia
D) Visual field deficits

Answer: A

Explanation: Basilar skull fractures present with characteristic signs: raccoon eyes (periorbital ecchymosis), Battle's sign (mastoid ecchymosis), hemotympanum (blood behind eardrum), or CSF otorrhea/rhinorrhea. These fractures can injure cranial nerves and vessels at skull base. Never insert NG tubes nasally in basilar skull fractures.

Question 49: Which medication is used for seizure prophylaxis in the first week after TBI?

A) Antibiotics
B) Steroids
C) Phenytoin or levetiracetam
D) Mannitol

Answer: C

Explanation: Phenytoin or levetiracetam are used for seizure prophylaxis in the first week after TBI to prevent early post-traumatic seizures, which increase ICP and worsen outcomes. Prophylaxis beyond one week hasn't been shown to prevent late seizures. Seizure prophylaxis is NOT given for all head injuries, only those at high risk.

Question 50: The primary difference between epidural and subdural hematoma on CT is:

A) Color
B) Shape (lens-shaped vs. crescent-shaped)
C) Size
D) Location in brain

Answer: B

Explanation: Epidural hematomas appear lens-shaped (lentiform/biconvex) and don't cross suture lines because dura is adherent to skull at sutures. Subdural hematomas appear crescent-shaped and cross suture lines because blood can spread along brain surface. Both appear bright (hyperdense) when acute, but shape distinguishes them.

Clinical Scenarios (6 Scenarios)

Clinical Scenario 1: Epidural Hematoma with Lucid Interval

A 22-year-old male was struck in the right temporal region during an assault 2 hours ago. He lost consciousness briefly at the scene but woke up within 1 minute. EMS brought him to the ED where he was alert (GCS 15), oriented, with only a scalp contusion. He was observed in the ED.

Thirty minutes later, the nurse notes he's "not acting right"—more confused, slower to respond. Current vitals: HR 68, BP 156/92, RR 14, SpO_2 98%. His GCS is now 12 (E3, V4, M5). Right pupil is 5 mm and sluggishly reactive; left pupil is 3 mm and reactive.

Questions:

1. What injury do you suspect based on mechanism and presentation?
2. What is happening with this patient's pupils and what does it indicate?
3. What are your immediate actions?
4. The patient's GCS drops to 8 (E2, V2, M4) and right pupil is now 7 mm and non-reactive. What does this represent and what's the urgency?

Answers:

1. **Suspected injury:** Epidural hematoma. Classic presentation: blow to temporal region, brief LOC, lucid interval where patient seems fine, then deterioration as hematoma expands. Temporal bone fracture likely lacerated middle meningeal artery, causing arterial bleeding that accumulated over time.
2. **Pupil findings:** Right pupil enlarging and becoming sluggish indicates developing uncal herniation on the right side. The expanding hematoma creates mass effect, pushing the uncus (part of temporal lobe) downward, compressing CN III (oculomotor nerve). This is an early warning sign of impending catastrophic herniation.
3. **Immediate actions:**
    - Call neurosurgery STAT—this is a neurosurgical emergency
    - Stat head CT (will show lens-shaped hyperdense collection not crossing suture lines)
    - Maintain adequate blood pressure (keep systolic >110 mmHg)—brain needs perfusion
    - Ensure adequate oxygenation
    - Elevate head of bed 30 degrees
    - Keep head midline
    - Prepare for immediate craniotomy
    - Consider osmotherapy (mannitol 1 g/kg or hypertonic saline) if neurosurgery delayed
    - Intubate if GCS continues dropping or airway compromise develops
    - Have OR ready—patient will need emergency craniotomy
    - Keep family informed
    - Document all findings with exact times
4. **GCS 8 with blown pupil significance:** This represents frank herniation—the uncus has herniated through the tentorial notch, completely compressing CN III. This is a surgical emergency requiring immediate intervention. Without emergency craniotomy to evacuate the hematoma and relieve pressure, the patient will die from progressive herniation causing brainstem compression.

Urgency level: IMMEDIATE. Minutes matter. Epidural hematomas are one of the few neurosurgical emergencies where perfect outcome is possible if treated promptly, but mortality approaches 100% if herniation progresses untreated.

Key teaching points from this scenario:

- Never dismiss head injury patients who initially appear fine—lucid intervals can be deceptive

- Temporal region impacts warrant close observation and often imaging even when patient seems well
- Pupillary changes are critical warning signs requiring immediate action
- GCS trends matter more than single assessments
- Early recognition and treatment lead to excellent outcomes; delayed treatment is catastrophic

Clinical Scenario 2: Subdural Hematoma in Elderly Patient on Anticoagulation

A 76-year-old female presents with confusion and difficulty walking that has worsened over the past 2 weeks. Family reports she fell at home about 3 weeks ago, hitting her head on a table, but "seemed fine afterward." She takes warfarin for atrial fibrillation.

She's confused, unable to state date or location (oriented only to person). Gait is unsteady. No focal weakness but seems slower on left side. Vitals: HR 88 (irregular), BP 148/82, RR 16, SpO_2 96%. GCS 14 (E4, V4, M6).

Questions:

1. What injury do you suspect and why is this patient at particularly high risk?
2. How does the presentation of chronic subdural hematoma differ from acute epidural hematoma?
3. What are your management priorities?
4. Family asks why a "minor fall" 3 weeks ago is causing problems now. How do you explain?

Answers:

1. **Suspected injury:** Chronic subdural hematoma. This patient has multiple risk factors:
    - **Age:** Elderly patients have brain atrophy, which stretches bridging veins, making them fragile and prone to tearing with minimal trauma
    - **Anticoagulation:** Warfarin increases bleeding risk dramatically. Even minor trauma can cause significant intracranial bleeding
    - **Mechanism:** Fall with head impact, though seemed minor
    - **Presentation:** Insidious onset of confusion and gait changes over weeks (classic for chronic subdural)

    Chronic subdurals develop slowly as venous blood gradually accumulates. In elderly patients with brain atrophy, there's more space for blood to accumulate before symptoms appear.

2. **Presentation differences:**

    Chronic Subdural:

    - Develops over weeks to months
    - Often from minor trauma or no remembered trauma
    - Gradual symptom onset: confusion, personality changes, gait instability

- May mimic dementia or stroke
- CT shows crescent-shaped hypodense (dark) collection
- Common in elderly, especially on anticoagulation

Acute Epidural:

- Develops over hours
- Usually from significant trauma
- Rapid symptom onset after lucid interval
- Obvious deterioration pattern
- CT shows lens-shaped hyperdense (bright) collection
- Common in younger patients with temporal bone fractures

The key is time course: chronic subdurals are insidious while epidurals are dramatic and rapid.

3. **Management priorities:**

Immediate:

- Stat head CT to confirm diagnosis and assess size/midline shift
- Labs: CBC, PT/INR (need to know anticoagulation status)
- Neurosurgery consultation
- Reverse anticoagulation:
  - Hold warfarin immediately
  - Give vitamin K 10 mg IV
  - Consider PCC (prothrombin complex concentrate) or FFP to rapidly reverse INR
  - Target INR <1.5
- Address atrial fibrillation risk (patient off anticoagulation temporarily—discuss with cardiology about stroke risk vs. bleeding risk)

Definitive treatment:

- Most chronic subdurals need burr hole drainage (less invasive than craniotomy)
- Procedure involves drilling small holes in skull and draining fluid
- May place temporary drain
- Can be done under local anesthesia in some cases

Post-procedure:

- Monitor for reaccumulation (chronic subdurals can recur)
- Gradual return to anticoagulation after discussing risks/benefits
- May need repeat imaging if symptoms recur
- Physical therapy for gait
- Close outpatient follow-up

4. **Explaining to family:**

"I understand it seems strange that a fall 3 weeks ago is causing problems now. Let me explain what happens in this type of brain bleeding.

When your mother fell and hit her head, it tore small veins on the surface of her brain. Because she takes blood thinners for her heart rhythm, these veins bled more than they would have otherwise. The bleeding was slow—just a little bit over time—so she didn't notice symptoms immediately.

As we age, our brains actually shrink slightly, creating more space inside the skull. This means blood can accumulate for a while before causing symptoms. Over the past few weeks, blood has been slowly collecting in the space around her brain.

Eventually, the collection got large enough to press on brain tissue, causing the confusion and walking problems you've noticed. The symptoms developed gradually because the bleeding was slow and the brain could compensate for a while.

The good news is that we can drain this blood collection with a relatively simple procedure. Many patients improve significantly after drainage. However, we need to balance her need for blood thinners for her heart with the risk of this happening again. We'll work with her cardiologist on the best plan going forward.

This situation is actually quite common in older adults taking blood thinners. Even minor bumps to the head can lead to this problem, which is why we encourage protective measures like removing fall hazards at home and being extra cautious."

Key teaching points:

- High suspicion for subdural in elderly patients with new confusion, especially on anticoagulation
- Minor trauma can cause significant bleeding in anticoagulated patients
- Chronic subdurals present insidiously—don't dismiss as "just dementia" or "just getting older"
- Balancing anticoagulation needs with bleeding risk is complex
- Falls prevention is critical in elderly patients on anticoagulation

Clinical Scenario 3: Cervical Spinal Cord Injury with Neurogenic Shock

A 28-year-old male dove into shallow water and struck his head on the bottom. Bystanders pulled him out, and he was moving only his arms. EMS immobilized him and brought him in.

On arrival: Alert and oriented, extremely anxious. Can move arms but not legs. No sensation below nipple line. Rectal exam shows no voluntary anal contraction. Vitals: HR 58, BP 84/52, RR 18, SpO2 97% on non-rebreather. Skin is warm and dry below the neck.

Questions:

1. What level of spinal cord injury does the examination suggest?

2. Explain why this patient has bradycardia and hypotension despite being alert and not having obvious bleeding.
3. What is your immediate management approach?
4. The patient asks if he'll walk again. How do you respond at this early stage?

Answers:

1. **Spinal cord injury level:** This patient has a complete spinal cord injury at approximately C6-C7 level based on:
   - Can move arms (indicates cervical level injury, not thoracic or lumbar)
   - No leg movement or sensation below nipples (nipple line is T4 dermatome, suggesting injury above this)
   - The diving mechanism (axial loading with neck flexion) commonly causes cervical injuries
   - Loss of sensation at nipple line suggests T4 sensory level, but motor level is likely C6-C7 (can move arms but not legs)
   - No voluntary anal contraction indicates complete injury (absence of sacral sparing)

   More detailed motor testing would refine the exact level (testing specific muscle groups), but this is a high cervical/low cervical complete spinal cord injury.

2. **Neurogenic shock explanation:**

   This patient has neurogenic shock, which is distinctly different from hypovolemic shock:

   Why bradycardia and hypotension occur:

   - Spinal cord injury above T6 disrupts sympathetic nervous system pathways (sympathetic outflow originates from T1-L2)
   - Loss of sympathetic tone causes:
     - **Vasodilation** (blood vessels dilate because no sympathetic-driven constriction) → blood pressure drops
     - **Loss of compensatory tachycardia** (heart rate normally increases in shock, but that requires sympathetic input) → instead get bradycardia from unopposed vagal tone
   - The warm, dry skin below injury confirms vasodilation (vessels dilated, blood flowing to periphery)

   Why he's alert despite low blood pressure:

   - His brain is getting adequate blood flow (injury is below the level of brain blood supply)
   - Blood pressure, while low, isn't critically low yet
   - He's not in hypovolemic shock—total blood volume is normal
   - The hypotension is from distributive problem (vessels too dilated) not volume problem

Critical distinction: This is NOT hypovolemic shock. Aggressive fluid resuscitation would cause pulmonary edema because the problem isn't volume—it's vascular tone. He needs vasopressors to restore vascular tone, not liters of fluid.

3. **Immediate management:**

Airway and breathing:

- High-flow oxygen (already in place)
- Close respiratory monitoring (C6-C7 injury preserves diaphragm but may affect intercostal muscles)
- Prepare for possible intubation if respiratory fatigue develops
- Consider arterial blood gas to assess adequacy of ventilation

Circulation—treating neurogenic shock:

- Large-bore IV access (two lines)
- Fluid resuscitation: Give 1-2 liters crystalloid CAREFULLY (but don't overdo it—these patients can't compensate for fluid overload)
- Start vasopressors EARLY (don't wait to see if fluids alone work):
    - Phenylephrine or norepinephrine to restore vascular tone
    - Target MAP 85-90 mmHg (maintain spinal cord perfusion)
- Atropine if bradycardia becomes severe (<45-50 bpm) or symptomatic
- Avoid aggressive fluid resuscitation (risks pulmonary edema)

Spinal cord protection:

- Maintain spinal immobilization (cervical collar, backboard)
- Stat CT cervical spine to identify fracture/injury
- MRI to assess cord injury and compression
- Neurosurgery consultation emergently

Preventing secondary injury:

- Maintain MAP 85-90 mmHg (spinal cord perfusion pressure)
- Ensure adequate oxygenation
- Prevent hypothermia (these patients can't thermoregulate—body temp matches environment)
- Methylprednisolone controversial (discuss with neurosurgery—many centers no longer use routinely)

Additional interventions:

- Foley catheter (bladder management—these patients lose bladder control)
- DVT prophylaxis (high risk for blood clots)
- Pressure ulcer prevention (turn every 2 hours, specialized mattress)
- Gastric decompression (NG tube—prevents aspiration)
- Pain management

- Psychological support (this is devastating news)

Surgical considerations:

- If fracture with cord compression, may need decompression surgery
- Stabilization of unstable fractures
- Timing controversial but trend toward early surgery (<24 hours)

4. **Responding to "will I walk again" question:**

This requires honesty balanced with appropriate hope at this early stage:

"I understand you're worried about whether you'll walk again, and that's a completely natural question. Let me explain what we know right now and what we need to learn over time.

You have a spinal cord injury at the level of your neck from the diving accident. Right now, you're not able to move your legs or feel sensation below your chest. We've also found that you don't have reflexes in your rectal area, which gives us information about the severity.

Here's what's important to understand: In the first 24-48 hours after spinal cord injury, your body goes through something called 'spinal shock,' where all the reflexes below the injury shut down temporarily. Until that resolves, we can't definitively determine whether your injury is complete or incomplete.

If the injury is complete (no nerve signals getting through), the chances of walking again are very low. I want to be honest with you about that.

If the injury is incomplete (some nerve signals still getting through), there's potential for recovery, though we can't predict how much. Some people with incomplete injuries regain significant function with intensive rehabilitation.

We won't know which category you fall into for at least 24-48 hours. Right now, our focus is on:

- Protecting your spine and preventing further injury
- Getting imaging to see exactly what's injured
- Possibly surgery to relieve pressure on your spinal cord
- Maintaining your blood pressure to keep blood flowing to the injured area
- Preventing complications

Over the coming days and weeks, we'll get a clearer picture of your potential for recovery. Regardless of the outcome, there are excellent rehabilitation programs that help people adapt and live full lives after spinal cord injuries. We'll support you every step of the way, whatever your recovery looks like.

I know this is overwhelming and scary. Do you have questions about what's happening right now or what comes next?"

Why this response works:

- Honest about severity without removing all hope
- Explains spinal shock concept so patient understands we can't predict yet
- Acknowledges both possibilities (complete vs. incomplete)
- Focuses on what's being done NOW
- Provides realistic timeline
- Offers support and resources
- Invites questions

Key teaching points:

- Neurogenic shock requires vasopressors, not just fluids
- Maintain high MAP (85-90) for spinal cord perfusion
- Can't determine complete vs. incomplete until spinal shock resolves
- Early honest communication while maintaining appropriate hope
- Diving injuries commonly cause cervical spine fractures

Clinical Scenario 4: Concussion with Delayed Symptoms

A 16-year-old high school football player took a hard hit during practice. He seemed dazed briefly but continued playing. Coach noticed he seemed "off" and pulled him out. He denied symptoms at the time.

Three hours later, his mother brings him to the ED. He has worsening headache, vomited twice, and "isn't acting like himself." On exam: GCS 15, oriented but seems slow to respond. Says his "head hurts really bad" and bright lights bother him. No focal neurological deficits. Vitals normal.

Questions:

1. What is your diagnosis and why are delayed symptoms concerning?
2. What red flags warrant imaging in this patient?
3. The coach asks if the player can return to the game next week. What's your response?
4. What education do you provide about second impact syndrome?

Answers:

1. **Diagnosis and concern about delayed symptoms:**

   Diagnosis: Concussion with post-concussion symptoms. However, the delayed onset and progression of symptoms (worsening headache, vomiting) are concerning red flags that warrant further evaluation.

   Why delayed symptoms are concerning:

   - Most concussion symptoms appear immediately or within minutes
   - Progressively worsening symptoms can indicate evolving intracranial injury

- Vomiting especially concerning (can indicate increased ICP)
- The combination of worsening headache + vomiting + altered behavior warrants ruling out more serious injury (epidural hematoma, subdural hematoma, cerebral contusion)

In this case:

- The impact was significant enough to make him dazed
- He continued playing (repeated head impacts possible)
- Symptoms worsened over 3 hours (evolution pattern)
- Vomiting is a red flag
- Behavior changes noted by family

While this may be "just" a concussion, the presentation requires imaging to rule out structural injury.

2. **Red flags warranting imaging:**

This patient has multiple red flags from standard concussion guidelines:

Red flags present:

- **Vomiting** (especially repeated)
- **Severe or worsening headache**
- **Behavior changes** ("not acting like himself")
- **Progressively worsening symptoms** over time

Other red flags to assess (ask about):

- Seizures (none reported)
- Focal neurological deficits (none found on exam)
- Severe mechanism (hard hit in football qualifies)
- Loss of consciousness >30 seconds (was "dazed" but unclear duration)

Recommendation: This patient needs CT scan of head to rule out intracranial hemorrhage or other structural injury.

If CT is normal: Diagnosis is concussion with post-concussion symptoms requiring observation, rest, and close follow-up.

If CT shows injury: Management depends on findings (hematoma may need neurosurgery, contusion needs monitoring, etc.)

3. **Response about returning to play:**

"Your player will not be able to return to football next week, and I want to explain why this is so important for his long-term health.

Right now, his brain has been injured—we call this a concussion. Even though we can't see it on a CT scan necessarily, there's real injury happening at the cellular level. His brain is in a vulnerable state where it's working hard to heal itself.

Here's what needs to happen before he can return to any sports:

First: All symptoms must completely resolve—no headaches, no dizziness, no concentration problems, no light sensitivity—while he's at rest. This typically takes 7-10 days minimum but can take longer.

Second: He needs medical clearance from a healthcare provider experienced in concussion management.

Third: He must successfully complete a graduated return-to-play protocol. This is a step-by-step process where he gradually increases activity over at least 5-6 days:

- Day 1: Light aerobic exercise only
- Day 2: Sport-specific drills
- Day 3: Non-contact practice
- Day 4-5: Full practice
- Day 6: Return to games

If symptoms return at ANY step, he stops, rests until symptom-free again, and starts back at the previous step.

Why this matters: If he returns to play while his brain is still recovering, he's at risk for second impact syndrome. This is a rare but potentially fatal condition where a second concussion during the vulnerable recovery period causes rapid brain swelling. Even impacts that seem minor can trigger this. It's deadly in about 50% of cases.

Additionally, repeated concussions before full recovery lead to:

- Longer recovery times
- More severe symptoms
- Increased risk of long-term cognitive problems
- Possible chronic traumatic encephalopathy (CTE) with repeated head trauma

I know missing games is disappointing, but his brain health and future are more important than any single game or season. If he follows the proper protocol, he can return safely when he's ready. If he rushes back, he risks his long-term health or even his life.

We'll provide documentation for school and coaching staff about his restrictions. He'll need academic accommodations too—reduced homework, extra time on tests, breaks during class—until symptoms resolve."

4. **Education about second impact syndrome:**

"Let me explain second impact syndrome because it's critical you understand this risk.

What it is: Second impact syndrome happens when someone with a concussion that hasn't fully healed gets another blow to the head. Even a seemingly minor impact—one that wouldn't normally cause problems—can trigger catastrophic brain swelling when the brain is still vulnerable from the first injury.

What happens: The second impact causes a loss of the brain's ability to regulate blood flow. The brain rapidly swells, increasing pressure inside the skull. This can lead to:

- Immediate collapse
- Rapid neurological deterioration
- Herniation
- Death or permanent severe disability in 50-100% of cases

How quickly it happens: Often within minutes of the second impact. Athletes might collapse on the field or shortly after.

Who's at risk: Young athletes (under 25) seem most vulnerable, possibly because their brains are still developing. High school and college athletes are at highest risk.

Prevention is simple but critical:

- **No return to sports** until completely symptom-free
- **Complete the full return-to-play protocol** without rushing
- **Get medical clearance** before returning
- **Report ANY symptoms** immediately—don't hide them to keep playing

Warning signs family should watch for:

- Worsening headache despite rest
- Repeated vomiting
- Increasing confusion
- Seizures
- Weakness or numbness
- Cannot be awakened
- Slurred speech

If any of these occur, call 911 immediately.

For schools and coaches: They need to understand that it's not safe to have players "tough it out" or hide symptoms to keep playing. Brain injuries are different from other sports injuries. A broken bone heals on a predictable timeline, but each brain is different. We can't rush brain healing.

The bottom line: Missing a few weeks of sports is temporary. Brain damage from second impact syndrome is permanent or fatal. The choice is clear, even though it's disappointing in the moment."

Key teaching points:

- Don't minimize concussions because imaging is normal
- Delayed or worsening symptoms warrant further evaluation
- Return-to-play protocols exist for athlete safety, not to be rushed
- Second impact syndrome is rare but devastating
- Proper education of athletes, parents, and coaches saves lives
- When in doubt, sit them out

Clinical Scenario 5: Increased ICP Management

A 34-year-old male was in a high-speed motor vehicle crash 2 hours ago. Initial GCS was 7 (E1, V2, M4), and he was intubated in the field. CT shows diffuse cerebral edema with small hemorrhagic contusions. ICP monitor was placed, reading 28 mmHg. Current MAP 75 mmHg.

Questions:

1. Calculate this patient's CPP and interpret the findings.
2. What is your tiered approach to managing elevated ICP?
3. The patient's ICP rises to 35 mmHg despite tier 1 interventions. What's your next step?
4. Explain why hyperventilation should be used cautiously and only temporarily.

Answers:

1. **CPP calculation and interpretation:**

   CPP = MAP - ICP CPP = 75 - 28 = 47 mmHg

   Interpretation: This CPP is critically low. Target CPP is 60-70 mmHg for adults with TBI. A CPP of 47 mmHg indicates inadequate cerebral perfusion—the brain isn't getting enough blood flow.

   This patient has two problems:

   - ICP too high (28 mmHg; normal <15 mmHg)
   - MAP too low for adequate CPP

   Immediate needs:

   - Reduce ICP through interventions
   - ALSO increase MAP (with vasopressors if needed) to improve CPP
   - Both problems must be addressed—just lowering ICP isn't enough if MAP remains low
2. **Tiered approach to elevated ICP:**

   Tier 1: Basic measures (always implement)

- **Head positioning:** Elevate head of bed 30 degrees, keep head midline (facilitates venous drainage)
- **Sedation:** Adequate sedation (propofol common) reduces metabolic demands and ICP
- **Analgesia:** Pain increases ICP—keep patient comfortable
- **Normothermia:** Treat fever aggressively (fever increases metabolic rate and ICP). Target 36-37°C
- **Oxygenation:** Keep PaO_2 >80 mmHg (hypoxia worsens brain injury)
- **Blood pressure support:** Target MAP >80 mmHg to maintain CPP 60-70 mmHg. Use vasopressors (norepinephrine) if needed
- **Avoid hypercapnia:** Keep $PaCO_2$ 35-40 mmHg (hypercapnia causes vasodilation and increases ICP)
- **Seizure prophylaxis:** Prevent seizures (phenytoin or levetiracetam) as seizures dramatically increase ICP

Tier 2: Osmotherapy (if tier 1 insufficient)

- **Mannitol:** 0.25-1 g/kg IV bolus, creates osmotic gradient pulling fluid from brain. Check serum osmolality (hold if >320 mOsm/L)
- **Hypertonic saline:** 23.4% bolus or 3% infusion. Also creates osmotic gradient, expands blood volume. Target sodium 145-155 mEq/L
- Either agent acceptable; hypertonic saline increasingly preferred

Tier 3: CSF drainage (if ventriculostomy in place)

- Drain CSF when ICP >20-22 mmHg
- Most effective immediate ICP reduction
- Monitor for infection

Tier 4: Controlled hyperventilation (temporary only)

- Lower $PaCO_2$ to 30-35 mmHg (causes vasoconstriction, reduces cerebral blood volume)
- Use ONLY for acute ICP crisis while preparing other interventions
- Don't use prophylactically
- Monitor with brain tissue oxygen if available

Tier 5: Barbiturate coma (refractory ICP)

- Pentobarbital suppresses metabolism
- Requires vasopressor support (causes hypotension)
- Continuous EEG monitoring for burst suppression
- Last medical option

Tier 6: Decompressive craniectomy (surgical)

- Remove skull bone to allow swelling
- Reduces ICP but doesn't guarantee good functional outcome
- Reserved for refractory cases

3. **ICP rises to 35 mmHg despite tier 1:**

   Immediate actions:

   - **Recheck tier 1 measures:** Ensure all are optimized (head position, sedation adequate, temperature normal, oxygenation good, no hypercapnia)
   - **Increase MAP:** If MAP is still 75, increase to 85-90 with vasopressors. Better CPP may help

   Escalate to tier 2:

   - **Give osmotherapy:** Either mannitol 1 g/kg IV push OR hypertonic saline 23.4% 30 mL IV push
   - Reassess ICP in 15-30 minutes

   If ventriculostomy present:

   - **Drain CSF:** Open drain to lower ICP

   If ICP remains >30 mmHg:

   - **Notify neurosurgery:** May need surgical intervention
   - **Consider repeat CT:** Rule out expanding hematoma or new bleeding requiring surgery

   If crisis with herniation signs (blown pupil, posturing):

   - **Hyperventilate temporarily:** Target $PaCO_2$ 30-35 mmHg while preparing for definitive intervention
   - This buys time but isn't a long-term solution

   Key principle: Escalate systematically through tiers. Don't jump to aggressive measures if simpler interventions haven't been tried. But also don't delay too long if patient deteriorating—escalate appropriately.

4. **Why hyperventilation should be used cautiously:**

   Mechanism: Lower $PaCO_2$ causes cerebral vasoconstriction, which reduces cerebral blood volume and ICP. Sounds good, right? But there are significant problems:

   Problems with hyperventilation:

   1. Reduces cerebral blood flow: Yes, this lowers ICP, but it also reduces oxygen and nutrient delivery to already-injured brain tissue. You're trading lower ICP for brain ischemia.

2. Effect is temporary: The body compensates within 24 hours by adjusting bicarbonate levels. The ICP-lowering effect wears off, but you've caused harm during that time.

3. Can worsen outcomes: Studies show prophylactic hyperventilation in TBI patients worsens outcomes, likely from cerebral ischemia.

4. Risk of excessive vasoconstriction: If $PaCO_2$ goes too low (<30 mmHg), severe vasoconstriction causes dangerous ischemia.

When to use hyperventilation:

- **ONLY for acute ICP crisis** with signs of herniation
- **Bridge therapy** while preparing for definitive intervention (surgery, tier 2/3 interventions)
- **Target $PaCO_2$ 30-35 mmHg** (never lower)
- **Monitor with brain tissue oxygen** if available
- **Time-limited:** Minutes to hours, not days

When NOT to use:

- Prophylactically in all TBI patients
- As primary/long-term ICP control
- Without other interventions in place
- In first 24 hours post-injury when cerebral blood flow already compromised

Teaching analogy: "Hyperventilation is like using a credit card in an emergency—it helps immediately but creates debt you'll pay later. Use it to get through the crisis, but have a real plan to address the underlying problem."

Key teaching points:

- CPP = MAP - ICP (both components matter)
- Systematic tier approach prevents over-treatment and under-treatment
- Simple measures first, escalate as needed
- Hyperventilation is rescue therapy, not maintenance therapy
- Balance ICP control with maintaining adequate cerebral perfusion

Clinical Scenario 6: Central Cord Syndrome

A 68-year-old male slipped on ice and fell backward, striking his occiput on concrete. He has a history of cervical spondylosis (arthritis in neck). On arrival, he's alert and complaining of neck pain. He can move his legs but has significant weakness in both arms and hands. Cannot grip well or move fingers much. Sensation intact to light touch but diminished in hands.

Vitals normal. No respiratory distress currently but respiratory rate is 22 and effort seems increased.

Questions:

1. What spinal cord syndrome does this presentation suggest and why?
2. Why is this mechanism (hyperextension) and history (cervical spondylosis) significant?
3. What are your respiratory concerns and why?
4. What is the typical recovery pattern for this syndrome?

Answers:

1. **Spinal cord syndrome:** Central cord syndrome

   Why this diagnosis fits:

   - **Classic presentation:** Arms much weaker than legs (can move legs but significant arm/hand weakness)
   - **Mechanism:** Hyperextension injury (fell backward striking occiput, causing neck to hyperextend)
   - **Demographics:** Elderly patient with pre-existing cervical stenosis (spondylosis)
   - **Sensory pattern:** Hand sensation diminished (cape-like distribution sometimes)

   Pathophysiology explanation:

   - Hyperextension caused spinal cord compression between vertebrae and infolding ligamentum flavum
   - Central gray matter and central white matter injured preferentially
   - Cervical motor fibers (to arms) located centrally in corticospinal tracts
   - Sacral/lumbar fibers (to legs) located peripherally
   - Central injury affects arms more than legs

   Why mechanism matters: Elderly patients with cervical stenosis (narrowed spinal canal from arthritis) have less room for the spinal cord. Hyperextension causes the already-narrow canal to narrow further, compressing the cord. Younger patients with normal spinal canals might have no injury from the same mechanism.

2. **Significance of mechanism and history:**

   Cervical spondylosis (degenerative arthritis):

   - Causes narrowing of spinal canal (stenosis)
   - Develops bone spurs that encroach on cord space
   - Makes spinal cord vulnerable to compression from relatively minor trauma
   - Common in elderly, often asymptomatic until traumatic event

Hyperextension mechanism:

- Posterior structures (ligamentum flavum, posterior vertebral bodies) compress cord from behind
- Anterior structures (bone spurs, disc material) compress from front
- Spinal cord gets squeezed between these structures
- Doesn't necessarily cause fracture (X-rays may be normal)
- MRI shows cord compression and often cord signal changes indicating injury

Why elderly are vulnerable:

- Pre-existing canal narrowing
- Decreased bone density (vertebrae more fragile)
- Decreased elasticity of ligaments
- Minor mechanisms can cause significant cord injury

Clinical implication: Ground-level falls in elderly with neck pain and neurological symptoms should prompt high suspicion for central cord syndrome even without obvious fracture.

Diagnosis requires:

- MRI (best for visualizing cord and soft tissue injury)
- CT cervical spine (evaluates bony structures, may be normal)
- Detailed neurological exam documenting extent of deficits

3. **Respiratory concerns:**

This patient has several respiratory risk factors that require close monitoring:

Why respiratory compromise is concerning in central cord syndrome:

Anatomical considerations:

- Diaphragm innervated by C3-C5 (phrenic nerve)
- Intercostal muscles innervated by thoracic nerves
- Accessory muscles of respiration innervated by cervical nerves
- Central cord injury at C5-C6 level can affect respiratory muscles

Specific concerns in this patient:

- **Increased respiratory rate (22) and effort:** Suggests he's working harder to breathe, indicating respiratory muscle weakness
- **Arm and hand weakness:** If injury extends to higher cervical levels or worsens, could affect diaphragm function
- **Potential for progression:** Cord edema can worsen over first 24-48 hours, causing ascending weakness
- **Secretion management:** Weak cough from intercostal weakness impairs ability to clear secretions, increasing pneumonia risk

- **Elderly patient:** Less respiratory reserve than younger patients

Monitoring needed:

- Serial respiratory assessments every 1-2 hours initially
- Measure vital capacity and negative inspiratory force (objective respiratory function measures)
- Arterial blood gas if concerns about adequacy of ventilation
- Continuous pulse oximetry
- Watch for declining vital capacity (<15 mL/kg suggests need for intubation)
- Monitor for increasing respiratory rate, use of accessory muscles, paradoxical breathing

Intervention thresholds:

- Vital capacity declining to <15-20 mL/kg → consider intubation
- Rising $PaCO_2$ or declining PaO_2 → ventilatory failure developing
- Unable to clear secretions → may need intubation for pulmonary toilet
- Patient exhaustion → don't wait until respiratory arrest

Key principle: Early elective intubation is safer than emergency intubation when patient crashes. If respiratory function declining, involve anesthesia/critical care early and have low threshold for intubation.

4. **Typical recovery pattern for central cord syndrome:**

Central cord syndrome has the best prognosis of all incomplete spinal cord injury syndromes. Understanding the recovery pattern helps set realistic expectations.

Recovery timeline and sequence:

First to recover (weeks to months):

- **Lower extremities:** Leg function typically returns first and most completely. Many patients regain ability to walk.
- **Bladder function:** Usually recovers, though may have some initial dysfunction requiring catheterization

Next to recover (months):

- **Proximal upper extremities:** Shoulder and elbow function improve before hand function
- **Sensation:** Generally improves in parallel with motor function

Last to recover and often incomplete (months to years):

- **Hand and finger function:** Fine motor control of hands is often the most persistent deficit
- **Intrinsic hand muscles:** May have lasting weakness affecting grip and dexterity

- Many patients have permanent hand dysfunction even with good recovery elsewhere

Prognosis statistics:

- About 90% of patients regain ability to walk independently or with minimal assistance
- 60-70% regain useful hand function, though often not to pre-injury level
- Younger patients generally recover better than elderly
- Early surgical decompression may improve outcomes (controversial but trend toward surgery within 24 hours)

Factors affecting prognosis:

- Age (younger better than older)
- Severity of initial deficit (less severe injuries recover better)
- Presence of other medical conditions
- Early vs. delayed surgical decompression
- Aggressive rehabilitation

Patient education about recovery:

"Let me explain what you can expect for recovery from this type of spinal cord injury.

Central cord syndrome, which is what you have, actually has the best prognosis of all spinal cord injuries. The pattern of recovery is fairly predictable:

Your legs will likely recover first and most completely. Most people with central cord syndrome regain the ability to walk, often within weeks to months. You may need physical therapy, but the outlook for leg function is very good.

Your bladder function should recover as well, though you might need a catheter temporarily.

Your arms and shoulders will improve next, typically over several months. Shoulder and elbow function usually gets quite good.

Your hands will be the slowest to recover and may not return to completely normal function. Hand and finger movements, especially fine motor tasks like buttoning shirts or writing, may remain challenging. This doesn't mean no recovery—just that hand function often doesn't get back to 100%.

The recovery process takes time. You'll see the most improvement in the first 6-12 months, but recovery can continue for up to 2 years. Intensive rehabilitation is crucial during this time.

What helps recovery:

- Possible surgery in the next 24 hours to relieve pressure on your spinal cord
- Aggressive physical and occupational therapy
- Preventing complications like pneumonia and blood clots

- Staying motivated and working hard in rehab

Most people with central cord syndrome regain independence with walking and self-care activities, though you may need adaptive equipment for some hand tasks. The key is starting rehabilitation early and staying committed to the process."

Management priorities:

- MRI to assess extent of cord compression
- Neurosurgery consultation for possible decompressive surgery
- ICU admission for close respiratory monitoring
- Early mobilization once spine cleared or stabilized
- Physical and occupational therapy consultation
- DVT prophylaxis
- Pressure ulcer prevention
- Bladder management (may need temporary catheterization)
- Pain management
- Psychological support

Key teaching points:

- Central cord syndrome has best prognosis of incomplete injuries
- Legs recover before arms; hands recover last and least
- Elderly with cervical stenosis at high risk from minor mechanisms
- Respiratory monitoring critical in cervical injuries
- Early surgery may improve outcomes
- Most patients regain ability to walk

Chapter 7 Summary and Key Concepts

You've now completed a comprehensive review of neurological trauma. Let's consolidate the most important concepts that will serve you both on the TCRN exam and throughout your trauma nursing career.

Core Principles That Guide All Neurological Trauma Care

Primary vs. Secondary Injury: The primary injury happens at impact and cannot be reversed. Every intervention we make targets preventing or minimizing secondary injury. This fundamental principle explains why we focus so intently on maintaining oxygenation, preventing hypotension, controlling ICP, and avoiding complications.

Time-Sensitivity: Neurological injuries are time-critical. An epidural hematoma caught early has excellent prognosis; caught late, it's fatal. Spinal cord perfusion pressure must be maintained immediately after injury. Every minute of hypoxia or hypotension worsens outcomes. Your rapid recognition and intervention directly impact whether patients walk, talk, and live independently.

Trends Over Single Values: A patient with GCS 13 who drops to 10 is deteriorating and needs immediate action. A stable GCS 10 over hours may be acceptable. A gradually enlarging pupil is more concerning than a stable dilated pupil. Watch the trajectory, not just the number.

Clinical Exam Trumps Imaging: A patient with severe symptoms but minimal CT findings still has severe injury (think diffuse axonal injury). A patient with significant CT findings but stable exam may be managed conservatively. Your neurological assessment skills are more valuable than any scan.

High-Yield Facts for Exam Success

GCS Scoring:

- 15 = Normal
- 13-14 = Mild TBI
- 9-12 = Moderate TBI
- ≤8 = Severe TBI (intubate)
- Motor score is most prognostically important

Critical Numbers:

- Normal ICP: <15 mmHg
- Target CPP: 60-70 mmHg
- CPP = MAP - ICP
- Mannitol dose: 0.25-1 g/kg
- Hyperventilation target (if used): $PaCO_2$ 30-35 mmHg
- MAP goal for spinal cord injury: 85-90 mmHg

Herniation Signs:

- Unilateral blown pupil = ipsilateral mass effect
- Cushing's triad = hypertension + bradycardia + irregular respirations (late sign!)
- Decreasing GCS + pupil changes = herniation until proven otherwise

Hemorrhage Types:

- Epidural: Lens-shaped, arterial, lucid interval, best prognosis if caught early
- Subdural: Crescent-shaped, venous, worse prognosis due to underlying brain injury
- Subarachnoid: Blood in sulci, risk of vasospasm days 3-14
- Intracerebral: Brain contusions, can expand over 24-48 hours

Spinal Cord Syndromes:

- Complete: No sacral sparing
- Central cord: Arms worse than legs (elderly, hyperextension)
- Anterior cord: Motor and pain/temp loss, proprioception intact (worst prognosis)
- Brown-Séquard: Ipsilateral motor/proprioception loss, contralateral pain/temp loss (best prognosis)
- Cauda equina: Lower motor neuron pattern, saddle anesthesia

Shock Patterns:

- Neurogenic shock: Hypotension + bradycardia + warm skin (injury above T6)
- Spinal shock: Temporary loss of all reflexes below injury
- These are different phenomena!

Common Pitfalls to Avoid

Pitfall 1: Waiting for imaging to act on deteriorating patient If a patient has rapidly declining GCS with blown pupil, they need immediate neurosurgical intervention. CT confirms what you already know clinically. Don't delay life-saving treatment for imaging when herniation is obvious.

Pitfall 2: Over-aggressive fluid resuscitation in neurogenic shock These patients need vasopressors to restore vascular tone, not liters of fluid. Excessive fluids cause pulmonary edema because they can't compensate for volume overload.

Pitfall 3: Prophylactic hyperventilation Hyperventilation reduces cerebral blood flow and worsens outcomes when used routinely. Reserve it for acute ICP crises only, and target $PaCO_2$ 30-35 mmHg, never lower.

Pitfall 4: Giving steroids for TBI Steroids don't help traumatic brain injury and may increase mortality. Don't confuse this with spinal cord injury (where steroids are controversial but sometimes used) or brain tumors (where steroids are standard).

Pitfall 5: Missing chronic subdural in elderly on anticoagulation Any elderly patient on anticoagulation with new confusion or neurological symptoms needs imaging, even if the fall was weeks ago and seemed minor. Chronic subdurals are subtle.

Pitfall 6: Dismissing concussion because CT is normal CT is typically normal in concussion. Diagnosis is clinical. Normal imaging doesn't mean the injury isn't real or doesn't need management.

Pitfall 7: Unnecessary spinal immobilization Not every trauma patient needs a collar and board. Use NEXUS criteria to identify low-risk patients who don't need immobilization. Prolonged immobilization causes pressure ulcers and delays care.

Pitfall 8: Allowing early return to play after concussion Second impact syndrome is rare but devastating. No return to sports until symptom-free at rest AND successful completion of graduated return-to-play protocol. When in doubt, sit them out.

Integration with Other Content

Neurological trauma doesn't exist in isolation. Connect these concepts to other chapters:

From Chapter 3 (Resuscitation):

- Hypotension is the most damaging preventable factor in TBI
- Avoid even single episodes of systolic BP <90 mmHg
- Maintain adequate oxygenation (hypoxia worsens brain injury)

From Chapter 4 (Thoracic Trauma):

- Cervical spine injuries affect respiratory function
- High cervical injuries can cause respiratory failure
- Pneumothorax can coexist with TBI (treat both)

From Chapter 5 (Abdominal Trauma):

- Abdominal injuries can coexist with head injuries
- Hypotension from abdominal bleeding worsens TBI outcomes
- Manage all injuries simultaneously

From Chapter 6 (Orthopedic Trauma):

- Long bone fractures can coexist with spinal injuries
- Fat embolism from fractures can cause neurological symptoms
- Proper immobilization prevents further spinal damage

Practical Application for Clinical Practice

Scenario Recognition Patterns:

When you see... Think...

- Temporal impact + lucid interval → Epidural hematoma
- Elderly on anticoagulation + new confusion → Chronic subdural
- Diving injury + can't move legs → Cervical spine injury
- Hypotension + bradycardia + warm skin → Neurogenic shock
- Decreased GCS + blown pupil → Herniation
- Sports injury + dazed appearance → Concussion
- Elderly fall + arms worse than legs → Central cord syndrome

Decision-Making Framework:

For every neurological trauma patient, ask:

1. Is the airway secure? (GCS ≤8 needs intubation)
2. Is oxygenation adequate? (Keep PaO_2 >80)
3. Is blood pressure adequate? (Avoid systolic <90)
4. Is the patient deteriorating? (Declining GCS, pupil changes)
5. Does imaging show operative lesion? (Evacuable hematoma)
6. Is ICP elevated? (Clinical signs, monitor if available)
7. Is spinal cord at risk? (Mechanism, exam findings)
8. What can I prevent? (Hypotension, hypoxia, hyperthermia, seizures)

Study Strategies for Mastery

For visual learners:

- Draw the brain with different hemorrhage locations and their CT appearances
- Sketch the spinal cord cross-section with tract locations
- Create flowcharts for ICP management tiers
- Diagram Cushing's triad and its physiological basis

For those who learn by teaching:

- Explain to a colleague why epidural hematomas have lucid intervals
- Teach the difference between neurogenic and spinal shock
- Describe how to calculate CPP and why it matters

For hands-on learners:

- Practice GCS scoring on every patient you see
- Perform thorough neurological exams regularly

- Document pupil assessments precisely
- Practice explaining NEXUS criteria

For pattern recognition:

- Create flashcards with injury syndromes on one side, presentations on the other
- Make a chart comparing hemorrhage types
- List spinal cord syndromes with their unique features

Final Preparation Tips

As you prepare for exam questions on neurological trauma:

1. **Read questions carefully for time course.** "Immediately after injury" suggests different pathology than "2 weeks after minor trauma."
2. **Look for mechanism clues.** Diving = cervical injury. Elderly fall = central cord or chronic subdural. Temporal impact = epidural.
3. **Calculate CPP when given MAP and ICP.** This is quick points if you know the formula.
4. **Don't overthink pupil questions.** Unilateral blown pupil = ipsilateral herniation. Bilateral pinpoint = pontine or drugs. Both dilated and fixed = severe injury or hypoxia.
5. **Remember the tier approach to ICP.** Simple measures first, escalate systematically.
6. **Know when NOT to do things.** No steroids in TBI. No prophylactic hyperventilation. No cervical collar on low-risk patients.
7. **Sacral sparing determines complete vs. incomplete.** Always assess this in spinal cord injuries.

You're Ready for This

Neurological trauma is complex, but you've now built a solid foundation. You understand not just what to do, but why you're doing it. You can recognize patterns, predict complications, and intervene appropriately. Most importantly, you understand that your actions in the first minutes and hours after neurological trauma can determine whether a patient returns to their normal life or faces permanent disability.

The knowledge you've gained here will serve you well beyond the exam. These are the skills that define expert trauma nursing—the ability to recognize subtle changes that herald disaster, the judgment to know when to act aggressively and when to observe, and the understanding of pathophysiology that lets you anticipate problems before they occur.

Trust your preparation. You've learned complex material and can apply it to clinical scenarios. When you see exam questions about blown pupils, GCS changes, spinal cord syndromes, or ICP management, you'll recognize the patterns and select the correct answers confidently.

Chapter 8: Burns and Environmental Trauma

Burns and environmental injuries present unique challenges in trauma care. Unlike traumatic injuries from blunt or penetrating mechanisms, these injuries involve complex physiological responses to heat, cold, chemicals, or electricity. Understanding burn pathophysiology, fluid resuscitation requirements, and environmental injury management is essential for preventing complications and optimizing outcomes.

This chapter covers thermal burns, inhalation injuries, hypothermia, heat-related illness, and electrical and chemical burns. Each type of injury has specific assessment criteria and management protocols that you need to master for both the TCRN exam and clinical practice.

Burn Classification and Assessment

Burn injuries damage the skin and sometimes deeper tissues through thermal, chemical, electrical, or radiation energy. The extent and depth of injury determine both immediate management and long-term prognosis.

Understanding Burn Pathophysiology

To properly assess and manage burns, you need to understand what's happening at the tissue level.

The skin's normal function: Skin is the body's largest organ, serving critical functions:

- Barrier against infection
- Temperature regulation through sweating and blood flow control
- Fluid retention (prevents evaporative losses)
- Sensory perception (pain, temperature, touch)
- Vitamin D synthesis
- Protection from environmental damage

What burns destroy: When burn injury occurs, these functions are compromised. Severe burns can lead to:

- Massive fluid loss through damaged skin (evaporative losses)
- Infection from loss of protective barrier
- Inability to regulate body temperature
- Loss of sensation in deeply burned areas
- Scarring and contractures as healing occurs

The zone model of burn injury: Burns don't uniformly destroy all tissue. Dr. Jackson's model describes three zones:

Zone of coagulation (center): This is the area of most severe damage where cells are destroyed immediately. Proteins denature from heat, blood vessels thrombose, and tissue becomes nonviable. This zone will definitely require debridement or will slough off naturally.

Zone of stasis (middle ring): This area has moderate damage with decreased blood flow. Cells are injured but not dead initially. With proper care (hydration, avoiding infection, preventing further injury), this zone can survive. With poor care, it can progress to full-thickness injury. This is why initial burn assessment may underestimate eventual depth—the zone of stasis can either recover or die over 48-72 hours.

Zone of hyperemia (outer ring): This outermost area has minimal damage with inflammation and increased blood flow. This zone typically recovers completely.

Clinical implication: Burns can appear to "get worse" over the first few days as the zone of stasis declares itself. Initial assessment provides a baseline, but serial assessments are necessary to determine true burn depth.

Burn Depth Classification

Burns are classified by depth, which determines treatment and healing potential.

Superficial (First-Degree) Burns:

Depth: Epidermis only (outermost skin layer)

Appearance:

- Red, dry, no blisters
- Blanches with pressure (capillaries intact)
- Minimal or no swelling

Sensation: Painful (nerve endings intact and irritated)

Healing: 3-7 days without scarring

Example: Mild sunburn

Management: Symptomatic care (cool compresses, moisturizers, pain relief). These burns aren't included in total body surface area (TBSA) calculations for fluid resuscitation because they don't cause significant capillary leak.

Superficial Partial-Thickness (Second-Degree Superficial) Burns:

Depth: Epidermis and upper dermis

Appearance:

- Red, moist, blistered
- Blanches with pressure
- May have clear fluid-filled blisters
- Appears wet or weeping

Sensation: Very painful (nerve endings exposed)

Healing: 7-21 days with minimal scarring if no infection occurs

Management: Clean, debride loose tissue, apply topical antimicrobials, dress appropriately. May not require grafting if infection prevented.

Deep Partial-Thickness (Second-Degree Deep) Burns:

Depth: Epidermis, upper and mid dermis. Some dermal appendages (hair follicles, sweat glands) survive and can regenerate skin.

Appearance:

- Red and white mottled appearance
- May or may not blanch
- Blisters present
- Less wet than superficial partial-thickness

Sensation: Painful but less than superficial partial-thickness (some nerve endings destroyed)

Healing: 21-35 days, often with hypertrophic scarring and contractures. High risk of poor cosmetic and functional outcomes without grafting.

Management: Often requires excision and grafting for optimal outcomes, especially over joints or cosmetically important areas.

Full-Thickness (Third-Degree) Burns:

Depth: Complete destruction of epidermis and dermis. May involve subcutaneous tissue.

Appearance:

- White, brown, black, or charred
- Leathery, dry texture (called eschar)
- Does not blanch
- Visible thrombosed vessels may be seen
- Waxy appearance

Sensation: Painless (nerve endings completely destroyed). Surrounding partial-thickness burns will hurt, but the full-thickness center feels nothing.

Healing: Cannot heal by regeneration (no dermal appendages remain). Requires grafting. Will contract and form severe scars if not grafted.

Management: Surgical excision and grafting required. Eschar may need escharotomy if circumferential and causing vascular compromise or chest restriction.

Fourth-Degree Burns:

Depth: Through all skin layers into muscle, tendon, or bone

Appearance:

- Charred, black
- Obviously deep injury
- May see exposed bone, tendon, or muscle

Sensation: Painless centrally

Healing: Requires extensive reconstruction, often multiple surgeries. May require amputation if limb involved.

Management: Complex surgical management, often in burn center.

Total Body Surface Area (TBSA) Calculation

Determining the percentage of body surface area burned is critical for fluid resuscitation and triage decisions.

Rule of Nines (adults):

This quick estimation method divides the body into areas representing 9% or multiples of 9%:

- **Head and neck:** 9%
- **Each arm:** 9% (front and back of entire arm)
- **Anterior trunk:** 18% (chest and abdomen)
- **Posterior trunk:** 18% (back)
- **Each leg:** 18% (entire leg, front and back)
- **Genitalia/perineum:** 1%
- **Total:** 100%

How to use it: For scattered burns, estimate what percentage of each region is burned, then add them up. For example, if the entire anterior trunk is burned (18%) plus the entire right arm (9%), that's 27% TBSA.

Modified Rule of Nines for children:

Children have proportionally larger heads and smaller legs:

- **Head:** 18% (larger because kids have proportionally bigger heads)
- **Each arm:** 9%
- **Anterior trunk:** 18%
- **Posterior trunk:** 18%
- **Each leg:** 14% (smaller than adults)

As children age, proportions gradually approach adult values.

Lund-Browder Chart:

This is the most accurate method, using a chart that shows body regions with percentages that vary by age. This accounts for changing body proportions from infancy through adulthood. Most burn centers use this method for precise calculation.

Palm method:

For small scattered burns, the patient's palm (not including fingers) represents approximately 1% TBSA. This works for quick estimation of small burns.

Important points:

- Only include partial-thickness and full-thickness burns in TBSA calculation
- Don't count superficial burns
- Overestimation and underestimation both cause problems (too much or too little fluid)
- Reassess over first 24-48 hours as burn depth declares itself

Burn Severity Classification

The American Burn Association classifies burns to guide triage and determine who needs burn center care.

Minor burns:

- <10% TBSA partial-thickness in adults
- <5% TBSA partial-thickness in children/elderly
- <2% TBSA full-thickness
- No involvement of face, hands, feet, genitalia, perineum, or major joints
- No inhalation injury, electrical injury, or complicating medical conditions

Management: Can be managed outpatient or in community hospital

Moderate burns:

- 10-20% TBSA partial-thickness in adults
- 5-10% TBSA in children/elderly
- 2-5% TBSA full-thickness not involving cosmetic or functional areas

Management: May require hospitalization but not necessarily burn center transfer

Major burns (require burn center transfer):

- 20% TBSA partial-thickness in adults
- 10% TBSA in children/elderly
- 5% TBSA full-thickness
- Burns involving face, hands, feet, genitalia, perineum, or major joints

- Circumferential burns
- Electrical burns including lightning
- Chemical burns
- Inhalation injury
- Burns with associated trauma where burn poses greatest risk
- Burns in patients with complicating medical conditions

Burn Assessment Process

Initial assessment follows standard trauma protocols:

Primary survey (ABCs): Burns don't exempt patients from standard trauma assessment. Ensure airway patency (especially critical with facial burns or inhalation injury), adequate breathing, and circulation. Control any bleeding from associated trauma.

Secondary survey specific to burns:

History:

- Mechanism (flame, scald, chemical, electrical, etc.)
- Enclosed space exposure (inhalation injury risk)
- Time of injury
- First aid performed
- Medical history and medications
- Tetanus status

Physical examination:

- **Assess burn depth:** Carefully examine all burned areas, noting appearance, blanching, and pain response
- **Calculate TBSA:** Use Rule of Nines or Lund-Browder chart
- **Identify circumferential burns:** Any burns that completely encircle a limb, neck, or chest require close monitoring for compartment syndrome or respiratory restriction
- **Look for associated injuries:** Burns often occur with other trauma (jumping from burning building, explosion with blast injuries, etc.)
- **Assess for inhalation injury:** Signs include facial burns, singed nasal hairs, carbonaceous sputum, hoarseness, stridor, respiratory distress
- **Check for other trauma:** Don't focus solely on burns and miss other injuries

Documentation: Photograph burns for baseline documentation. This helps track progression and provides medicolegal documentation.

Fluid Resuscitation for Burns

Major burns cause massive fluid shifts from intravascular space into burned tissue and third spaces. Without aggressive fluid resuscitation, burn shock leads to organ failure and death.

Understanding Burn Shock Pathophysiology

What happens after major burns:

Local response: Heat damages capillaries, causing increased permeability. Fluid, electrolytes, and proteins leak from blood vessels into interstitial space (the space between cells).

Systemic response: With burns >20% TBSA, the inflammatory response becomes systemic. Inflammatory mediators released from burned tissue travel throughout the body, causing capillary leak everywhere, not just at burn sites. This means fluid shifts into tissue throughout the body.

The result:

- Intravascular volume drops (hypovolemia)
- Tissue edema increases massively (third-spacing)
- Cardiac output decreases
- Organ perfusion decreases
- Without resuscitation: shock, organ failure, death

Time course: Capillary leak is worst in the first 8-12 hours post-burn, then gradually improves over 24-48 hours as inflammatory response resolves. By 48-72 hours, capillaries begin to heal and fluid starts shifting back into vessels (mobilization phase).

Fluid Resuscitation Formulas

Several formulas guide initial fluid resuscitation. The most commonly used is the Parkland (Baxter) formula.

Parkland Formula:

Calculation: 4 mL × patient weight (kg) × % TBSA burned = total fluid volume for first 24 hours

Example: 70 kg patient with 30% TBSA burn

- 4 × 70 × 30 = 8,400 mL for first 24 hours

Administration schedule:

- Give half the calculated volume in the first 8 hours from time of burn (not from time of arrival)
- Give the second half over the next 16 hours

Example continued:

- Total: 8,400 mL
- First 8 hours: 4,200 mL
- Next 16 hours: 4,200 mL

Fluid type: Lactated Ringer's solution is preferred. It's isotonic and contains some lactate that can be metabolized to bicarbonate, helping with acidosis.

Important considerations:

Start time: The 24-hour clock starts at time of burn, not time of arrival. If a patient arrives 3 hours post-burn, the first 8-hour period has only 5 hours remaining. You need to calculate how much fluid they should have received by now and play catch-up.

Example: Patient burned at 1800, arrives at 2100 (3 hours post-burn). The first 8 hours ends at 0200 (8 hours from 1800). Patient should have received 4,200 mL by 0200, but has received nothing. You have 5 hours (2100-0200) to give 4,200 mL = 840 mL/hour.

These are starting estimates only: The formula provides initial rates, but actual fluid needs vary based on patient response. You must titrate fluids based on clinical response.

Monitoring Resuscitation Adequacy

The goal isn't to give a specific amount of fluid—it's to maintain adequate perfusion. Monitor these parameters:

Urine output (most important):

- **Adults:** Target 0.5-1 mL/kg/hr (roughly 30-50 mL/hr for average adult)
- **Children:** Target 1-2 mL/kg/hr
- **Electrical burns or myoglobinuria:** Target higher output (75-100 mL/hr) to prevent renal damage from myoglobin

Rationale: Adequate urine output indicates adequate renal perfusion, which suggests adequate overall perfusion.

What to do:

- If urine output too low: Increase fluid rate
- If urine output too high (>1 mL/kg/hr in adults): Decrease fluid rate slightly to avoid over-resuscitation

Other perfusion indicators:

- **Mental status:** Awake and oriented (adequate cerebral perfusion)
- **Heart rate:** Decreasing toward normal (compensatory tachycardia resolving)
- **Blood pressure:** Maintaining adequate pressure (though BP is late indicator)
- **Peripheral pulses:** Present (adequate peripheral perfusion)
- **Capillary refill:** <2 seconds
- **Lactate:** Decreasing (improving tissue perfusion)
- **Base deficit:** Improving (resolving acidosis from poor perfusion)

Laboratory monitoring:

- Electrolytes every 4-6 hours initially (sodium can rise or fall, potassium can rise from cell injury)
- Hematocrit every 6-12 hours (rises initially from hemoconcentration, then drops as fluid mobilizes)
- Monitor for compartment syndrome with circumferential burns

Complications of Fluid Resuscitation

Under-resuscitation:

- Acute kidney injury from inadequate renal perfusion
- Conversion of partial-thickness to full-thickness burns (zone of stasis dies from inadequate perfusion)
- Multi-organ failure
- Death

Over-resuscitation:

- Excessive edema (including pulmonary edema, cerebral edema, compartment syndrome)
- Abdominal compartment syndrome (massive fluid causes bowel edema, increasing intra-abdominal pressure)
- Prolonged mechanical ventilation
- Increased infection risk
- Worse outcomes

The key: Titrate fluids to maintain adequate perfusion (monitored by urine output) without excessive administration. This requires frequent reassessment and adjustment.

The Second 24 Hours and Beyond

After the first 24 hours, capillary integrity begins restoring and fluid requirements change.

Colloid administration: Many burn centers begin colloid (albumin or fresh frozen plasma) after 12-24 hours once capillary leak begins resolving. Colloids stay in vessels better than crystalloids, helping maintain intravascular volume with less total fluid.

Decreased rates: Total fluid needs decrease in the second 24 hours as leak resolves.

Mobilization phase (48-72 hours): Edema fluid starts shifting back into vessels. This can cause:

- Increased urine output (good—body eliminating excess fluid)
- Risk of volume overload if continuing aggressive fluid administration
- Need for diuretics in some patients if mobilization causes pulmonary edema

Maintenance fluids: By day 3-5, patients transition from resuscitation mode to maintenance fluids plus replacement of ongoing losses (from burn wounds, drains, etc.).

Inhalation Injuries

Inhalation injury significantly increases burn mortality. Patients with combined burns and inhalation injury have worse outcomes than either injury alone.

Types of Inhalation Injury

Supraglottic (upper airway) injury:

Mechanism: Direct thermal injury to mouth, pharynx, and upper airway from hot air or steam

Why it matters: The upper airway is very efficient at cooling inhaled air, so thermal injury usually doesn't extend below the vocal cords. However, steam carries much more heat than dry air and can cause thermal injury deeper into airways.

Result: Edema of face, oropharynx, and larynx, causing airway obstruction

Signs:

- Facial burns
- Singed nasal hairs, eyebrows, facial hair
- Carbonaceous sputum (black, sooty)
- Oral or pharyngeal burns
- Hoarseness
- Stridor (ominous—indicates significant airway narrowing)

Time course: Edema worsens over 12-24 hours, then peaks and begins resolving over several days.

Management: Early intubation before edema becomes severe. Once edema is severe, intubation may be impossible, requiring emergency surgical airway. Don't wait for obvious respiratory distress—if signs of inhalation injury and you're questioning whether to intubate, intubate now. It's much easier and safer before edema progresses.

Infraglottic (lower airway) injury:

Mechanism: Chemical injury from smoke particles and toxic gases, not heat

Substances causing injury:

- Carbon particles (carbonaceous material)
- Toxic gases (carbon monoxide, hydrogen cyanide, aldehydes, nitrogen oxides)
- Chemicals from burning synthetic materials

Result: Chemical tracheobronchitis (inflammation of lower airways), mucosal sloughing, increased secretions, bronchospasm, decreased mucociliary clearance, pneumonia risk

Signs:

- May have no immediate signs (presents over hours to days)
- Wheezing or bronchospasm
- Increased secretions
- Hypoxemia
- Respiratory distress developing over time
- Carbonaceous sputum
- Abnormal chest X-ray (initially may be normal, progresses to show infiltrates)

Diagnosis: Bronchoscopy shows carbonaceous material in airways, erythema, edema, mucosal sloughing

Management:

- Intubation and mechanical ventilation often required
- Aggressive pulmonary toilet (suctioning, chest physiotherapy)
- Bronchodilators for bronchospasm
- Antibiotics if pneumonia develops (not prophylactically)
- Supportive care
- May progress to acute respiratory distress syndrome (ARDS)

Systemic toxicity (poisoning):

Smoke contains toxic gases that cause systemic poisoning separate from direct airway injury.

Carbon monoxide (CO) poisoning:

Mechanism: CO binds hemoglobin with 200-250 times the affinity of oxygen, forming carboxyhemoglobin (COHb). This prevents oxygen binding and transport.

Why it's dangerous: Patients can have tissue hypoxia despite normal oxygen saturation on pulse oximetry (pulse ox can't differentiate oxyhemoglobin from carboxyhemoglobin, showing falsely normal readings).

Signs/symptoms:

- Headache
- Dizziness, confusion
- Nausea
- Cherry-red skin color (classic but rare)
- Syncope, seizures
- Coma, death

Diagnosis: COHb level on blood gas analysis (not pulse oximetry)

- <10%: Normal (smokers may have 5-10% baseline)
- 10-20%: Mild symptoms (headache)
- 20-40%: Moderate symptoms (confusion, nausea)
- 40-60%: Severe symptoms (seizures, coma)
- 60%: Often fatal

Treatment:

- 100% oxygen (displaces CO from hemoglobin)

- Half-life of COHb: 4-6 hours on room air, 90 minutes on 100% O2, 20-30 minutes on hyperbaric oxygen
- Hyperbaric oxygen therapy considered for severe poisoning (COHb >25-40% or significant symptoms)

Cyanide poisoning:

Mechanism: Cyanide (from burning synthetic materials, wool, silk) inhibits cellular cytochrome oxidase, preventing cells from using oxygen even when oxygen is present (cellular hypoxia despite adequate oxygen delivery)

Signs: Similar to CO poisoning but also causes metabolic acidosis with elevated lactate

Diagnosis: High suspicion based on mechanism (enclosed space fire with synthetic materials), metabolic acidosis despite resuscitation, elevated lactate

Treatment:

- Supportive care
- Hydroxocobalamin (preferred) or sodium thiosulfate (cyanide antidotes)
- Most patients recover with supportive care alone if suspected early

Assessment for Inhalation Injury

History clues:

- Enclosed space fire (building, car, etc.)
- Prolonged exposure
- Loss of consciousness at scene
- Explosion

Physical examination:

- Facial burns
- Singed nasal hairs, eyebrows
- Carbonaceous sputum
- Hoarseness, stridor
- Respiratory distress
- Wheezing
- Altered mental status

Diagnostic tests:

- Arterial blood gas with COHb level
- Chest X-ray (may be initially normal)
- Bronchoscopy (diagnostic for lower airway injury)
- Lactate (elevated with CO or cyanide poisoning)

Key point: Assume inhalation injury with facial burns or history of enclosed space exposure until proven otherwise. The stakes are too high to miss this.

Hypothermia

Hypothermia occurs when core body temperature drops below 35°C (95°F). It can result from environmental exposure or medical conditions that impair thermoregulation.

Classification of Hypothermia

Mild hypothermia: 32-35°C (89.6-95°F)

- Shivering (body's attempt to generate heat)
- Tachycardia, tachypnea initially
- Vasoconstriction (cold, pale skin)
- Confusion, poor judgment ("paradoxical undressing"—confused patients remove clothes)
- Ataxia (uncoordinated movements)

Moderate hypothermia: 28-32°C (82.4-89.6°F)

- Shivering stops (body exhausted)
- Bradycardia
- Hypotension
- Hypoventilation
- Decreased level of consciousness
- Arrhythmias begin appearing on ECG (Osborn or J waves)
- Pupils dilated, sluggish

Severe hypothermia: <28°C (82.4°F)

- Profound bradycardia or cardiac arrest
- Ventricular fibrillation risk high
- Appears dead (cold and stiff, pupils fixed and dilated, no detectable vital signs)
- Minimal or no respiration
- Profound hypotension

Key principle: "No one is dead until they're warm and dead." Don't pronounce death in hypothermic patients until they've been rewarmed and remain pulseless. People have survived prolonged cardiac arrest from severe hypothermia because cold protects the brain from hypoxic injury.

Pathophysiology

How the body loses heat:

- Radiation (heat radiates from warm body to cooler environment)
- Conduction (direct contact with cold surfaces)
- Convection (air or water moving across skin surface)
- Evaporation (wet skin or clothing accelerates cooling)
- Respiration (breathing cold air)

Physiologic effects:

- Decreased metabolic rate (slows all body processes)
- Myocardial depression (heart contracts less effectively)
- Arrhythmias (cold heart is electrically unstable)
- Coagulopathy (clotting factors don't work well when cold)
- Leftward shift of oxygen-hemoglobin dissociation curve (hemoglobin holds oxygen tighter, releasing less to tissues)

Management of Hypothermia

Assessment:

- Core temperature (rectal, esophageal, or bladder probe—not oral or tympanic)
- Full trauma assessment (hypothermia often accompanies trauma)
- ECG monitoring (watch for arrhythmias)
- Labs (glucose, electrolytes, blood gas, coagulation studies)

General principles:

- Handle patient gently (rough handling can trigger ventricular fibrillation in cold, irritable myocardium)
- Remove wet clothing
- Insulate from further heat loss
- Monitor continuously

Rewarming methods:

Passive external rewarming (mild hypothermia):

- Remove from cold environment
- Remove wet clothes, dry patient
- Cover with blankets
- Warm environment
- Body generates own heat, blankets prevent further loss

Active external rewarming (mild to moderate hypothermia):

- Forced-air warming blankets (Bair Hugger)
- Warm water immersion (if patient alert and shivering)
- Heat packs to trunk (not extremities—can cause peripheral vasodilation and core temperature afterdrop)

Active core rewarming (moderate to severe hypothermia):

- Warm IV fluids (38-42°C)
- Heated humidified oxygen
- Warm gastric, bladder, or peritoneal lavage
- Hemodialysis or continuous venovenous hemofiltration with warmed blood
- Extracorporeal membrane oxygenation (ECMO) or cardiopulmonary bypass (most effective for severe hypothermia with cardiac arrest)

Rewarming rate:

- No faster than 1-2°C per hour for moderate to severe hypothermia (faster rates can cause complications)
- Afterdrop: Core temperature can initially drop further during rewarming as cold blood from extremities returns to core—expect this

Cardiac arrest management:

- Standard ACLS protocols apply but with modifications
- Continue CPR (brain protected by hypothermia, can tolerate longer arrest times)
- Defibrillation may be ineffective until core temperature >30°C
- Medications may not work until rewarmed (can accumulate and cause toxicity once warm)
- Rewarm to at least 32-35°C before terminating resuscitation efforts

Complications to watch for:

- Arrhythmias during rewarming
- Hypotension as peripheral vessels dilate

- Hypoglycemia (cold impairs gluconeogenesis)
- Acidosis
- Rhabdomyolysis (if prolonged immobility)
- Frostbite of extremities

Hyperthermia and Heat Stroke

Heat-related illnesses range from mild heat cramps to life-threatening heat stroke. Understanding the spectrum helps you recognize when simple cooling isn't enough.

Heat Illness Spectrum

Heat cramps:

- Muscle cramps (usually legs, arms, abdomen) from salt and water loss through sweating
- Patient alert, normal vital signs except maybe mild tachycardia
- Core temperature normal or mildly elevated

Management: Rest, oral rehydration with electrolyte solution, gentle stretching

Heat exhaustion:

- Inadequate cardiovascular compensation for heat stress
- Core temperature 37-40°C (98.6-104°F)
- Profuse sweating (still able to sweat)
- Weakness, fatigue
- Headache, dizziness
- Nausea, vomiting
- Tachycardia, hypotension possible
- Normal mental status

Management: Remove from heat, rest, oral or IV fluids, cooling measures. Usually improves quickly with treatment.

Heat stroke:

- Life-threatening failure of thermoregulation
- Core temperature >40°C (104°F)
- Altered mental status (hallmark—confusion, aggression, seizures, coma)
- May have hot, dry skin (classic heat stroke) OR may still be sweating (exertional heat stroke)
- Tachycardia, hypotension
- Tachypnea
- Multi-organ dysfunction

Two types:

Classic (non-exertional) heat stroke:

- Affects elderly, chronically ill, very young
- Develops over days during heat wave
- Impaired physiologic response to heat
- Usually hot, dry skin (lost ability to sweat)

Exertional heat stroke:

- Affects young, healthy people exercising in heat
- Develops rapidly (hours)
- Overwhelming heat production exceeds body's cooling capacity
- May still be sweating

Pathophysiology of Heat Stroke

Normal thermoregulation: Hypothalamus maintains core temperature around 37°C through:

- Sweating and evaporation
- Vasodilation (shunts blood to skin for cooling)
- Behavioral changes (seeking shade, removing clothes)

What happens in heat stroke:

1. Heat production or environmental heat overwhelms cooling mechanisms
2. Core temperature rises uncontrollably
3. At 40-41°C, cellular proteins denature
4. Multi-organ dysfunction begins:
    - Brain: Cerebral edema, neuronal death (explains altered mental status)
    - Heart: Myocardial injury, arrhythmias
    - Liver: Hepatocellular necrosis (elevated liver enzymes)
    - Kidneys: Acute kidney injury from dehydration and direct thermal injury
    - Muscles: Rhabdomyolysis (muscle breakdown releasing myoglobin)
    - Blood: Coagulopathy (DIC possible)
5. Without rapid cooling, progression to death

Management of Heat Stroke

This is a medical emergency requiring immediate aggressive cooling.

Initial assessment:

- Core temperature (rectal most accurate)
- Mental status
- Full set of vital signs
- Assess for trauma (people with heat stroke have altered mental status and may fall or have seizures)

Immediate interventions:

Cooling (priority):

Goal: Reduce core temperature to <39°C (102.2°F) as quickly as possible. Every minute of hyperthermia causes ongoing organ damage.

Methods:

- Remove all clothing
- Evaporative cooling: Spray/mist patient with tepid water while using fans to blow air over them (most practical and effective in most settings)
- Ice packs to groin, axillae, neck (major vessels close to surface)

- Cold water immersion (very effective but difficult to monitor patient and provide care)
- Cooling blankets
- Cold IV fluids
- Avoid antipyretics (Tylenol, NSAIDs)—these don't work for heat stroke because problem isn't the hypothalamic set point

Stop cooling at 39°C to prevent overshoot hypothermia

Supportive care:

- Airway protection (intubate if GCS <8 or unable to protect airway)
- IV access and fluid resuscitation (dehydrated from sweating, may be hypotensive)
- Supplemental oxygen
- Continuous monitoring (cardiac, temperature, oxygen saturation)
- Seizure management (benzodiazepines if seizures occur)

Laboratory monitoring:

- Comprehensive metabolic panel (electrolytes, renal function, liver enzymes)
- CBC
- Coagulation studies (watch for DIC)
- Creatine kinase (rhabdomyolysis)
- Urinalysis (myoglobin)
- Arterial blood gas

Treat complications:

- Rhabdomyolysis: Aggressive IV fluids to maintain urine output >200 mL/hr, alkalinize urine if severe
- Acute kidney injury: Fluids, may need dialysis
- DIC: Blood products as needed
- Seizures: Benzodiazepines
- Arrhythmias: Standard ACLS but address hypothermia first

ICU admission: All heat stroke patients need ICU-level care for close monitoring and management of multi-organ dysfunction.

Prevention Education

For patients being discharged after heat illness or community education:

- Gradual acclimatization to heat (takes 1-2 weeks)
- Adequate hydration before, during, and after activity
- Avoid exercise during hottest parts of day
- Wear light-colored, loose clothing
- Take breaks in shade or air conditioning
- Recognize early symptoms

- Higher risk: elderly, infants, athletes, outdoor workers, certain medications (anticholinergics, diuretics, beta-blockers)

Electrical and Chemical Burns

Electrical and chemical burns have unique mechanisms causing injury patterns different from thermal burns. Understanding these differences is critical for proper assessment and management.

Electrical Burns

Electrical injuries occur when electrical current passes through the body, causing tissue damage along the path of current flow. These injuries are deceptive because external burns may appear minor while internal damage is extensive.

Understanding electrical injury mechanisms:

When electricity contacts the body, it enters at one point (contact point) and exits at another (ground point), taking the path of least resistance through the body. Tissues with low resistance (nerves, blood vessels, muscles) conduct electricity well and sustain more damage. Tissues with high resistance (bone, fat, skin) resist current flow but generate heat as electricity passes through, causing thermal injury.

The iceberg effect: What you see on the surface represents only a small portion of the total injury. Like an iceberg where most of the mass is underwater, most electrical injury damage is deep and invisible from the surface.

Types of electrical injury:

Low-voltage injuries (<1000 volts):

- Usually household current (110-220 volts)
- Causes local burns at contact points
- Can cause cardiac arrhythmias
- Generally less severe but not benign

High-voltage injuries (>1000 volts):

- Power lines, industrial accidents, lightning
- Causes extensive deep tissue damage
- High risk of cardiac arrest
- Multiple organ system involvement
- Severe complications common

Lightning strikes:

- Extremely high voltage (millions of volts) but very brief duration
- Usually causes cardiac arrest from ventricular fibrillation
- If patient survives initial arrest, prognosis can be good
- Can cause unique injury patterns (Lichtenberg figures—fern-like skin patterns)

Pathophysiology of electrical injury:

Direct effects:

- Tissue destruction from heat generated by current resistance
- Muscle necrosis deep within limbs (largest concern)
- Vascular thrombosis from vessel wall damage

- Nerve injury from direct current effects

Secondary effects:

- Cardiac arrhythmias (ventricular fibrillation, asystole)
- Respiratory arrest from tetanic contraction of respiratory muscles or central nervous system injury
- Falls or trauma from being thrown by electrical force
- Compartment syndrome from deep muscle injury and edema

Assessment of electrical injuries:

Initial assessment priorities:

- Ensure scene safety (power source off, patient no longer in contact)
- Cardiac monitoring immediately (arrhythmias can occur anytime)
- ABCDE assessment
- Look for entrance and exit wounds (may be multiple)
- Assess for associated trauma (falls, blast injuries)

Entrance wounds:

- Usually on hands (person grabbed electrical source)
- May appear as charred, leathery burns
- Often smaller than exit wounds

Exit wounds:

- Usually on feet (current exits to ground)
- Often larger and more explosive in appearance
- May have surrounding blast injury

Path of current: The most dangerous paths cross the heart or brain:

- Hand-to-hand (across chest and heart)—very dangerous
- Hand-to-foot (through heart)—very dangerous
- Foot-to-foot (doesn't cross heart)—less immediately dangerous but can cause severe leg damage

Hidden injuries to assess for:

- Myocardial injury (chest pain, ECG changes, elevated troponin)
- Muscle necrosis and rhabdomyolysis (myoglobin in urine making it tea-colored, elevated creatine kinase)
- Compartment syndrome (from deep muscle injury causing edema)
- Vascular injury (check all pulses carefully)
- Nerve injury (assess motor and sensory function)
- Fractures (from falls or violent muscle contractions)
- Intra-abdominal injury (current path through abdomen)
- Spinal injury (from falls or violent muscle contractions)

Laboratory and diagnostic studies:

- ECG (baseline and continuous monitoring for 24 hours minimum)
- Cardiac biomarkers (troponin if ECG abnormal or chest pain)
- Creatine kinase (elevated indicates muscle damage)
- Comprehensive metabolic panel (potassium, renal function)
- Urinalysis (myoglobin indicates rhabdomyolysis)
- Coagulation studies
- Imaging as indicated by exam findings

Management principles:

Immediate care:

- Cardiac monitoring (continue for at least 24 hours)
- IV access and aggressive fluid resuscitation
- Urine output goal: 75-100 mL/hr if myoglobinuria present (higher than standard burn resuscitation)
- Alkalinize urine if severe rhabdomyolysis (prevents myoglobin precipitation in renal tubules)
- Pain management
- Tetanus prophylaxis
- Wound care (debride obviously dead tissue, but extensive damage may not be apparent initially)

Monitoring for compartment syndrome:

- High index of suspicion with electrical injuries to extremities
- Serial neurovascular checks
- Early fasciotomy if any signs develop
- Don't wait for absent pulses

Surgical management:

- Early debridement of obviously necrotic tissue
- May need multiple operations as extent of necrosis declares itself over several days
- Amputation sometimes necessary if limb has extensive vascular or muscle damage
- Fasciotomy for compartment syndrome

Complications:

- Cardiac arrhythmias (immediate or delayed)
- Rhabdomyolysis with acute kidney injury
- Compartment syndrome
- Infection (extensive devitalized tissue)
- Neurological sequelae (peripheral nerve injury, spinal cord injury, cognitive changes)
- Cataracts (can develop months to years later)
- Vascular thrombosis causing delayed tissue loss

Admission criteria:

- High-voltage exposure (all require admission)
- Cardiac arrhythmia or abnormal ECG
- Loss of consciousness
- Significant tissue injury
- Myoglobinuria
- Any patient with concerning mechanism even if initially appears well

Chemical Burns

Chemical burns result from skin contact with acids, alkalis (bases), or other corrosive substances. The severity depends on the chemical agent, concentration, duration of contact, and amount involved.

Mechanisms of injury:

Acids (low pH):

- Cause coagulation necrosis (proteins denature and coagulate)
- Forms eschar that limits further penetration
- Examples: sulfuric acid (battery acid), hydrochloric acid, nitric acid

- Injury depth often self-limiting because eschar acts as barrier

Alkalis (high pH):

- Cause liquefaction necrosis (saponification of fats, protein denaturation)
- Continues penetrating deeper into tissue
- No eschar formation, so damage continues as long as chemical present
- More dangerous than acid burns for this reason
- Examples: sodium hydroxide (lye, drain cleaner), potassium hydroxide, cement (contains lime)

Organic compounds:

- Petroleum products (gasoline, tar)
- Phenols
- Various industrial chemicals
- Each has unique injury pattern

Assessment:

History (critical for treatment):

- What chemical? (get exact name if possible)
- How much?
- How long was contact before decontamination started?
- What area of body affected?
- Was patient in enclosed space (inhalation exposure)?
- What first aid was performed?

Physical examination:

- Extent of burns (calculate TBSA like thermal burns)
- Depth of burns (may not be initially apparent)
- Associated injuries (trauma, inhalation injury)
- Systemic effects (some chemicals cause systemic toxicity)

Special chemical burns and their unique concerns:

Hydrofluoric acid (HF):

- Used in glass etching, rust removal, electronics manufacturing
- Extremely dangerous despite sometimes appearing as minor burn
- Fluoride ion penetrates deeply and binds calcium, causing severe pain and potentially fatal hypocalcemia and hyperkalemia
- Pain out of proportion to visible injury
- Can cause cardiac arrhythmias from electrolyte disturbances

Management: Calcium gluconate gel topically, calcium gluconate injection into wound margins or intra-arterially, monitor calcium and potassium closely, cardiac monitoring

White phosphorus:

- Military munitions, fireworks, fertilizers
- Ignites spontaneously on contact with air
- Causes thermal and chemical burns
- Particles embedded in skin continue burning

Management: Remove particles under water (prevents ignition), debride embedded particles, cover with wet dressings, copper sulfate sometimes used to identify remaining particles (turns them black)

Phenol:

- Industrial cleaners, chemical peels
- Lipid soluble, absorbs systemically
- Can cause CNS depression, cardiac arrhythmias, hepatic and renal toxicity

Management: Decontaminate with polyethylene glycol (if available) or copious water, monitor for systemic toxicity

Cement/concrete:

- Contains calcium oxide (lime), which is alkaline
- Often prolonged contact because people don't realize it's burning them
- Can cause full-thickness burns over large areas

Management: Immediate copious irrigation, debridement, standard burn care

Management principles for all chemical burns:

Immediate decontamination (most important):

The first and most critical step is removing the chemical from the skin. For most chemicals, this means copious water irrigation.

Steps:

1. **Remove patient from source** (ensure safety of rescuers—don't become victims)
2. **Remove all clothing and jewelry** (chemicals can be trapped in fabric, continuing to burn)
3. **Brush off dry chemicals** before irrigation (some chemicals react with water, but for most, immediate irrigation is still correct)
4. **Irrigate with copious water or normal saline** (15-30 minutes minimum, longer for alkalis)
    - Use lukewarm water if possible (cold water can cause hypothermia)

    - Ensure runoff doesn't contact other body areas
    - Pay special attention to skin folds, between fingers/toes, under nails
5. **Continue irrigation until pain improves** (with alkalis, may need hours of irrigation)
6. **Check pH if alkali or acid** (litmus paper)—continue irrigation until pH normalizes

Exceptions to water irrigation:

- Certain reactive metals (sodium, potassium, lithium, magnesium)—react violently with water, producing heat and sometimes igniting. Brush off thoroughly, then use mineral oil if available, or small amounts of water if necessary.
- Check chemical MSDS (Material Safety Data Sheet) for specific decontamination recommendations when possible

After decontamination:

- Assess burn depth and TBSA
- Wound care (similar to thermal burns but may need more aggressive debridement)
- Pain management
- Tetanus prophylaxis
- Monitor for systemic effects of specific chemical
- Ophthalmology consult for eye exposures (chemicals in eyes require immediate and prolonged irrigation—30 minutes minimum)

Systemic management:

- IV access and fluid resuscitation based on TBSA (use Parkland formula)
- Laboratory monitoring (electrolytes, renal function, specific tests for chemical involved)
- Specific antidotes for certain chemicals (calcium for HF, specific chelators for heavy metals)
- Monitor for inhalation injury if enclosed space exposure

Wound management:

- Debridement of devitalized tissue
- Topical antimicrobials
- Dressings
- May require grafting for deep burns
- Chemical burns often deeper than initially apparent—reassess over 48-72 hours

Special considerations:

Eye exposures:

- Ophthalmologic emergency
- Immediate continuous irrigation (30-60 minutes) with eye irrigation solution or normal saline
- Check pH of tears—continue irrigation until neutral

- Ophthalmology consultation
- May need topical antibiotics, cycloplegics, pain management
- Alkali burns to eyes are particularly devastating

Inhalation exposures:

- Some chemicals produce toxic fumes (chlorine, ammonia, acid fumes)
- Can cause chemical pneumonitis or pulmonary edema
- Assess for respiratory symptoms, monitor oxygen saturation
- May need intubation and mechanical ventilation
- Supportive care (bronchodilators, oxygen, PEEP if pulmonary edema)

Ingestions:

- Some chemical burns occur from ingestion (drain cleaner, other household chemicals)
- Can cause esophageal and gastric burns
- DO NOT induce vomiting (re-exposes tissues to chemical)
- May need endoscopy to assess extent of injury
- May require surgical intervention if perforation occurs

Prevention and safety:

- Proper protective equipment when handling chemicals
- MSDS readily available for all chemicals in workplace
- Training on chemical hazards and first aid
- Emergency eyewash stations and safety showers in areas with chemical hazards
- Proper chemical storage and labeling

Chapter 8 Practice Questions

Question 1: Using the Rule of Nines for adults, a burn involving the entire anterior trunk and the entire right arm represents what percentage TBSA?

A) 18%
B) 27%
C) 36%
D) 45%

Answer: B

Explanation: Anterior trunk = 18%, entire right arm = 9%, total = 27% TBSA. The Rule of Nines divides the body into areas of 9% or multiples thereof for quick burn size estimation.

Question 2: Which burn depth is characterized by painless wounds with a white, leathery appearance?

A) Superficial
B) Superficial partial-thickness
C) Deep partial-thickness
D) Full-thickness

Answer: D

Explanation: Full-thickness burns destroy all skin layers including nerve endings, making them painless. They appear white, brown, black, or leathery. Deep partial-thickness burns are painful, and superficial burns are very painful.

Question 3: According to the Parkland formula, a 70 kg patient with 40% TBSA burn should receive how much fluid in the first 8 hours?

A) 5,600 mL
B) 8,400 mL
C) 11,200 mL
D) 14,000 mL

Answer: A

Explanation: Parkland formula: 4 mL × 70 kg × 40% = 11,200 mL total for 24 hours. Give half (5,600 mL) in the first 8 hours from time of burn, the other half over the next 16 hours.

Question 4: What is the primary indicator used to assess adequacy of burn resuscitation?

A) Blood pressure
B) Heart rate
C) Urine output
D) Central venous pressure

Answer: C

Explanation: Urine output is the best indicator of adequate resuscitation. Target 0.5-1 mL/kg/hr in adults (roughly 30-50 mL/hr). Adequate urine output indicates adequate organ perfusion. Adjust fluid rates based on urine output response.

Question 5: Which finding most strongly suggests inhalation injury?

A) Mild facial erythema
B) Singed nasal hairs and carbonaceous sputum
C) Cough
D) Mild hoarseness

Answer: B

Explanation: Singed nasal hairs and carbonaceous (black, sooty) sputum are classic signs of inhalation injury indicating that hot gases and smoke particles entered the airway. This warrants close monitoring and consideration for early intubation.

Question 6: Carbon monoxide poisoning is best diagnosed by:

A) Pulse oximetry
B) Chest X-ray
C) Carboxyhemoglobin level on blood gas
D) Oxygen saturation on ABG

Answer: C

Explanation: Carboxyhemoglobin (COHb) level on blood gas is diagnostic for CO poisoning. Pulse oximetry cannot differentiate between oxyhemoglobin and carboxyhemoglobin, showing falsely normal readings. Always measure COHb level if CO exposure suspected.

Question 7: A patient with facial burns and hoarseness should:

A) Receive oral fluids and observe
B) Be considered for early intubation before airway edema worsens
C) Receive nebulized treatments only
D) Wait for respiratory distress before intervention

Answer: B

Explanation: Facial burns with hoarseness indicate supraglottic injury with developing edema. Airway edema worsens over 12-24 hours. Early intubation before severe edema develops is safer than waiting until the airway is critically narrowed and intubation becomes difficult or impossible.

Question 8: Which type of chemical burn typically causes deeper injury?

A) Acid burns
B) Alkali burns
C) Both cause equal depth
D) Neither penetrates deeply

Answer: B

Explanation: Alkali burns cause liquefaction necrosis and continue penetrating deeper without forming a protective eschar, making them more dangerous than acid burns. Acids cause coagulation necrosis with eschar formation that limits penetration.

Question 9: The immediate treatment for most chemical burns is:

A) Apply neutralizing agent
B) Cover with petroleum jelly
C) Copious water irrigation
D) Apply dry dressing

Answer: C

Explanation: Copious water irrigation for 15-30 minutes (longer for alkalis) is the immediate treatment for most chemical burns. Remove all clothing first. Don't waste time searching for neutralizing agents—dilution and removal by irrigation is key.

Question 10: A patient with electrical injury has tea-colored urine. This indicates:

A) Urinary tract infection
B) Myoglobinuria from muscle breakdown
C) Hematuria
D) Normal finding

Answer: B

Explanation: Tea-colored or cola-colored urine indicates myoglobinuria from rhabdomyolysis (muscle breakdown). Electrical current causes deep muscle damage releasing myoglobin, which can precipitate in renal tubules causing kidney injury. Requires aggressive hydration targeting urine output 75-100 mL/hr.

Question 11: Burns that require transfer to a burn center include:

A) 5% TBSA partial-thickness in an adult
B) Burns involving the hands or face
C) Superficial burns only
D) Minor burns in healthy adults

Answer: B

Explanation: Burns involving face, hands, feet, genitalia, perineum, or major joints require burn center care due to functional and cosmetic importance. Other burn center criteria include >10% TBSA in children/elderly, >20% TBSA in adults, full-thickness burns, electrical/chemical burns, and inhalation injury.

Question 12: Core body temperature of 30°C indicates:

A) Mild hypothermia
B) Moderate hypothermia
C) Severe hypothermia
D) Normal for cold environment

Answer: B

Explanation: Moderate hypothermia is 28-32°C (82.4-89.6°F). At this temperature, shivering stops, level of consciousness decreases, and cardiac arrhythmias begin. Mild is 32-35°C, severe is <28°C.

Question 13: The most important principle in managing heat stroke is:

A) Administering antipyretics
B) Rapid cooling to <39°C
C) IV fluid resuscitation
D) Antibiotics

Answer: B

Explanation: Rapid cooling is the priority in heat stroke. Every minute of hyperthermia causes ongoing organ damage. Cool to <39°C using evaporative cooling, ice packs, and cold fluids. Antipyretics don't work for heat stroke because the problem isn't the hypothalamic set point.

Question 14: Which distinguishes heat stroke from heat exhaustion?

A) Elevated temperature
B) Altered mental status
C) Sweating
D) Tachycardia

Answer: B

Explanation: Altered mental status (confusion, aggression, seizures, coma) is the hallmark of heat stroke distinguishing it from heat exhaustion. Heat stroke is a medical emergency with multi-organ dysfunction, while heat exhaustion patients have normal mental status.

Question 15: In hypothermic cardiac arrest, resuscitation efforts should continue until:

A) 15 minutes of ACLS
B) 30 minutes of ACLS
C) Patient is rewarmed to at least 32-35°C
D) First defibrillation attempt fails

Answer: C

Explanation: "No one is dead until they're warm and dead." Hypothermia protects the brain from hypoxic injury, and people have survived prolonged arrests. Continue resuscitation while actively rewarming to at least 32-35°C before terminating efforts.

Question 16: Electrical injuries are most dangerous when the current path crosses:

A) Between fingers
B) Through a single limb
C) The heart or brain
D) The abdomen only

Answer: C

Explanation: Hand-to-hand or hand-to-foot paths cross the heart and are most dangerous, risking immediate ventricular fibrillation or asystole. Paths crossing the brain can cause respiratory arrest. Foot-to-foot paths avoid vital organs but can cause severe leg damage.

Question 17: The 24-hour fluid resuscitation clock for burns starts:

A) When patient arrives at hospital
B) When IV is established
C) At time of burn injury
D) When transfer to burn center occurs

Answer: C

Explanation: The resuscitation clock starts at time of burn injury, not arrival time. If a patient burned at 6 PM arrives at 9 PM (3 hours post-burn), they should have received some of their first 8-hour fluids already. Calculate catch-up fluid rates accordingly.

Question 18: Escharotomy is performed to:

A) Remove burned tissue
B) Relieve constriction from circumferential burns
C) Prepare for skin grafting
D) Treat infection

Answer: B

Explanation: Escharotomy is an emergent bedside incision through eschar to relieve constriction from circumferential full-thickness burns. This restores circulation to limbs or allows chest wall expansion for breathing. It's not the same as surgical debridement or excision.

Question 19: Over-resuscitation in burns can cause:

A) Improved outcomes
B) Decreased edema
C) Abdominal compartment syndrome and excessive edema
D) Faster wound healing

Answer: C

Explanation: Over-resuscitation causes excessive edema throughout the body, including bowel edema that can lead to abdominal compartment syndrome. It also increases infection risk and prolongs recovery. Titrate fluids to maintain adequate urine output without excess.

Question 20: Hydrofluoric acid burns require special treatment with:

A) Immediate surgical debridement
B) Calcium gluconate topically and/or injected
C) Antibiotics only
D) Standard burn care only

Answer: B

Explanation: Hydrofluoric acid burns require calcium gluconate treatment because fluoride ions penetrate deeply and bind calcium, causing severe pain and potentially fatal hypocalcemia and hyperkalemia. Apply calcium gluconate gel topically or inject into wound margins. Monitor electrolytes and cardiac rhythm closely.

Question 21: Superficial burns are included in TBSA calculations for fluid resuscitation:

A) True
B) False
C) Only if >10% TBSA
D) Only if painful

Answer: B

Explanation: False. Superficial burns (first-degree) are NOT included in TBSA calculations for fluid resuscitation because they don't cause significant capillary leak. Only partial-thickness and full-thickness burns are counted when calculating fluid needs.

Question 22: A patient with moderate hypothermia (30°C) would exhibit:

A) Vigorous shivering
B) Cessation of shivering with decreased consciousness
C) Normal vital signs
D) Hyperthermia

Answer: B

Explanation: Moderate hypothermia (28-32°C) features cessation of shivering (body exhausted), decreased level of consciousness, bradycardia, and risk of arrhythmias. Shivering occurs in mild hypothermia but stops as temperature drops further.

Question 23: The zone of stasis in burn injury:

A) Is definitely dead tissue
B) Is undamaged tissue
C) Can survive with proper care or progress to necrosis
D) Always requires grafting

Answer: C

Explanation: The zone of stasis has moderate injury with decreased blood flow. Cells are injured but not initially dead. With adequate resuscitation and care, this zone can survive. With poor care, infection, or hypoperfusion, it progresses to full-thickness injury. This is why burns can appear to worsen over 48-72 hours.

Question 24: Inhalation injury significantly increases burn mortality because it:

A) Increases fluid requirements
B) Impairs gas exchange and increases infection risk
C) Causes immediate death
D) Only affects the nose

Answer: B

Explanation: Inhalation injury damages airways, impairs gas exchange, increases secretions, and dramatically increases pneumonia risk. Combined burn and inhalation injury has significantly higher mortality than either alone. Lower airway injury can progress to ARDS.

Question 25: The best method for cooling a heat stroke patient is:

A) Antipyretics like acetaminophen
B) Evaporative cooling with misting and fans
C) Covering with blankets to prevent shivering
D) Slow cooling over 24 hours

Answer: B

Explanation: Evaporative cooling (misting patient with tepid water while fans blow air over them) is most practical and effective in most settings. Cold water immersion is effective but makes patient monitoring difficult. Cool rapidly to <39°C. Antipyretics don't work for heat stroke.

Question 26: In electrical injuries, the extent of internal damage:

A) Matches external burns
B) Is less than external appearance
C) Can be far more extensive than external burns suggest
D) Only affects the skin

Answer: C

Explanation: Electrical injuries are deceptive—extensive deep muscle, nerve, and vascular damage can exist with minimal external burns (iceberg effect). Electricity follows path of least resistance through internal tissues, causing damage not visible externally. Always assume significant internal injury.

Question 27: Cement burns are particularly dangerous because:

A) They cause immediate pain
B) They're alkaline and people often don't realize they're burning
C) They only affect small areas
D) They heal quickly

Answer: B

Explanation: Cement contains calcium oxide (lime), which is alkaline. Prolonged contact often occurs because people don't realize cement is caustic and burning them. This can result in full-thickness burns over large areas. Immediate copious irrigation is essential.

Question 28: A patient requires monitoring for cardiac arrhythmias after electrical injury for at least:

A) 6 hours
B) 12 hours
C) 24 hours
D) No monitoring needed if initial ECG normal

Answer: C

Explanation: Cardiac monitoring for at least 24 hours is standard after electrical injury because arrhythmias can develop in a delayed fashion. High-voltage injuries, loss of consciousness, abnormal ECG, or chest pain require admission for monitoring.

Question 29: Which statement about alkali burns is correct?

A) They form protective eschar
B) They cause coagulation necrosis

C) They cause liquefaction necrosis and continue penetrating
D) They require minimal irrigation

Answer: C

Explanation: Alkali burns cause liquefaction necrosis without eschar formation, allowing continued deep penetration. They're more dangerous than acid burns for this reason and require prolonged irrigation (sometimes hours) until pH normalizes.

Question 30: The purpose of adding colloids (albumin) in later burn resuscitation is to:

A) Provide nutrition
B) Help maintain intravascular volume after capillary leak resolves
C) Decrease fluid needs initially
D) Treat infection

Answer: B

Explanation: Colloids like albumin are added after 12-24 hours once capillary leak begins resolving. Colloids stay in vessels better than crystalloids, helping maintain intravascular volume with less total fluid. Given earlier, they leak into tissues and worsen edema.

Question 31: Lightning strike victims should be resuscitated:

A) In standard triage priority (treat worst first)
B) Using reverse triage (treat those appearing dead first)
C) Only if pulse present
D) After other patients stabilized

Answer: B

Explanation: Lightning strikes use reverse triage: treat those who appear dead first. Lightning can cause cardiac and respiratory arrest, but immediate CPR may be successful because the heart often recovers. Those who survive initial strike and are breathing will likely continue surviving.

Question 32: White phosphorus burns require special management including:

A) Keeping wound dry
B) Removing particles under water to prevent ignition
C) Immediate surgical excision
D) No special treatment

Answer: B

Explanation: White phosphorus ignites spontaneously on contact with air. Remove embedded particles under water to prevent re-ignition, then debride and cover with wet dressings. Copper sulfate can identify remaining particles (turns them black) but is toxic and less commonly used now.

Question 33: A burn patient in the mobilization phase (48-72 hours post-burn) may develop:

A) Decreased urine output
B) Increased edema
C) Pulmonary edema from fluid shifting back into vessels
D) Worsening shock

Answer: C

Explanation: During mobilization phase, capillaries heal and edema fluid shifts back into vessels. This increases urine output (good—body eliminating excess fluid) but can cause volume overload and pulmonary edema if fluid administration isn't decreased. Some patients need diuretics.

Question 34: Phenol burns should be decontaminated with:

A) Water alone
B) Polyethylene glycol or isopropyl alcohol,

then water
C) Vinegar
D) No decontamination needed

Answer: B

Explanation: Phenol is lipid-soluble. If available, polyethylene glycol or isopropyl alcohol removes it more effectively than water alone, followed by water irrigation. Phenol can cause systemic toxicity (CNS depression, arrhythmias, organ damage), so complete decontamination is critical.

Question 35: The most important factor determining chemical burn severity is:

A) Type of chemical
B) Concentration and duration of contact
C) Location on body
D) Patient age

Answer: B

Explanation: While chemical type matters, concentration and duration of contact are most critical. High concentration chemicals cause more damage, and prolonged contact (delayed decontamination) allows deeper penetration. This emphasizes the importance of immediate copious irrigation.

Clinical Scenarios

Clinical Scenario 1: Major Thermal Burn with Fluid Resuscitation

A 45-year-old male was trapped in a house fire for several minutes before rescue. He has burns to his entire anterior and posterior trunk, entire right arm, and entire right leg. He also has facial burns with singed nasal hairs. He's conscious but anxious. Vitals: HR 118, BP 108/72, RR 22, SpO_2 97% on non-rebreather mask. He weighs 80 kg.

Questions:

1. Calculate his TBSA burn percentage using Rule of Nines
2. Calculate his first 24-hour fluid requirement using Parkland formula
3. What is your immediate concern regarding his airway?
4. Six hours post-burn, his urine output has been 20 mL/hr for the past two hours. What action should you take?

Answers:

1. **TBSA calculation using Rule of Nines:**
    - Anterior trunk: 18%
    - Posterior trunk: 18%
    - Entire right arm: 9%
    - Entire right leg: 18%
    - **Total: 63% TBSA**

    (Don't count facial burns in TBSA unless partial or full-thickness, and the question specifies burns, not just erythema)

2. **Parkland formula calculation:**

- Formula: 4 mL × weight (kg) × % TBSA
- 4 × 80 × 63 = 20,160 mL total for 24 hours
- First 8 hours: 10,080 mL (half of total)
- Next 16 hours: 10,080 mL (second half)

Rate for first 8 hours: 10,080 mL ÷ 8 hours = 1,260 mL/hour

Important: If patient arrives hours after burn, adjust timing. Clock starts at time of burn, not arrival.

3. **Immediate airway concerns:**

This patient has HIGH risk for airway compromise:

- Facial burns
- Singed nasal hairs (indicates inhalation of hot gases)
- Enclosed space exposure (house fire)
- Likely inhalation injury

Immediate actions:

- Assess for other inhalation injury signs: hoarseness, stridor, carbonaceous sputum, respiratory distress
- Check COHb level on arterial blood gas
- Consider early intubation BEFORE airway edema worsens
- Don't wait for respiratory distress—edema progresses over 12-24 hours
- If signs of significant inhalation injury present, intubate now while it's still possible
- Once severe edema develops, intubation becomes extremely difficult or impossible, requiring surgical airway

Why early intubation matters: Upper airway edema from thermal injury peaks at 12-24 hours post-burn. The window for safe intubation closes as edema progresses. It's much safer to intubate early than to wait until the patient crashes.

4. **Urine output 20 mL/hr for past two hours:**

Target urine output: 0.5-1 mL/kg/hr (for this 80 kg patient: 40-80 mL/hr)

Current output: 20 mL/hr is INADEQUATE (below 0.5 mL/kg/hr)

What this means: Inadequate urine output indicates insufficient renal perfusion, suggesting overall inadequate tissue perfusion. The patient needs more fluid.

Actions to take:

- INCREASE IV fluid rate by 20-30% initially
- Reassess urine output hourly

- Continue adjusting fluid rate based on response
- If increasing to 1,500 mL/hr, recheck output after 1-2 hours
- If output improves to target range, continue current rate
- If still inadequate, increase further
- Monitor for other perfusion indicators (mental status, heart rate, blood pressure, lactate)

Important principle: The Parkland formula provides a starting estimate only. Actual fluid needs vary tremendously between patients. Some need more, some need less. Always titrate based on physiologic response (primarily urine output), not rigid adherence to calculated rates.

Why some patients need more:

- Deeper burns than estimated
- Inhalation injury (increases fluid needs by 30-50%)
- Delayed resuscitation
- Calculation errors
- Individual physiologic variation

Key learning points from this scenario:

- Burn TBSA calculation is fundamental for fluid resuscitation
- Parkland formula is a starting point, not a fixed prescription
- Urine output is the primary guide for adjusting fluid rates
- Early intubation in inhalation injury prevents airway crisis
- Enclosed space fires carry high inhalation injury risk
- Aggressive but carefully monitored resuscitation is essential for survival

---

Clinical Scenario 2: Electrical Injury with Hidden Damage

A 32-year-old electrician was working on high-voltage power lines when he received a shock. Co-workers saw him thrown backward off the ladder (10-foot fall). He was briefly unconscious but is now awake and alert. You note a small charred area on his right palm and a larger wound on his right foot.

Vitals: HR 108, BP 118/76, RR 20, SpO2 96% on room air. He complains of right arm and leg pain. His urine appears dark, tea-colored.

Questions:

1. What is the path of electrical current in this patient and why does it matter?
2. What does the tea-colored urine indicate and how should it be managed?
3. Despite relatively small external burns, what internal injuries must you assess for?
4. The patient asks if he can go home since he feels okay. How do you respond?

Answers:

1. **Current path and significance:**

   Path: Right hand (entrance) → through arm → across chest → down right leg → right foot (exit)

   Why this matters critically:

   - This path crosses the HEART (hand-to-foot is one of the most dangerous paths)
   - High risk of cardiac arrhythmias including ventricular fibrillation
   - Current traveled through large muscle masses (arm, chest, leg), causing extensive deep muscle damage despite small external burns
   - Path through chest may have caused myocardial injury

   Other significant factors:

   - High voltage (power lines = thousands of volts)
   - Fall from 10 feet adds trauma injuries to assess
   - Brief loss of consciousness suggests either cardiac arrest (successfully resuscitated by co-workers) or head injury

   Immediate implications:

   - MUST have continuous cardiac monitoring for at least 24 hours
   - High suspicion for deep muscle injury throughout current path
   - Need imaging to rule out fractures or internal injuries from fall
   - Neurological assessment (loss of consciousness could indicate head injury or transient cardiac arrest)
2. **Tea-colored urine indicates rhabdomyolysis:**

   What's happening: Electrical current caused deep muscle damage throughout the right arm and leg. Damaged muscle releases myoglobin (muscle protein) into bloodstream. Kidneys filter myoglobin, turning urine tea or cola-colored. Myoglobin can precipitate in renal tubules, causing acute kidney injury.

   Management priorities:

   - **Aggressive IV fluid resuscitation:** Target urine output 75-100 mL/hr (higher than standard burn resuscitation)
   - Rationale: High urine flow prevents myoglobin from precipitating in renal tubules
   - **Consider alkalinizing urine:** IV sodium bicarbonate to achieve urine pH >6.5 makes myoglobin more soluble, reducing precipitation risk
   - **Monitor creatine kinase (CK):** Severely elevated CK confirms rhabdomyolysis severity
   - **Monitor renal function:** Serial creatinine, BUN, electrolytes (especially potassium—cell death releases potassium, causing hyperkalemia)

- **Monitor for compartment syndrome:** Deep muscle injury causes swelling; watch for pain out of proportion, pain with passive stretch
- **Avoid nephrotoxic medications:** NSAIDs, aminoglycosides, contrast dye if possible
- **Watch for hyperkalemia:** Can cause cardiac arrhythmias; treat with calcium, insulin/glucose, possibly dialysis if severe

3. **Hidden internal injuries to assess:**

Despite small external burns, assume EXTENSIVE internal damage:

Cardiovascular:

- Myocardial injury (check troponin if chest pain or ECG changes)
- Cardiac arrhythmias (continuous monitoring essential)
- Vascular thrombosis (assess all pulses carefully and repeatedly)

Musculoskeletal:

- Deep muscle necrosis throughout current path (right arm, chest, right leg)
- Compartment syndrome (monitor closely, measure compartment pressures if concerning signs)
- Fractures from fall (cervical spine, skull, extremities)—obtain imaging
- Bone injuries (electricity superheats bone, causing injury)

Neurological:

- Peripheral nerve injury along current path
- Spinal cord injury (from electrical injury or fall)
- Brain injury (from loss of consciousness—was it cardiac arrest or head trauma from fall?)
- Assess motor and sensory function carefully

Renal:

- Acute kidney injury from myoglobinuria (already identified)
- Monitor urine output, creatinine, electrolytes

Other:

- Internal organ injuries from fall
- Intra-abdominal injuries if current path crossed abdomen

Diagnostic workup:

- ECG immediately and continuous cardiac monitoring
- Cardiac biomarkers (troponin) if any cardiac symptoms or ECG changes
- Creatine kinase (CK), comprehensive metabolic panel, CBC
- Urinalysis (myoglobin)

    - CT head (loss of consciousness)
    - Cervical spine imaging (fall mechanism)
    - X-rays of any painful areas
    - Consider CT chest/abdomen/pelvis if significant trauma from fall
4. **Response to discharge request:**

    Provide clear education about why admission is mandatory:

    "I understand you feel okay right now, and that's actually common with electrical injuries. However, I need to explain why you absolutely cannot go home today:

    Hidden danger: The small burns on your hand and foot are just the tip of the iceberg. Electricity traveled through your entire arm, across your chest and heart, and down your leg. This caused damage to deep muscles and potentially your heart that we can't see from the outside.

    Heart risk: The electrical current crossed your heart. You're at risk for serious heart rhythm problems that can happen anytime in the next 24-48 hours. These arrhythmias can be fatal. You need continuous heart monitoring to catch any problems immediately.

    Kidney risk: Your dark urine shows that damaged muscle is releasing protein that can damage your kidneys. You need IV fluids and close monitoring to prevent kidney failure.

    Muscle damage: You likely have significant muscle damage in your arm and leg that will declare itself over the next few days. This can require surgery if compartment syndrome develops.

    The fall: You fell 10 feet and lost consciousness. We need to make sure you don't have head injury, neck injury, or internal injuries.

    What we're doing: You'll be admitted for at least 24 hours of cardiac monitoring, aggressive IV fluids, frequent assessments, and treatment of any complications that develop. Most electrical injury patients stay 2-5 days.

    Why it matters: Electrical injuries can look minor but be life-threatening. People have died after going home because no one monitored for delayed complications. We're keeping you here to prevent that.

    I know this isn't what you wanted to hear, but your safety is our priority. Do you have any questions about why this is necessary?"

    Key points to emphasize:

    - Electrical injuries are deceptive
    - Cardiac monitoring is non-negotiable for at least 24 hours
    - Multiple organ systems at risk
    - Delayed complications are common
    - Hospital admission is standard of care for high-voltage injuries

Key learning points:

- External burns don't reflect internal damage with electrical injuries
- Current path through heart or brain is most dangerous
- Myoglobinuria requires aggressive hydration targeting high urine output
- All high-voltage injuries require admission and cardiac monitoring
- Compartment syndrome risk is very high
- Multiple organ system assessment and monitoring essential

Clinical Scenario 3: Chemical Burn with Systemic Effects

A 28-year-old laboratory technician spilled hydrofluoric acid on her right hand and forearm while working. The spill occurred 30 minutes ago. She initially rinsed with water for 2-3 minutes but continued working because "it didn't look that bad." Now she's in severe pain despite the burn appearing relatively minor—slight erythema with a few small blisters on the dorsum of her hand.

Vitals: HR 98, BP 124/78, RR 18, SpO2 98%. She rates her pain as 9/10, describing it as deep, burning pain that seems disproportionate to the appearance.

Questions:

1. Why is the pain out of proportion to the visible injury with hydrofluoric acid burns?
2. What immediate treatment is required?
3. What life-threatening complication can occur with HF burns?
4. Why was the initial 2-3 minutes of water irrigation inadequate?

Answers:

1. **Pain out of proportion with HF burns:**

   Hydrofluoric acid is uniquely dangerous among chemical burns:

   Mechanism of injury:

   - HF penetrates deeply into tissues despite causing minimal surface damage
   - Fluoride ions bind calcium at the cellular level, causing:
     - Cellular death (calcium necessary for cellular function)
     - Severe pain from nerve stimulation
     - Bone decalcification if burn reaches bone
     - Deep tissue necrosis that's not visible externally

   Why pain is so severe:

   - Fluoride ions penetrate deeply and continue damaging tissue for hours
   - Nerve endings are directly stimulated by fluoride-calcium interaction

- Pain is described as deep, boring, excruciating, unrelieved by standard pain medications
- Pain severity doesn't match visible injury—this is the hallmark of HF burns

Time course:

- Concentrated HF (>50%): Pain immediate, visible damage develops quickly
- Dilute HF (<20%): Pain may be delayed hours, visible damage minimal initially, but deep injury progresses
- Continued pain despite appearing minor should always raise suspicion for HF exposure

2. **Immediate treatment required:**

HF burns require specific urgent treatment beyond standard burn care:

Decontamination (should continue):

- Continue copious water irrigation for 30 minutes minimum (she only did 2-3 minutes—inadequate)
- Remove any contaminated jewelry or clothing
- Goal: Remove all remaining acid

Calcium gluconate treatment (specific antidote):

Topical treatment:

- Apply calcium gluconate gel liberally to entire affected area
- Calcium binds free fluoride ions, stopping the injury process
- Apply every 15 minutes or keep continuously covered
- Continue until pain resolves
- This should provide some pain relief within 30-60 minutes if effective

Injection treatment (if topical ineffective or for deeper burns):

- Inject calcium gluconate 10% solution subcutaneously around and under the burn
- Small amounts (0.5 mL) injected throughout affected area using 27-30 gauge needle
- Provides calcium directly to tissue where fluoride ions are binding calcium
- Usually provides dramatic pain relief
- May need repeated injections

Intra-arterial calcium gluconate (for severe hand/finger burns):

- Anesthesiologist or interventional radiologist places arterial catheter
- Calcium gluconate infused directly into arterial supply of affected limb
- Reserved for severe burns or when other methods fail
- Most effective for maintaining tissue calcium levels

Pain management:

- Systemic analgesia (opioids)—but pain often resistant until calcium treatment given
- Regional anesthesia (nerve blocks) may help

Monitoring:

- Continuous cardiac monitoring (fluoride can cause arrhythmias)
- Serial calcium levels (hypocalcemia risk)
- Serial potassium levels (hyperkalemia risk)
- ECG monitoring for QT prolongation

Surgical consultation:

- Hand surgery evaluation (HF commonly affects hands)
- May need debridement of necrotic tissue
- Severe cases may require amputation of affected digits

3. **Life-threatening complications:**

Systemic fluoride toxicity causing severe electrolyte disturbances:

Hypocalcemia:

- Fluoride ions bind calcium systemically if absorbed in sufficient quantity
- Severe hypocalcemia can cause:
  - Tetany
  - Seizures
  - Cardiac arrhythmias (QT prolongation, torsades de pointes, ventricular fibrillation)
  - Death

Hyperkalemia:

- Cell death from fluoride releases intracellular potassium
- Severe hyperkalemia causes:
  - Peaked T waves
  - Widened QRS
  - Cardiac arrest

Hypomagnesemia:

- Often accompanies hypocalcemia
- Worsens cardiac instability

When to worry about systemic toxicity:

- Burns >2-3% TBSA with concentrated HF (>50%)

- Any burn with highly concentrated HF (>70%)
- Inhalation exposure
- Ingestion
- Signs of toxicity: cardiac arrhythmias, tetany, altered mental status

Monitoring and treatment:

- Continuous cardiac monitoring
- Frequent electrolyte checks (calcium, potassium, magnesium)
- IV calcium replacement (calcium chloride or calcium gluconate)
- Treat hyperkalemia aggressively if present
- ICU admission for significant exposures

This patient's risk: Small burn area (<1% TBSA likely) makes systemic toxicity less likely but still possible. Monitor cardiac rhythm and check electrolytes. The 30-minute delay before treatment increases risk.

4. **Why 2-3 minutes irrigation was inadequate:**

HF penetrates rapidly and deeply:

- Unlike most chemicals that act on surface, HF penetrates through intact skin within minutes
- Short irrigation doesn't remove fluoride ions that have already penetrated
- Continued tissue damage occurs from these penetrated ions

Standard irrigation protocol for HF:

- MINIMUM 30 minutes of continuous irrigation
- Some protocols recommend up to 2 hours for concentrated HF
- Continue until pain improves
- Goal: Remove surface chemical and dilute penetrated ions

Her 2-3 minute irrigation:

- Removed some surface chemical
- Did NOT remove fluoride that had already penetrated (30 minutes elapsed before treatment)
- Fluoride continued penetrating and binding calcium
- This delay explains severe pain and why she needs calcium treatment now

Teaching point: Chemical exposure requires immediate, prolonged irrigation. "A quick rinse" is never adequate. This is why safety showers in labs have 15-minute timers—that's minimum time needed.

Current treatment plan:

- Irrigate again now with water or saline

- Apply calcium gluconate gel immediately and continuously
- If pain doesn't improve within 30-60 minutes, proceed to calcium injection
- Don't wait for pain to become unbearable before escalating treatment
- Consider intra-arterial calcium for hand burns if other methods insufficient

Key learning points:

- HF burns are medical emergencies requiring specific treatment
- Pain out of proportion to visible injury is characteristic
- Calcium gluconate (topical, injection, or intra-arterial) is specific antidote
- Systemic toxicity can be life-threatening
- Immediate prolonged irrigation is essential for all chemical burns
- Never underestimate chemical burns based on appearance alone
- Occupational exposures require knowledge of specific chemical hazards

---

Clinical Scenario 4: Heat Stroke in Athlete

A 22-year-old male collapsed during football practice on a hot, humid day (95°F, 80% humidity). He was practicing in full pads for 2 hours. Teammates report he was "acting weird" for the last 15 minutes before collapse—stumbling, not responding appropriately to commands, appearing confused.

On your arrival, he's lying on the field, responsive only to painful stimuli. His skin is hot and flushed, still sweating. Vitals: HR 132, BP 98/62, RR 26, rectal temperature 41.2°C (106.2°F), SpO2 94% on room air.

Questions:

1. What distinguishes heat stroke from heat exhaustion in this case?
2. What are your immediate treatment priorities and specific actions?
3. Why is this case considered exertional heat stroke, and how does it differ from classic heat stroke?
4. What complications should you monitor for as you treat this patient?

Answers:

1. **Heat stroke vs. heat exhaustion:**

   This patient has HEAT STROKE (medical emergency) based on:

   Core temperature >40°C (104°F):

   - His temperature is 41.2°C (106.2°F)
   - This exceeds heat stroke threshold
   - Heat exhaustion: temperature <40°C

Altered mental status:

- Responds only to painful stimuli
- Teammates noted confusion, inappropriate responses before collapse
- Mental status alteration is the HALLMARK differentiating heat stroke from exhaustion
- Heat exhaustion: normal mental status

Cardiovascular compromise:

- Tachycardia and relative hypotension
- Indicates significant physiologic stress

Why distinction matters:

- Heat exhaustion: serious but responsive to fluids and rest
- Heat stroke: life-threatening emergency requiring immediate aggressive cooling
- Heat stroke causes multi-organ dysfunction if not treated immediately
- Mortality can be 10-50% depending on severity and treatment delay
- Every minute of hyperthermia causes ongoing cellular damage

2. **Immediate treatment priorities:**

Priority 1: RAPID COOLING (most important)

Goal: Reduce core temperature to <39°C (102.2°F) as quickly as possible

Immediate cooling methods (use multiple simultaneously):

On the field/immediately:

- Move to shade or air-conditioned area
- Remove ALL clothing and equipment (pads trap heat)
- Start evaporative cooling immediately:
  - Spray/mist body with tepid water
  - Use fans to blow air over patient
  - This is most practical and effective method in most settings
- Apply ice packs to groin, axillae, neck (major vessels near surface)
- If ice bath available and can monitor patient: cold water immersion (very effective but makes assessment difficult)

During transport/in ED:

- Continue evaporative cooling
- Cold IV fluids (as cold as available)
- Cooling blankets if available
- Continue ice packs to major vessels
- Monitor temperature continuously (rectal probe most accurate)
- **STOP cooling at 39°C** to prevent overshoot hypothermia

DO NOT:

- Use antipyretics (acetaminophen, NSAIDs)—they don't work for heat stroke
- Pack in ice (causes vasoconstriction, reducing cooling effectiveness)
- Use rubbing alcohol (toxic if absorbed, evaporation can cause shivering)

Priority 2: Airway/Breathing/Circulation

Airway:

- Assess airway patency
- Position to maintain airway (recovery position if spontaneous breathing adequate)
- Consider intubation if GCS ≤8, unable to protect airway, or seizures
- Supplemental oxygen

Circulation:

- Large-bore IV access (two lines)
- IV fluid resuscitation (aggressive but monitor carefully—balance dehydration with risk of pulmonary edema)
- Normal saline or Lactated Ringer's
- Monitor for hypotension, tachycardia

Priority 3: Immediate transport

- EMS activation if not already done
- Continue cooling during transport
- Continuous monitoring

Priority 4: Supportive care

- Continuous cardiac monitoring
- Monitor oxygen saturation
- Manage seizures if occur (benzodiazepines)
- Position appropriately (left lateral if vomiting risk)

Time is critical: Studies show mortality dramatically increases with time above 40°C. Cooling within first 30 minutes of collapse improves outcomes significantly. Don't delay cooling for anything except life-threatening airway/breathing issues.

3. **Exertional vs. classic heat stroke:**

This patient has EXERTIONAL heat stroke:

Characteristics:

- Affects young, healthy, fit individuals

- Occurs during strenuous physical activity in hot conditions
- Heat production from exercise overwhelms body's cooling capacity
- Develops rapidly (over minutes to hours)
- May still be sweating (common misconception that heat stroke always means dry skin)
- Core temperature often >41°C (105.8°F)
- High risk of rhabdomyolysis, acute kidney injury, DIC

Classic (non-exertional) heat stroke:

- Affects elderly, very young, chronically ill, or people with impaired thermoregulation
- Occurs during heat waves in people who can't escape heat
- Develops over days of heat exposure
- Typically NOT sweating (lost ability to sweat)
- Core temperature usually 40-41°C
- Skin hot and DRY

Why distinction matters clinically:

Rhabdomyolysis risk:

- Much higher in exertional heat stroke due to muscle damage from exercise
- Monitor CK, myoglobin in urine
- Requires aggressive hydration

DIC risk:

- Higher in exertional heat stroke
- Monitor coagulation studies closely

Recovery:

- Young exertional heat stroke patients may recover fully if treated rapidly
- Elderly classic heat stroke patients often have residual deficits

Prevention:

- Different strategies needed
- Athletes: acclimatization, hydration, rest breaks, avoid hottest times
- Elderly: air conditioning access, checking on vulnerable people during heat waves

4. **Complications to monitor:**

Heat stroke causes multi-organ dysfunction. Monitor for:

Neurological:

- Persistent altered mental status or coma
- Seizures (treat with benzodiazepines)
- Cerebral edema (can cause increased intracranial pressure)
- Long-term: cognitive impairment, cerebellar dysfunction, personality changes
- Serial GCS assessments

Cardiovascular:

- Hypotension requiring vasopressor support
- Myocardial injury (check troponin)
- Arrhythmias (from electrolyte disturbances or direct thermal myocardial injury)
- Monitor: continuous cardiac monitoring, serial troponins if indicated

Renal:

- Acute kidney injury from:
    - Direct thermal injury to kidneys
    - Rhabdomyolysis (myoglobin damaging tubules)
    - Hypovolemia
- Monitor: urine output, creatinine, BUN
- Treatment: aggressive fluids, target urine output 100-200 mL/hr if rhabdomyolysis

Hepatic:

- Hepatocellular injury (heat damages liver cells)
- Elevated AST, ALT, bilirubin
- Can progress to liver failure in severe cases
- Monitor: serial liver function tests

Hematologic:

- Disseminated intravascular coagulation (DIC)
- Thrombocytopenia
- Elevated PT/PTT, D-dimer
- Treatment: blood products as needed
- Monitor: serial coagulation studies, platelet count

Musculoskeletal:

- Rhabdomyolysis (very common in exertional heat stroke)
- Elevated CK (often >10,000, sometimes >100,000)
- Myoglobinuria (tea-colored urine)
- Can cause acute kidney injury
- Treatment: aggressive IV hydration, alkalinize urine
- Monitor: CK, urine myoglobin, urine color

Metabolic:

- Hypoglycemia (increased glucose utilization, impaired gluconeogenesis)
- Hyperkalemia or hypokalemia
- Metabolic acidosis (lactic acidosis from poor tissue perfusion)
- Monitor: frequent electrolytes, glucose, lactate, blood gas

Respiratory:

- Acute respiratory distress syndrome (ARDS)
- Pulmonary edema
- Aspiration pneumonia (if vomited while unconscious)
- May require intubation and mechanical ventilation
- Monitor: oxygen saturation, respiratory rate, chest X-ray

Gastrointestinal:

- Nausea, vomiting (from direct GI thermal injury and ischemia)
- GI bleeding
- Bowel ischemia
- Monitor: abdominal exam, stool for blood

Laboratory monitoring schedule:

- Initially: comprehensive metabolic panel, CBC, coagulation studies, CK, lactate, blood gas, urinalysis
- Repeat: every 4-6 hours initially, then every 12-24 hours as patient stabilizes
- Trend values to identify developing complications

ICU admission: All heat stroke patients require ICU-level care for close monitoring and management of multi-organ dysfunction.

Key learning points:

- Heat stroke is defined by core temperature >40°C AND altered mental status
- Immediate rapid cooling is the definitive treatment
- Exertional heat stroke can occur in young, healthy athletes
- Still sweating doesn't rule out heat stroke
- Multi-organ dysfunction is common and requires intensive monitoring
- Every minute of hyperthermia causes ongoing damage
- Prevention through acclimatization, hydration, and environmental modifications is ideal

Chapter 8 Summary: Key Concepts to Master

You've completed an extensive review of burns and environmental trauma. Let's consolidate the most critical concepts for exam success and clinical practice.

Burns - Essential Knowledge:

1. **Burn depth determines treatment:**
   - Superficial: not counted in TBSA
   - Partial-thickness: painful, may heal without grafting
   - Full-thickness: painless, always requires grafting
   - Remember: burns evolve over 48-72 hours
2. **TBSA calculation:**
   - Rule of Nines for quick estimation
   - Only count partial and full-thickness burns
   - Accurate calculation guides fluid resuscitation
3. **Fluid resuscitation:**
   - Parkland formula: 4 mL × kg × % TBSA
   - Half in first 8 hours, half in next 16 hours
   - Clock starts at time of burn
   - Titrate to urine output 0.5-1 mL/kg/hr
   - Formula is starting point—adjust based on response
4. **Inhalation injury:**
   - Significantly increases mortality
   - Upper airway: thermal injury, causes edema
   - Lower airway: chemical injury, causes pneumonitis
   - Early intubation before edema worsens
   - Carbon monoxide poisoning: check COHb level
   - Signs: facial burns, singed hairs, carbonaceous sputum, hoarseness
5. **Burn center criteria:**
   - 20% TBSA adults, >10% children/elderly
   - Burns to face, hands, feet, genitals, joints
   - Full-thickness burns
   - Electrical, chemical, inhalation injury
   - Circumferential burns
   - Burns with other trauma

Electrical Injuries - Critical Points:

1. **Hidden damage exceeds visible injury**
2. **Current path through heart most dangerous**
3. **Myoglobinuria requires aggressive hydration (75-100 mL/hr)**
4. **Cardiac monitoring mandatory 24 hours minimum**
5. **High compartment syndrome risk**
6. **All high-voltage injuries require admission**

Chemical Burns - Key Concepts:

1. **Immediate copious irrigation (30+ minutes)**
2. **Alkalis more dangerous than acids (liquefaction necrosis)**
3. **HF burns require calcium gluconate**
4. **Don't waste time seeking neutralizing agents—irrigate**

5. **Eye exposures: immediate irrigation 30-60 minutes**

Environmental Injuries - Must-Know:

1. **Hypothermia:**
   - <35°C core temperature
   - Mild: 32-35°C (shivering)
   - Moderate: 28-32°C (shivering stops, confusion)
   - Severe: <28°C (appears dead, high VF risk)
   - Rewarm carefully, continue CPR until warm
2. **Heat stroke:**
   - 40°C + altered mental status = heat stroke
   - Rapid cooling to <39°C is definitive treatment
   - Multi-organ dysfunction common
   - Exertional (athletes) vs. classic (elderly)
   - Still sweating doesn't rule out heat stroke

High-Yield Exam Topics:

- Calculating fluid resuscitation
- Recognizing inhalation injury
- Burn center transfer criteria
- Electrical injury complications
- Chemical burn specific treatments
- Hypothermia management
- Heat stroke vs. heat exhaustion

Study Tips for This Material:

1. Practice TBSA calculations until automatic
2. Memorize Parkland formula and how to apply it
3. Understand burn depth characteristics (don't just memorize)
4. Know specific treatments for specific chemicals
5. Recognize time-sensitive emergencies (heat stroke, inhalation injury)
6. Connect pathophysiology to clinical presentation

You're building competence in managing some of the most challenging trauma scenarios. Burns and environmental injuries require rapid assessment, aggressive intervention, and careful monitoring. The systematic approaches you've learned here will serve you throughout your trauma nursing career.

Chapter 9: Maxillofacial and Ocular Trauma

Facial and eye injuries can be deceptive. They often look dramatic with significant bleeding and swelling, yet the patient may be relatively stable. However, these injuries can also hide life-threatening airway compromise or vision-threatening damage. Understanding maxillofacial and ocular trauma means recognizing when injuries are purely cosmetic versus when they threaten critical functions like breathing, sight, or neurological integrity.

This chapter covers facial bone fractures, dental injuries, eye trauma, and injuries to the ears, nose, and throat. You'll learn to identify patterns that indicate specific fractures, recognize when airway management becomes critical, and understand which eye injuries require emergency intervention to preserve vision.

Facial Fractures

The facial skeleton is complex, containing multiple bones that protect the brain, eyes, and sinuses while allowing for eating, breathing, and facial expression. Understanding common fracture patterns helps you anticipate complications and guide appropriate treatment.

Mandible Fractures

The mandible (lower jaw) is the most commonly fractured facial bone because it's prominent and relatively unsupported. Think of it as a horseshoe-shaped bone with multiple potential weak points.

Common fracture locations:

- **Condyle** (where mandible articulates with skull): Most common site, often from blows to chin
- **Angle** (back corner where jaw turns upward): Common with direct lateral blows
- **Body** (main horizontal portion): From direct trauma
- **Symphysis** (midline where two halves fuse): Less common, usually high-energy trauma

Why location matters: Fractures often occur at two points because force travels through the bone. A blow to one side of the jaw often causes fractures on both that side and the opposite condyle (called a contralateral fracture). Always examine the entire mandible, not just the obvious injury site.

Clinical presentation:

- Pain with jaw movement or speaking

- Malocclusion (teeth don't fit together properly—patient notices immediately)
- Visible step-off or asymmetry of jaw line
- Loose or missing teeth at fracture site
- Inability to open mouth fully (trismus)
- Numbness of lower lip (if inferior alveolar nerve injured)
- Drooling (can't manage secretions due to pain)

Assessment technique: Ask patient to bite down—they'll report pain at fracture site. Check dental occlusion by asking if teeth feel "normal" when biting. Palpate along entire jaw for tenderness, step-offs, or crepitus.

Airway considerations: Most mandible fractures don't immediately threaten the airway, but complications can develop:

- Bilateral body fractures can allow tongue to fall backward (floor of mouth loses structural support)
- Significant swelling may progress to obstruct airway
- Blood and secretions pool if patient can't manage them due to pain
- Hematoma in floor of mouth can push tongue up and back

Initial management:

- Assess and secure airway (position patient upright if possible to allow secretions to drain forward)
- Control bleeding (usually from oral lacerations or dental injuries)
- Pain management
- Soft diet or NPO if surgery planned
- Antibiotics if fracture communicates with oral cavity (most do)
- Avoid manual manipulation of unstable segments

Definitive treatment:

- Closed reduction with maxillomandibular fixation (wiring jaws together) for stable fractures
- Open reduction with internal fixation (plates and screws) for displaced or unstable fractures
- Liquid diet for 4-6 weeks during healing

Complications:

- Malocclusion if not properly reduced
- Infection (oral bacteria contaminate fracture)
- TMJ dysfunction
- Facial nerve injury (rare)

Midface Fractures (Le Fort Fractures)

Le Fort fractures are classified patterns of midface fractures described over a century ago but still clinically relevant. Understanding these patterns helps you recognize injury severity and predict associated complications.

The Le Fort classification separates the midface from the skull base in predictable patterns:

Le Fort I (Horizontal maxillary fracture):

- Fracture line runs horizontally above the teeth, through the maxilla
- Essentially separates the upper teeth and palate from rest of face
- Least severe Le Fort fracture

Clinical findings:

- Mobile upper teeth/palate (grasp upper teeth and gently pull—entire segment moves)
- Malocclusion
- Epistaxis (nosebleed)
- Facial swelling

Le Fort II (Pyramidal fracture):

- Fracture extends from nasal bridge down and laterally through orbital floor and across upper jaw
- Creates pyramid-shaped mobile segment including nose and maxilla
- More severe than Le Fort I

Clinical findings:

- Mobile midface (nose and upper jaw move together)
- Significant facial edema
- Epistaxis
- Subconjunctival hemorrhage (blood in white of eye)
- CSF rhinorrhea possible if cribriform plate involved
- Orbital floor fractures may cause enophthalmos (sunken eye) or diplopia

Le Fort III (Craniofacial separation):

- Complete separation of entire midface from cranium
- Fracture extends through nasal bridge, orbits, and zygomatic arches
- Most severe, often life-threatening

Clinical findings:

- Entire face mobile when upper teeth grasped
- Massive facial swelling ("beaten with baseball bat" appearance)

- Raccoon eyes (periorbital ecchymosis)
- Dish-face deformity (midface retrusion makes face look concave)
- CSF rhinorrhea common
- Airway compromise likely
- Often associated with severe head injury

Critical assessment: Test for midface mobility by grasping the upper incisors and gently attempting to move the maxilla. Stable = no Le Fort fracture. Movement = Le Fort fracture present (degree of movement helps classify which type).

Airway management with Le Fort fractures:

These fractures create unique airway challenges:

- Massive swelling can obstruct nasopharynx and oropharynx
- Blood accumulates in posterior pharynx
- Displaced bone fragments may compromise airway
- Le Fort III fractures frequently require intubation

Intubation considerations:

- Oral intubation is preferred when possible
- Nasal intubation relatively contraindicated (may pass through cribriform plate fracture into brain)
- Surgical airway may be necessary if oral intubation fails
- Some Le Fort fractures make bag-mask ventilation ineffective (no facial structure to seal against)

Initial management:

- Secure airway (early intubation often needed for Le Fort II and III)
- Control hemorrhage (can be massive)
- Elevate head of bed to reduce swelling and facilitate venous drainage
- Ice to reduce swelling
- Antibiotics (all communicate with sinuses)
- Ophthalmology consultation (orbital involvement common)
- Neurosurgery if CSF leak present
- Maxillofacial surgery consultation

Definitive treatment:

- Open reduction internal fixation with plates and screws
- Timing depends on swelling and other injuries
- Often delayed 3-7 days to allow swelling to decrease
- Maxillomandibular fixation during healing

Orbital Fractures

The orbit (eye socket) is a bony cavity that protects the eye. Fractures can occur from direct trauma or from pressure transmitted through the eye to the thin orbital floor.

Orbital floor fractures (blowout fractures):

These occur when blunt trauma to the eye increases intraorbital pressure, causing the thin orbital floor to fracture and herniate orbital contents (fat, muscles) into the maxillary sinus below.

Classic mechanism: Fist, ball, or other blunt object strikes the eye. The eye compresses but can't rupture (it's tough), so pressure transmits to the weakest point—the orbital floor—which gives way.

Clinical presentation:

- Periorbital ecchymosis and swelling
- Subconjunctival hemorrhage
- **Enophthalmos** (eye appears sunken because orbital contents herniated into sinus)
- **Diplopia** (double vision, especially with upward gaze—inferior rectus muscle trapped in fracture)
- **Infraorbital hypesthesia** (numbness of cheek, upper lip, side of nose—infraorbital nerve runs in orbital floor and gets injured)
- Restricted eye movement, particularly looking up (muscle entrapment)

Physical examination:

- Check visual acuity in both eyes
- Test extraocular movements (ask patient to track your finger through all fields of gaze)
- Assess sensation over cheek and upper lip
- Palpate orbital rims for step-offs or crepitus
- **Never press on the globe itself** if orbital fracture suspected

Imaging: CT scan is gold standard—shows fracture, herniated orbital contents, and air in orbit (from sinus communication).

When is blowout fracture an emergency?

Most are managed semi-urgently, but two situations require immediate surgery:

1. **White-eyed blowout fracture (pediatric emergency):**

- Occurs in children whose bones are more elastic
- Bone fractures like a trapdoor, snapping back and trapping muscle
- Minimal external signs ("white eye" without much bruising)
- Severe nausea/vomiting and bradycardia from oculocardiac reflex (vagal stimulation from trapped muscle)

- Requires surgery within 24-48 hours to release muscle and prevent permanent restriction and vision loss

2. **Acute orbital compartment syndrome:**

- Retrobulbar hematoma increases pressure in orbit
- Compresses optic nerve and retinal blood supply
- Causes blindness if not immediately relieved
- Covered in detail in eye injuries section below

Non-emergent management:

- Ice and elevation
- Antibiotics (orbit now communicates with sinus)
- Avoid nose blowing (can force air from sinus into orbit, worsening swelling)
- Decongestants to reduce sinus congestion
- Ophthalmology and maxillofacial surgery consultation
- Surgical repair timing controversial (early versus delayed to allow swelling to resolve)

Zygoma Fractures (Cheekbone)

The zygoma (cheekbone) articulates with multiple facial bones, so fractures often involve multiple sites.

Zygomatic arch fracture: Simple fracture of the arch that extends laterally from zygoma toward ear.

Clinical findings:

- Flattened cheek contour
- Pain with jaw opening (fractured arch impinges on temporalis muscle and coronoid process)
- Limited jaw opening
- Palpable step-off over arch

Zygomaticomaxillary complex (ZMC) fracture (tripod fracture): The zygoma separates from surrounding bones at multiple articulation points.

Clinical findings:

- Flattened malar eminence (cheek)
- Periorbital ecchymosis
- Subconjunctival hemorrhage
- Infraorbital hypesthesia (nerve runs through this area)
- Epistaxis
- Trismus (limited jaw opening)
- Step-offs palpable at:
    - Inferior orbital rim
    - Lateral orbital rim
    - Zygomatic arch

Management:

- Similar to other facial fractures
- Surgical reduction and fixation if displaced
- Restore facial contour and function

Nasal Fractures

The most common facial fracture, usually from direct frontal blow.

Clinical presentation:

- Epistaxis
- Nasal deformity or deviation
- Periorbital ecchymosis
- Nasal bone tenderness and crepitus
- Nasal obstruction

Assessment:

- Inspect for external deformity
- Check nasal patency (occlude one nostril, ask patient to breathe through other)
- Look inside nose for septal hematoma (bluish bulge on septum—surgical emergency)
- Palpate nasal bones gently for crepitus

Septal hematoma: Blood collection between septal cartilage and its overlying perichondrium. This is an emergency because:

- Cartilage gets blood supply from perichondrium
- Hematoma separates cartilage from blood supply
- Cartilage dies (avascular necrosis)
- Results in saddle nose deformity (nasal bridge collapses)

Management: Immediate drainage and packing to prevent reaccumulation

Nasal fracture management:

- Most don't require immediate reduction
- Ice and analgesia
- Head elevation
- Definitive reduction performed 3-7 days after injury (after swelling decreases but before healing begins)
- Some heal well without intervention

CSF rhinorrhea: If clear fluid drains from nose after facial trauma, suspect CSF leak (fracture through cribriform plate or ethmoid). Test fluid:

- Halo sign: Drop of fluid on gauze shows central blood spot with clear halo (CSF and blood separate)
- Beta-2 transferrin test: Lab test specific for CSF
- Glucose test: CSF contains glucose, but so does mucus (less reliable)

Management: Neurosurgery consultation, antibiotics to prevent meningitis, head elevation, avoid straining/nose blowing

Dental Trauma

Dental injuries range from minor chips to complete tooth avulsion. Proper immediate management can mean the difference between saving and losing a tooth.

Tooth Fractures

Ellis classification:

Class I: Enamel only

- Smooth fracture, no sensitivity
- Non-urgent dental follow-up
- Rough edges can be smoothed

Class II: Enamel and dentin exposed	Class III: Pulp exposed
• Yellow dentin visible • Tooth sensitive to air and temperature • Dental follow-up within 24 hours • Cover exposed dentin with calcium hydroxide paste or temporary filling material if available	• Pink pulp visible or bleeding from tooth • Severe pain and sensitivity • Urgent dental care needed (within hours) • Keep tooth moist, cover if possible • Antibiotics and pain management

Tooth Avulsion (Complete Tooth Knocked Out)

Time is critical—tooth survival depends on time outside socket:

Immediate management (at scene or ED):

1. **Find the tooth**—time matters
2. **Handle correctly:**
    - Hold by crown only (never touch root)
    - Don't scrub or remove attached tissue
    - Gently rinse if dirty (use saline or milk, not tap water)
3. **Reimplant immediately if possible:**
    - Best outcomes if reimplanted within 20 minutes
    - Rinse tooth and socket gently
    - Press tooth firmly into socket
    - Have patient bite on gauze to hold in place
    - Immediate dental referral
4. **If can't reimplant, preserve the tooth:**
    - Best: Place in socket (as above)
    - Second best: Place in Hank's Balanced Salt Solution (special preservation medium—some EDs stock it)
    - Good options: Cold milk, patient's saliva (have them hold in mouth against cheek)
    - Poor option but better than dry: Saline
    - Never: Tap water (damages root cells), dry storage

Why these fluids? The periodontal ligament cells on the tooth root must stay alive for successful reimplantation. Proper pH and osmolarity are critical. Milk has appropriate osmolarity. Saliva is acceptable. Tap water is hypotonic and kills cells.

In the ED:

- Reimplant if not already done (even hours later—worth attempting)
- Splint tooth to adjacent teeth
- Antibiotics (amoxicillin or penicillin)
- Tetanus if needed
- Pain management
- Soft diet
- Urgent dental follow-up

- Inform patient that root canal will likely be needed

Primary (baby) teeth: Don't reimplant (can damage permanent tooth bud). Dental follow-up to ensure permanent tooth development not affected.

Tooth Luxation

Tooth loosened or displaced but still in socket.

Types:

- **Subluxation:** Loose but in normal position
- **Extrusive luxation:** Tooth appears longer (partially out of socket)
- **Lateral luxation:** Tooth displaced to side
- **Intrusive luxation:** Tooth pushed into socket (appears shorter)

Management:

- Gently reposition if significantly displaced
- Splint to adjacent teeth
- Soft diet
- Dental follow-up
- May need root canal later

Alveolar Ridge Fracture

Segment of jaw containing teeth is fractured.

Clinical presentation:

- Multiple teeth move as unit
- Malocclusion
- Gingival laceration
- Palpable mobile bone segment

Management:

- Reposition segment
- Splinting
- Soft diet
- Antibiotics
- Maxillofacial surgery referral

Eye Injuries

Eye injuries range from minor corneal abrasions to devastating globe ruptures. Your assessment determines whether the patient keeps their vision.

Globe Rupture (Open Globe Injury)

A full-thickness injury to the cornea or sclera. This is an ophthalmologic emergency.

Mechanisms:

- High-velocity projectiles (hammering metal on metal, grinding)
- Sharp penetrating trauma
- Blunt trauma with high energy (can burst globe like grape)

Clinical presentation:

Obvious signs:

- Visible laceration of cornea or sclera
- Prolapsed iris (looks like dark tissue coming through defect)

- Prolapsed vitreous (looks like clear jelly)
- Irregular or peaked pupil (iris pulled toward laceration)
- Hyphema (blood in anterior chamber)
- Severe subconjunctival hemorrhage (may hide underlying rupture)
- Significantly decreased vision

Subtle signs (can look like simple injury):

- Shallow anterior chamber (compared to other eye—fluid leaked out)
- Soft eye (reduced intraocular pressure from fluid loss)
- Conjunctival hemorrhage hiding scleral rupture
- 360-degree subconjunctival hemorrhage (blood all around limbus suggests scleral rupture)

What NOT to do:

- **Don't press on the eye** (extrudes intraocular contents)
- **Don't attempt to remove foreign bodies**
- **Don't instill anything in eye** until ruled out
- **Don't allow patient to bend over or perform Valsalva** (increases intraocular pressure)

Management:

- Protect the eye immediately: rigid eye shield (Fox shield or bottom of paper cup—something that doesn't touch globe)
- NPO (going to OR)
- Head of bed elevated 30 degrees
- Avoid anything that increases IOP (straining, coughing, vomiting)
- Antiemetics if needed
- IV antibiotics (broad spectrum including coverage for Bacillus cereus if vegetative matter involved)
- Tetanus
- Pain management (avoid anything causing vomiting)
- Stat ophthalmology consultation
- Urgent surgical repair (primary closure)

Intraocular foreign body: If penetrating trauma suspected, imaging (CT) identifies foreign body. Never try to remove in ED—ophthalmology does this in OR with proper technique.

Hyphema

Blood in the anterior chamber (space between cornea and iris). Appears as layer of blood settling inferiorly when patient upright, or diffuse redness throughout chamber.

Causes:

- Blunt trauma (most common)
- Penetrating trauma
- Spontaneous (rare, in patients with bleeding disorders)

Grading:

- Grade I: <1/3 of anterior chamber
- Grade II: 1/3 to 1/2
- Grade III: >1/2 but not total
- Grade IV: Total (8-ball hyphema—entire chamber filled)

Why it matters:

- Can increase intraocular pressure (blood cells block drainage)
- Risk of rebleed (usually days 3-5 post-injury—worse than initial bleed)
- Blood staining of cornea if not treated
- Vision loss if IOP not controlled

Assessment:

- Visual acuity
- Examine with pen light (see layering of blood)
- Check IOP if equipment available (may be elevated)
- Rule out globe rupture before manipulating
- Assess for associated injuries (traumatic cataract, lens dislocation, retinal injury)

Management:

- Elevate head of bed 30-45 degrees (allows blood to settle away from visual axis)
- Eye shield (protect from further trauma)
- Limit activity (bed rest initially)
- Topical steroids (reduce inflammation)
- Cycloplegic drops (paralyze ciliary muscle, reduce pain)
- IOP control if elevated (topical medications, rarely systemic)
- Avoid antiplatelet agents/NSAIDs (increase rebleed risk)
- Ophthalmology follow-up (daily initially to monitor for rebleed and elevated IOP)
- Admit for observation if:
    - Large hyphema (grade III-IV)
    - Elevated IOP
    - Sickle cell trait or disease (higher complication risk)
    - Poor compliance anticipated

Complications:

- Rebleeding (3-5 days post-injury)
- Glaucoma (acute or chronic)
- Corneal blood staining
- Vision loss

Retrobulbar Hematoma and Orbital Compartment Syndrome

Blood accumulates behind the globe in the confined orbital space, increasing pressure and compromising optic nerve blood supply. This causes blindness if not immediately relieved.

Causes:

- Orbital fractures
- Penetrating trauma to orbit
- Severe blunt periorbital trauma
- Retrobulbar injections (iatrogenic)

Clinical presentation:

- **Proptosis** (eye pushed forward out of socket—compare to other side)
- **Tense, firm eyelids** (swollen and hard to touch)
- **Severe eye pain**
- **Decreased visual acuity or loss of vision**
- **Afferent pupillary defect** (pupil doesn't constrict appropriately when light shined in that eye)
- **Ophthalmoplegia** (can't move eye—muscles compressed)
- **Increased IOP** (>40 mmHg)

This is an emergency: Minutes matter for saving vision.

Management:

Immediate (if ophthalmology not immediately available):

Lateral canthotomy and cantholysis (ED procedure to decompress orbit):

1. Anesthetize lateral canthus (1% lidocaine with epinephrine)
2. Clamp lateral canthus with hemostat for 1-2 minutes (achieve hemostasis)
3. Cut through full thickness of clamped tissue with scissors (canthotomy—opens lateral corner of eyelid)
4. Grasp lower lid, pull away from globe
5. Identify inferior canthal tendon (feels like guitar string)
6. Cut inferior canthal tendon (cantholysis—releases lower lid completely)
7. This decompresses orbit by allowing eye to move forward

Goal: Drop IOP and improve optic nerve perfusion. Effect should be immediate if successful.

Additional measures:

- Elevate head of bed
- Mannitol 1-2 g/kg IV (osmotic agent reduces swelling)
- Acetazolamide (reduces aqueous humor production)
- Stat ophthalmology consultation
- Consider steroids
- Prepare for OR drainage if no improvement

Key concept: Don't wait for ophthalmology if vision threatened and they're not immediately available. Lateral canthotomy/cantholysis is sight-saving and must be done urgently.

Corneal Abrasion

Scratch or defect in corneal epithelium. Common and painful but usually not vision-threatening.

Mechanisms:

- Foreign body (dust, dirt, contact lens)
- Fingernail scratch
- Tree branch
- Welding without proper eye protection (UV burn)

Clinical presentation:

- Severe eye pain (cornea is exquisitely sensitive)
- Foreign body sensation ("something in my eye")
- Tearing
- Photophobia (light hurts)
- Blepharospasm (can't keep eye open)

Assessment:

- Visual acuity (usually normal or mildly decreased)
- Fluorescein staining: Apply fluorescein drops, examine with cobalt blue light—abrasion lights up bright green
- Evert upper eyelid to check for foreign body (often hidden under lid)
- Check for penetrating injury (be sure it's just superficial abrasion)

Management:

- Remove foreign body if present (irrigation or cotton swab)
- Topical antibiotic ointment or drops (erythromycin or polymyxin-bacitracin)
- Pain management (topical NSAIDs like ketorolac effective; oral analgesics)
- **No topical anesthetics for home use** (delay healing, can cause corneal damage)
- **No eye patching** (doesn't improve healing, increases infection risk)
- Follow-up in 24-48 hours
- Contact lens wearers: Pseudomonas coverage (fluoroquinolone), no lens wear until healed

Healing: Most corneal abrasions heal in 24-48 hours. Epithelium regenerates quickly.

Red flags suggesting more serious injury:

- Vision loss beyond what pain/tearing explain
- Deep or large abrasion
- Central location (over pupil)
- Associated trauma mechanism suggesting penetration
- Rust ring (metallic foreign body left rust deposit—needs removal)

Chemical Burns

Chemical exposure to eyes is an emergency requiring immediate treatment.

Types:

- **Alkali burns** (drain cleaner, cement, lye): Worse than acids—penetrate deeper, liquefy tissues, continue damaging for hours
- **Acid burns** (battery acid, pool chemicals): Painful but usually less severe—coagulate proteins, limiting penetration

Immediate management—Time is vision:

Copious irrigation:

- Start immediately—don't wait for anything
- Use normal saline or lactated Ringer's (if unavailable, tap water is acceptable—don't delay)
- Topical anesthetic first (allows patient to open eye)
- Remove contact lenses if present
- Evert eyelids and irrigate fornices (chemicals hide in crevices)
- Minimum 30 minutes continuous irrigation (alkali burns may need hours)
- Check pH after irrigation (normal is 7.0-7.4)—continue until normalized

- If solid chemical particles visible, remove them (they continue releasing chemical)

After irrigation:

- Check visual acuity
- Fluorescein to assess corneal damage
- Examine for conjunctival blanching (white areas where blood supply destroyed—very poor prognostic sign)
- Assess anterior chamber for inflammation
- Check IOP

Management:

- Continue irrigation if pH not normalized
- Topical antibiotics
- Cycloplegic drops (reduce ciliary spasm pain)
- Topical steroids (controversial—may use initially then stop to avoid delayed healing)
- Pain management
- Urgent ophthalmology consultation
- Admit for severe burns

Prognosis:

- Mild burns: Full recovery expected
- Moderate burns: May have some scarring
- Severe burns: Risk of vision loss, corneal opacity, glaucoma, symblepharon (scarring between lid and globe)

Ear, Nose, and Throat Trauma

Auricular Hematoma (Cauliflower Ear)

Blood collection between perichondrium and cartilage of external ear, usually from blunt trauma.

Why it matters:

- Cartilage gets blood supply from perichondrium
- Hematoma separates cartilage from blood supply
- Cartilage dies and becomes fibrotic
- Results in "cauliflower ear" deformity (permanent if not drained)

Clinical presentation:

- Fluctuant swelling of ear (usually on anterior surface)
- History of trauma (boxing, wrestling, assault)
- Pain

Management:

- Drain hematoma (incision and drainage or needle aspiration)
- Apply pressure dressing to prevent reaccumulation (dental rolls or cotton secured with through-and-through sutures)
- Antibiotics (perichondritis can occur)
- ENT follow-up in 24-48 hours

- Re-drain if reaccumulates

If untreated: Permanent deformity as cartilage dies and scars.

Tympanic Membrane Perforation

Hole in eardrum from trauma.

Mechanisms:

- Direct: Cotton swab, pencil, bobby pin inserted in ear
- Blast injury: Explosion creates pressure wave
- Barotrauma: Diving, flying with URI
- Temporal bone fracture

Clinical presentation:

- Hearing loss (conductive)
- Ear pain (initially, often improves after perforation)
- Bloody otorrhea (drainage from ear)
- Tinnitus (ringing)
- Vertigo (if ossicles or inner ear involved)

Assessment:

- Otoscopic exam: visualize perforation
- Hearing assessment (whisper test, tuning forks)
- Check for CSF otorrhea (clear fluid suggests temporal bone fracture with dural tear)
- Assess facial nerve function (temporal bone fracture can injure facial nerve)

Management:

- Keep ear dry (no water)
- Antibiotics if contaminated or CSF leak present
- Pain management
- No ear drops unless specifically prescribed (some are ototoxic if they reach middle ear)
- ENT follow-up
- Most perforations heal spontaneously (4-8 weeks)
- Tympanoplasty if doesn't heal

Epistaxis (Nosebleed)

Common presentation, usually from anterior nasal septum (Kiesselbach's plexus).

Anterior versus posterior bleeding:

Anterior (90%):

- Usually visible bleeding from nostril
- Bleeding site often visible on septal mucosa
- Easier to control

Posterior (10%):

- Blood drains posteriorly into pharynx
- Patient swallows or spits blood
- More difficult to control
- More common in elderly, hypertensives

Initial management:

1. **Position:** Sit upright, lean forward (prevents swallowing blood)
2. **Pinch nose:** Continuous pressure on soft part of nose for 10-15 minutes (actually time it)
3. **Topical vasoconstrictors:** Oxymetazoline (Afrin) or

phenylephrine on cotton pledget inserted in nose
4. **Ice:** To bridge of nose (questionable efficacy but traditional)

If initial measures fail:

Anterior packing:

- Petroleum gauze or nasal tampon (Rapid Rhino, Merocel)
- Leave 2-3 days
- Antibiotics while packed (prevent toxic shock syndrome)

Posterior packing:

- Foley catheter inserted in nose, inflated in nasopharynx, pulled forward to tamponade
- Or commercial posterior packing devices
- Requires admission (can cause hypoxia, arrhythmias)
- Very uncomfortable

ENT consultation if:

- Can't control with packing
- Recurrent severe bleeds
- Posterior packing needed

Definitive treatment for refractory cases:

- Cauterization (silver nitrate or electrocautery)
- Arterial ligation (rare)
- Angiographic embolization

Chapter 9 Practice Questions

Question 1: A patient presents with malocclusion, drooling, and numbness of the lower lip after assault. What injury do these findings suggest?

A) Nasal fracture
B) Mandible fracture
C) Maxillary fracture
D) Zygomatic fracture

Answer: B

Explanation: Malocclusion (teeth don't fit together properly), drooling (difficulty managing secretions due to pain), and lower lip numbness (inferior alveolar nerve injury) are classic signs of mandible fracture. Patients immediately notice when their bite feels wrong.

Question 2: When testing for Le Fort fractures, you should grasp the upper teeth and attempt to move the maxilla. If the entire face moves, this indicates:

A) Le Fort I
B) Le Fort II
C) Le Fort III
D) No fracture

Answer: C

Explanation: Le Fort III (craniofacial separation) presents with the entire midface mobile when upper teeth are grasped and pulled. Le Fort I shows only palate/teeth mobile; Le Fort II shows nose and upper jaw mobile together. This test helps classify severity.

Question 3: A patient has an orbital floor fracture with diplopia when looking upward and numbness of the cheek. These findings indicate:

A) Optic nerve injury
B) Inferior rectus muscle entrapment and infraorbital nerve injury
C) Superior rectus muscle injury
D) Zygomatic arch fracture

Answer: B

Explanation: Diplopia with upward gaze indicates inferior rectus muscle entrapment in the orbital floor fracture. Cheek numbness indicates infraorbital nerve injury (nerve runs in the orbital floor). These are classic findings of orbital blowout fracture.

Question 4: What is the immediate management priority for suspected globe rupture?

A) Visual acuity testing
B) Tonometry to check intraocular pressure
C) Protect eye with rigid shield without applying pressure
D) Irrigate eye thoroughly

Answer: C

Explanation: Suspected globe rupture requires immediate eye protection with a rigid shield (Fox shield or paper cup bottom) that doesn't touch the globe. Never apply pressure, instill medications, or perform tonometry as these can extrude intraocular contents. Visual acuity can be checked if it doesn't require manipulating the eye.

Question 5: A patient has a tooth completely knocked out. The best storage medium until reimplantation is:

A) Tap water
B) Cold milk or Hank's solution
C) Dry gauze
D) Alcohol

Answer: B

Explanation: Cold milk or Hank's Balanced Salt Solution best preserve periodontal ligament cells on the tooth root. These fluids have appropriate pH and osmolarity. Tap water is hypotonic and kills cells. Dry storage destroys cells quickly. Alcohol damages tissue. The tooth should be reimplanted within 20 minutes for best outcomes.

Question 6: Septal hematoma is a complication of nasal fracture that requires immediate drainage to prevent:

A) Epistaxis
B) CSF leak
C) Saddle nose deformity from cartilage necrosis
D) Vision loss

Answer: C

Explanation: Septal hematoma separates cartilage from its blood supply (perichondrium), causing avascular necrosis. The cartilage dies and collapses, resulting in permanent saddle nose deformity. Immediate incision and drainage prevents this complication.

Question 7: A patient with orbital trauma develops proptosis, severe eye pain, decreased vision, and a tense orbit. This indicates:

A) Simple orbital fracture
B) Retrobulbar hematoma requiring immediate decompression
C) Corneal abrasion
D) Conjunctivitis

Answer: B

Explanation: Retrobulbar hematoma causes orbital compartment syndrome with proptosis (eye pushed forward), tense orbit, pain, and vision loss. This is an emergency requiring immediate lateral canthotomy and cantholysis to decompress the orbit and save vision. Minutes matter for preventing permanent blindness.

Question 8: Which Le Fort fracture represents complete craniofacial separation?

A) Le Fort I
B) Le Fort II
C) Le Fort III

D) All Le Fort fractures separate the face from skull

Answer: C

Explanation: Le Fort III represents complete separation of the entire midface from the cranium. When you grasp the upper teeth and pull, the entire face moves. This is the most severe Le Fort fracture, often requiring intubation and frequently associated with severe head injury and CSF leaks.

Question 9: A chemical splash to the eye requires:

A) Immediate ophthalmology consultation before treatment
B) Immediate copious irrigation for at least 30 minutes
C) Application of neutralizing agent
D) Eye patching and observation

Answer: B

Explanation: Chemical eye injuries require immediate copious irrigation with saline, LR, or even tap water if nothing else available. Don't wait for anything—start irrigating immediately. Continue for at least 30 minutes and until pH normalized. Alkali burns may need hours of irrigation. Time is vision.

Question 10: Hyphema is blood in the:

A) Vitreous humor
B) Anterior chamber
C) Posterior chamber
D) Subconjunctival space

Answer: B

Explanation: Hyphema is blood in the anterior chamber (space between cornea and iris). It appears as a layer of blood settling inferiorly when the patient is upright or diffuse redness throughout the chamber. Complications include increased IOP, rebleeding, and corneal blood staining.

Question 11: The most common facial bone fracture is:

A) Mandible
B) Nasal bone
C) Zygoma
D) Maxilla

Answer: B

Explanation: Nasal fractures are the most common facial fractures due to the nose's prominent, unprotected position. Mandible is the most commonly fractured facial bone requiring surgery, but nasal fractures occur more frequently overall. Most nasal fractures don't require immediate treatment.

Question 12: A patient with mandible fracture reports that their teeth "don't fit together right." This describes:

A) Trismus
B) Malocclusion
C) Subluxation
D) Ankylosis

Answer: B

Explanation: Malocclusion means the teeth don't occlude (fit together) properly. Patients with mandible fractures immediately notice this abnormality and will report that their bite feels wrong. This is one of the most reliable signs of jaw fracture.

Question 13: Which statement about tooth avulsion is correct?

A) Primary teeth should be reimplanted
B) Handle the tooth by the root for cleaning
C) Reimplant immediately or store in milk
D) Scrub the tooth thoroughly before reimplanting

Answer: C

Explanation: Avulsed permanent teeth should be reimplanted immediately (within 20 minutes) or stored in cold milk, Hank's solution, or saliva. Never touch the root, scrub the tooth, or use tap water for storage. Primary (baby) teeth should NOT be reimplanted as this can damage the permanent tooth bud.

Question 14: A white-eyed blowout fracture in a child is concerning because:

A) It indicates no significant injury
B) The muscle can be trapped causing severe complications requiring urgent surgery
C) It always requires immediate enucleation
D) It indicates globe rupture

Answer: B

Explanation: White-eyed blowout fractures in children occur when the elastic pediatric bone fractures like a trapdoor, trapping the extraocular muscle with minimal external signs. This causes severe nausea, vomiting, bradycardia (oculocardiac reflex), and requires surgery within 24-48 hours to prevent permanent muscle damage.

Question 15: CSF rhinorrhea after facial trauma suggests:

A) Simple nasal fracture
B) Fracture through cribriform plate or skull base
C) Sinus infection
D) Severe epistaxis

Answer: B

Explanation: Clear fluid draining from nose after trauma suggests CSF leak from fracture through the cribriform plate or skull base. This requires neurosurgery consultation, antibiotics to prevent meningitis, and avoiding nose blowing or straining. Test fluid with halo sign or beta-2 transferrin.

Question 16: Management of corneal abrasion includes all EXCEPT:

A) Topical antibiotic
B) Topical anesthetic for home use
C) Fluorescein staining for diagnosis
D) Pain management

Answer: B

Explanation: Never prescribe topical anesthetics for home use—they delay healing and can cause severe corneal damage. Corneal abrasions need topical antibiotics, pain management (topical NSAIDs or oral analgesics), and follow-up in 24-48 hours. Eye patching is no longer recommended.

Question 17: Auricular hematoma requires drainage to prevent:

A) Hearing loss
B) Infection
C) Permanent cauliflower ear deformity
D) Tympanic membrane rupture

Answer: C

Explanation: Auricular hematoma separates cartilage from its blood supply (perichondrium), causing cartilage death and fibrosis that creates permanent cauliflower ear deformity. Immediate drainage and pressure dressing prevent this. If left untreated, the deformity is permanent.

Question 18: A patient has an orbital fracture with diplopia when looking upward. The affected muscle is most likely:

A) Superior rectus
B) Inferior rectus
C) Medial rectus
D) Lateral rectus

Answer: B

Explanation: Diplopia with upward gaze indicates inferior rectus muscle entrapment in an orbital floor fracture. The muscle gets caught in the fracture, restricting upward eye movement. This is a classic finding of orbital blowout fracture.

Question 19: The primary reason alkali burns are more serious than acid burns to the eye is:

A) Alkalis are more painful
B) Alkalis penetrate deeper and continue damaging tissue
C) Acids require surgery
D) Alkalis cause immediate blindness

Answer: B

Explanation: Alkali burns penetrate deeper into ocular tissues and continue causing damage for hours by liquefying proteins. Acid burns coagulate proteins, limiting penetration. Alkali burns (drain cleaner, cement, lye) require prolonged irrigation and have worse prognosis than acid burns.

Question 20: A patient with mandible fracture has bilateral body fractures. The primary airway concern is:

A) Laryngeal edema
B) Tongue falling backward due to loss of floor of mouth support
C) Nasal obstruction
D) Foreign body aspiration

Answer: B

Explanation: Bilateral mandible body fractures destabilize the floor of the mouth, allowing the tongue to fall backward and obstruct the airway. This is the primary airway concern with this fracture pattern. Position patient upright, consider jaw thrust, and prepare for possible intubation.

Question 21: Hyphema patients are at risk for rebleeding, which typically occurs:

A) Within the first 6 hours
B) Days 3-5 post-injury
C) After 2 weeks
D) Rebleeding doesn't occur

Answer: B

Explanation: Hyphema rebleeding typically occurs 3-5 days post-injury and is often worse than the initial bleed. This is why patients need close ophthalmology follow-up during this period. Avoid antiplatelet agents and NSAIDs that increase rebleed risk.

Question 22: The infraorbital nerve runs through the orbital floor. Injury causes:

A) Vision loss
B) Inability to close eye
C) Numbness of cheek, upper lip, and side of nose
D) Ptosis

Answer: C

Explanation: The infraorbital nerve provides sensation to the cheek, upper lip, and side of nose. Orbital floor fractures often injure this nerve, causing numbness in these areas. This is a classic finding helping diagnose orbital floor fractures.

Question 23: Which finding indicates a tooth fracture has exposed the pulp (Ellis Class III)?

A) Rough enamel edge
B) Yellow dentin visible
C) Pink tissue visible or bleeding from tooth
D) Tooth mobility

Answer: C

Explanation: Pink pulp visible or bleeding from the tooth indicates Ellis Class III fracture with pulp exposure. This requires urgent dental care within hours. Class I shows only enamel damage; Class II exposes yellow dentin. Pulp exposure is painful and risks infection.

Question 24: A patient cannot open their mouth fully after zygomatic arch fracture. This is caused by:

A) Masseter muscle spasm
B) Fractured arch impinging on coronoid process/temporalis muscle
C) TMJ dislocation
D) Facial nerve injury

Answer: B

Explanation: Zygomatic arch fractures cause limited jaw opening (trismus) because the depressed fractured arch impinges on the coronoid process of the mandible and temporalis muscle during jaw opening. This mechanical obstruction limits movement.

Question 25: Lateral canthotomy and cantholysis is performed for:

A) Ectropion repair
B) Retrobulbar hematoma decompression
C) Globe rupture repair
D) Corneal transplant

Answer: B

Explanation: Lateral canthotomy (cutting lateral corner of eyelid) and cantholysis (releasing inferior canthal tendon) decompress the orbit in retrobulbar hematoma/orbital compartment syndrome. This emergent procedure can be performed in the ED to save vision when ophthalmology isn't immediately available.

Question 26: Tympanic membrane perforation requires which instruction?

A) Use ear drops three times daily
B) Keep ear dry—no swimming or water exposure
C) Clean ear canal daily with cotton swabs
D) Apply heat to affected ear

Answer: B

Explanation: Keep ear dry with tympanic membrane perforation to prevent infection. No swimming, showering should protect ear from water, no ear drops unless specifically prescribed (some are ototoxic if they reach middle ear). Most perforations heal spontaneously in 4-8 weeks.

Question 27: A patient with facial trauma has clear fluid draining from the nose. The halo sign test involves:

A) Shining light through nose to see fluid
B) Placing drop of fluid on gauze to see if blood and CSF separate
C) Testing fluid pH
D) Culturing the fluid

Answer: B

Explanation: The halo sign (or target sign) appears when a drop of bloody fluid is placed on gauze or filter paper. CSF and blood separate, showing a central blood spot with a clear halo around it. This suggests CSF leak, though beta-2 transferrin testing is more specific.

Question 28: Which injury commonly occurs with posterior hip dislocation but is also seen with mandibular fractures?

A) Sciatic nerve injury and inferior alveolar nerve injury respectively
B) Femoral nerve injury and facial nerve injury
C) Obturator nerve injury and hypoglossal nerve injury
D) Common peroneal nerve and glossopharyngeal nerve

Answer: A

Explanation: Posterior hip dislocations risk sciatic nerve injury. Mandible fractures risk inferior alveolar nerve injury (causing lower lip numbness). Understanding nerve-injury patterns helps you anticipate and assess for specific neurological deficits with certain fractures.

Question 29: A patient has significant facial swelling 24 hours after Le Fort II fracture. The priority intervention is:

A) Ice application only
B) Monitor airway closely and prepare for possible intubation
C) Immediate surgical repair
D) Discharge with follow-up

Answer: B

Explanation: Facial swelling from Le Fort fractures can progress and compromise the airway. Close airway monitoring is essential, with low threshold for early intubation before swelling makes it difficult or impossible. Don't wait until the patient is in distress—act early.

Question 30: The most important factor determining success of tooth reimplantation is:

A) Patient's age
B) Time out of socket (ideally <20 minutes)
C) Tooth cleaning technique
D) Antibiotic choice

Answer: B

Explanation: Time is the most critical factor for tooth reimplantation success. Periodontal ligament cells on the root die quickly when dry. Best outcomes occur with reimplantation within 20 minutes. After 2 hours, success rates drop dramatically. This is why immediate action at the scene is crucial.

Clinical Scenarios

Clinical Scenario 1: Complex Facial Fractures with Airway Compromise

A 28-year-old male arrives after high-speed motor vehicle crash. He was unrestrained and struck the windshield with his face. He's sitting upright, leaning forward, drooling blood-tinged saliva. His face is massively swollen with obvious deformity. You note bilateral periorbital ecchymosis ("raccoon eyes") and blood draining from both nostrils.

Vitals: HR 108, BP 142/88, RR 24, SpO2 94% on non-rebreather mask. He's anxious and having difficulty speaking. When he tries to talk, his words are muffled and unclear.

Questions:

1. Based on the presentation, what facial fracture pattern do you suspect?
2. What is your most immediate concern and why?
3. How do you assess for midface fractures in this patient?
4. The patient's oxygen saturation drops to 88% and his respiratory effort increases. What interventions should you prepare for and why?

Answers:

1. **Suspected fracture pattern:** This presentation strongly suggests **Le Fort II or III fractures** based on:
    - High-energy mechanism (unrestrained, windshield impact)
    - Massive facial swelling
    - Raccoon eyes (periorbital ecchymosis suggests skull base involvement)
    - Epistaxis from both nostrils (midface fractures communicate with sinuses)
    - Facial deformity
    - Speech difficulty (structural disruption affecting articulation)

    The bilateral periorbital ecchymosis particularly suggests Le Fort III or associated skull base fractures. The massive swelling ("beaten with baseball bat" appearance) is classic for severe midface trauma.

2. **Most immediate concern—Airway:**

    This patient has multiple signs of impending airway compromise:

    - Sitting upright, leaning forward (tripod positioning indicates respiratory distress)
    - Drooling (can't manage secretions—either too painful or anatomically can't swallow)
    - Blood in posterior pharynx (from epistaxis)
    - Massive facial swelling (can progress to obstruct nasopharynx/oropharynx)
    - Muffled speech (airway narrowing or structural disruption)
    - Increased work of breathing (tachypnea, increased effort)
    - Oxygen requirement despite supplemental oxygen

    Why airway is critical in midface fractures:

    - Displaced bone fragments can narrow or obstruct airway
    - Blood pools in posterior pharynx
    - Progressive swelling continues for 24-48 hours
    - Le Fort fractures can destabilize facial structure, making bag-mask ventilation ineffective
    - Once airway lost, it may be impossible to regain with traditional methods

    Key principle: Secure the airway early, before it becomes impossible. Don't wait for complete obstruction—by then you've lost your window.

3. **Assessing for midface fractures:**

    Inspection:

    - Facial symmetry and contour (note deformities)
    - Periorbital ecchymosis, subconjunctival hemorrhage
    - Epistaxis (suggests sinus involvement)
    - Clear nasal drainage (CSF rhinorrhea from skull base fracture)
    - Dish-face deformity (midface retrusion)

Palpation:

- Palpate facial bones for step-offs, crepitus, mobility
- Check orbital rims for irregularities
- Assess zygomatic arches

Midface mobility test (key diagnostic maneuver):

- Explain procedure to patient
- Wearing gloves, grasp upper central incisors firmly
- Gently attempt to move maxilla forward and back
- Observe what moves:
  - **Normal:** Firm, no movement
  - **Le Fort I:** Only upper teeth/palate move
  - **Le Fort II:** Nose and upper jaw move together as pyramid
  - **Le Fort III:** Entire midface moves separately from cranium

However, in this patient: Given massive swelling, testing may be difficult and findings unreliable. Also, aggressive manipulation risks worsening fractures or causing more bleeding. Clinical suspicion based on mechanism, appearance, and associated findings may be sufficient for initial management decisions.

Additional assessments:

- Examine for CSF leak (halo sign if bloody drainage present)
- Assess vision and extraocular movements (orbital involvement common)
- Check for skull base fracture signs (Battle's sign, hemotympanum)
- Neurological exam (often have associated head injury)

4. **Deteriorating respiratory status—Immediate interventions:**

Desaturation to 88% with increased work of breathing indicates impending airway failure. Prepare for:

First-line: Rapid sequence intubation (RSI):

- Call for most experienced intubator available (anesthesia, ED attending, or ICU)
- Prepare all equipment: multiple laryngoscope blades, video laryngoscopy if available, multiple ET tube sizes, stylet, bougie
- Preoxygenate maximally
- Position patient optimally (may need to remain upright initially due to blood/secretions)
- Have suction ready (massive amounts likely needed)
- Medications ready for RSI

Intubation challenges anticipated:

- Massive swelling distorts anatomy
- Blood obscures view

- Displaced fractures alter normal landmarks
- Bag-mask ventilation may be ineffective (no stable facial structure to seal against)

Backup plan: Surgical airway (have equipment ready):

- If oral intubation fails, will need immediate cricothyrotomy
- Equipment prepped and within reach
- Someone designated to perform if needed
- Don't attempt multiple intubations—if first attempt fails and patient deteriorating, proceed to surgical airway

Why surgical airway may be necessary:

- Facial fractures can make traditional intubation impossible
- Bleeding and swelling obscure view
- Anatomical disruption prevents normal intubation landmarks
- Can't ventilate with bag-mask due to facial instability

Immediate actions while preparing:

- Keep patient upright if tolerated (helps drain blood/secretions forward)
- Continuous suction available
- 100% oxygen
- Have patient lean forward to allow drainage
- Minimize agitation (worsens oxygen consumption and bleeding)
- Consider small dose of anxiolytic if time permits and patient not hypoxic

After securing airway:

- Obtain facial CT scan to define fractures
- Neurosurgery evaluation for CSF leak
- Maxillofacial surgery consultation
- Ophthalmology if orbital involvement
- Continued airway protection (likely needs to stay intubated through acute swelling phase)

Key learning points:

- Le Fort fractures create unique airway challenges requiring early intervention
- Don't wait for complete obstruction—secure airway when you anticipate problems
- Have backup plan (surgical airway) ready before attempting intubation
- Massive facial swelling indicates high-energy trauma warranting evaluation for other injuries
- Clear nasal drainage after facial trauma = CSF leak until proven otherwise

Clinical Scenario 2: Globe Rupture with Penetrating Injury

A 35-year-old construction worker was using a hammer and chisel when a metal fragment struck his right eye. He reports immediate severe pain and vision loss. He's holding a towel over his eye.

On examination, after gently removing the towel, you see severe subconjunctival hemorrhage, a peaked pupil pointing toward the 10 o'clock position, and what appears to be dark tissue (possibly iris) visible in a small laceration at the corneal-scleral junction.

Vitals: HR 96, BP 138/84, RR 16, SpO_2 98%. Patient is alert, in pain, but cooperative.

Questions:

1. What injury has occurred and what findings support this diagnosis?
2. What should you absolutely NOT do in your assessment or management?
3. What immediate interventions are necessary?
4. The patient asks about his prognosis for vision. How do you respond?

Answers:

1. **Diagnosis: Open globe injury (globe rupture) with possible intraocular foreign body**

Findings supporting this diagnosis:

- **Mechanism:** High-velocity metal fragment from hammering (classic for penetrating eye injury and intraocular foreign body)
- **Immediate severe vision loss:** Suggests serious injury to globe
- **Peaked pupil pointing toward laceration:** Iris is pulled toward the defect, classic sign of globe rupture
- **Visible dark tissue in wound:** Likely prolapsed iris tissue coming through the laceration
- **Corneal-scleral junction laceration:** This is the actual full-thickness penetrating injury
- **Severe subconjunctival hemorrhage:** Can hide underlying scleral rupture; 360-degree hemorrhage particularly suspicious

Additional findings you might see with globe rupture:

- Shallow anterior chamber (aqueous humor leaked out)
- Hyphema (blood in anterior chamber)
- Prolapsed vitreous (clear jelly-like material)
- Soft eye (reduced IOP from fluid loss)
- Visible foreign body penetrating globe

Why this mechanism is high-risk: Metal-on-metal hammering creates high-velocity fragments that easily penetrate the eye. These injuries often have intraocular foreign bodies requiring removal. Any "hammering metal on metal" or grinding without eye protection should raise immediate suspicion for penetrating eye injury.

2. **What absolutely NOT to do:**

DO NOT:

- **Press on or palpate the globe:** Extrudes intraocular contents through the rupture
- **Attempt to remove any foreign body:** Removed in OR by ophthalmology under controlled conditions
- **Measure intraocular pressure:** Tonometry applies pressure to globe
- **Instill any drops or ointment:** Until globe rupture ruled out
- **Apply direct pressure to eye:** Use rigid shield only
- **Irrigate the eye:** Can worsen injury
- **Evert eyelids aggressively:** Gentle examination only
- **Perform detailed eye examination:** Basic assessment only until ophthalmology present
- **Allow patient to bend over, strain, or Valsalva:** Increases IOP and extrudes contents

Rationale: Any pressure on a ruptured globe can extrude intraocular contents (iris, lens, vitreous, retina) through the defect, worsening injury and reducing chance of vision preservation.

3. **Immediate interventions:**

Protect the eye:

- Apply rigid eye shield immediately (Fox shield or improvise with bottom of paper cup)
- Shield must not touch globe
- Tape securely but avoid pressure
- Protect from any further trauma

Patient positioning and activity:

- Elevate head of bed 30 degrees
- Keep patient calm and still
- Strict bed rest
- No bending, straining, or Valsalva
- Limit movement and talking if possible

Prevent increased IOP:

- Antiemetics if any nausea (vomiting increases IOP)
- Pain control (but avoid medications that cause nausea)
- Keep patient calm (anxiety increases IOP)
- Avoid anything causing coughing or straining

Medical management:

- NPO immediately (going to OR)
- IV access
- **Broad-spectrum IV antibiotics:**
    - Vancomycin (gram-positive coverage including MRSA)
    - Ceftazidime or fluoroquinolone (gram-negative coverage)
    - If vegetative matter involved: Add coverage for Bacillus cereus
- Tetanus prophylaxis if needed
- Pain management (IV opioids, avoid NSAIDs until ophthalmology clears)

Consultations and diagnostics:

- STAT ophthalmology consultation (this is a true emergency)
- CT scan of orbits (identifies intraocular foreign body, extent of injury)
    - **Important:** Patient must remain still during CT
    - Get images in both axial and coronal planes
    - Thin cuts through orbits
- Do NOT get MRI if metallic foreign body suspected (magnet will move metal fragment, causing further damage)

Surgical preparation:

- Consent for emergency surgery
- OR team notification
- Anticipate primary closure of globe, possible foreign body removal, possible vitrectomy

Documentation:

- Visual acuity if possible without touching eye (may only be able to document light perception or hand motion)
- Detailed description of injury
- Mechanism documentation (important for ophthalmology surgical planning)
- Time of injury
- Photos if possible without manipulating eye

4. **Prognosis discussion with patient:**

Provide honest but supportive information:

"I know you're worried about your vision, and that's completely understandable. What happened is a serious injury to your eye—we call it an open globe injury, which means the wall of your eye has been penetrated. There also may be a small piece of metal inside your eye from the chisel.

Immediate plan: The eye specialist is on their way now, and you'll need emergency surgery to repair your eye. The surgeon will close the opening in your eye and remove any foreign material. This surgery needs to happen as soon as possible—we're treating this as an emergency.

About your vision: It's too early to know exactly what your final vision will be. Several factors affect the outcome:

- The location and extent of the injury
- Whether important structures like the lens or retina are damaged
- How quickly we get you to surgery (you're getting excellent care quickly, which helps)
- Whether infection develops (we're giving antibiotics to prevent this)
- Any damage from the metal fragment

Possible outcomes:

- Best case: With successful surgery and healing, some people recover good vision
- Some people have partial vision recovery—enough to function but not perfect
- In severe cases, despite our best efforts, vision may be significantly limited
- The eye specialist will be able to give you more specific information after examining you and seeing what's found during surgery

What we know: Getting you to treatment quickly gives you the best chance for a good outcome. You did the right thing coming in immediately and not touching or rubbing your eye. The specialist will do everything possible to save your vision.

What happens next: You'll have surgery today. After surgery, you'll need close follow-up with the eye specialist, probably multiple visits over the coming weeks. There may be additional procedures needed depending on what's found.

I know this is scary and not the answer you were hoping for, but I want you to know you're in good hands, we're moving quickly, and we're doing everything possible to give you the best outcome."

Key communication points:

- Be honest about uncertainty
- Provide realistic expectations without destroying hope
- Emphasize rapid, appropriate treatment occurring
- Explain why immediate surgery is necessary
- Prepare for possibility of poor outcome while noting possibility of recovery
- Acknowledge emotional impact
- Demonstrate care team is coordinated and acting quickly

Follow-up the conversation might include:

- Occupational injury implications (worker's compensation, safety equipment discussion)
- Importance of eye protection (prevent injury to other eye)
- Family notification and support
- Resources for coping with potential vision loss if outcome is poor

This scenario emphasizes the critical nature of open globe injuries, importance of avoiding any pressure on the eye, and need for immediate ophthalmologic surgical intervention. The prognosis discussion demonstrates how to provide honest information while maintaining hope and showing empathy for the patient's situation.

Clinical Scenario 3: Dental Avulsion in Child

An 8-year-old boy arrives after being hit in the mouth with a baseball. His mother brings him in with the tooth wrapped in a paper towel. The incident occurred about 30 minutes ago at a baseball field 15 minutes away. The tooth appears to be a permanent central incisor, and it's completely out of the socket. The boy is crying, blood is coming from the socket, and his mother is very anxious.

On examination, there's an empty socket where the right central incisor should be. The tooth is intact, with root visible, and has been wrapped dry in the paper towel.

Questions:

1. What are your immediate actions regarding the tooth and socket?
2. The mother asks if this tooth will be okay or if it's lost. What factors determine success?
3. How do you manage this case from dental perspective?
4. What education do you provide to prevent future dental trauma?

Answers:

1. **Immediate actions for tooth and socket:**

Assess the tooth:

- Inspect to confirm it's a permanent tooth (check with mother—at age 8, likely permanent central incisor)
- Examine tooth for fractures or damage
- Note: Root appears intact, which is good
- Problem: Tooth has been stored dry in paper towel for 30 minutes

Handle the tooth properly:

- Pick up tooth by crown only (never touch the root—damages periodontal ligament cells)
- DO NOT scrub, clean, or remove tissue from root
- Gently rinse tooth if dirty: Use saline or milk (NOT tap water which is hypotonic and kills cells)
- Keep root moist at all times from this point forward

Prepare the socket:

- Gently irrigate socket with saline to remove any blood clot and debris
- Do NOT curette or scrub socket (destroys remaining periodontal ligament cells in socket)

- Ensure no bone fragments or foreign material in socket
- Control bleeding if excessive (gentle pressure with gauze)

Reimplant the tooth immediately:

Even though 30 minutes dry time has passed, reimplantation should still be attempted:

Technique:

- Ensure tooth is oriented correctly (convex surface faces forward)
- Gently but firmly press tooth into socket
- Tooth should seat fully to level of adjacent teeth
- Have patient (or parent) hold tooth in place by gently biting on gauze
- If tooth won't seat easily:
    - Check for clot in socket (remove with irrigation)
    - Check for bone fragment (may need gentle manipulation)
    - Don't force—if significant resistance, stop and wait for dentist

Why reimplant even with dry time:

- Success rate drops significantly after 20 minutes dry time, but some teeth still survive
- Even if tooth eventually fails, it maintains alveolar bone while permanent solution is considered
- Always worth attempting—nothing to lose
- Sooner reimplanted, better the chance

Immediate post-reimplantation care:

- Have patient bite gently on gauze to hold tooth in place
- Keep tooth moist with saline-soaked gauze until splinting
- Do NOT test if tooth is solid (wiggling damages healing)
- Prepare for splinting by dental professional

2. **Factors determining success:**

Provide honest but hopeful information to the mother:

"I know this is scary, and you're worried about whether we can save your son's tooth. Let me explain what affects whether the tooth will be okay:

Factors that help:

- It's a permanent tooth (we definitely want to save it)
- The tooth is intact—the root isn't broken
- You brought him in quickly (30 minutes is longer than ideal, but we can still try)
- We're reimplanting it right now
- Your son is healthy and young (children's bodies heal well)

Factors that make it challenging:

- The tooth was stored dry in a paper towel—ideally it should have been kept in milk or back in his mouth
- It's been out of the socket for 30 minutes (best outcomes are when reimplanted within 20 minutes)
- The longer a tooth is dry, the more periodontal ligament cells die, and those cells are crucial for the tooth to reattach

What this means:

- We're going to reimplant the tooth and splint it to the neighboring teeth
- Some teeth in this situation survive and function normally for years
- Others may need a root canal or eventually be replaced with an implant
- We won't know the final outcome for several weeks or months as the tooth heals
- Even if the tooth doesn't survive long-term, keeping it in place now helps maintain the bone and gum tissue

Best case: The tooth reattaches successfully and functions normally. Your son will likely need a root canal, but the tooth stays.

Realistic expectation: Because of the dry storage time, there's a significant chance the tooth may eventually need to be replaced, but we're giving it the best chance by reimplanting now.

The dentist will follow up closely and monitor for any signs that the tooth isn't healing properly. We'll know more in the coming weeks."

Key teaching moment for future injuries: "For any future dental injuries—whether for your son or anyone else—here's what to do:

- Find the tooth immediately
- Hold it by the crown (white part), never touch the root
- If dirty, rinse very gently with milk or saline—NOT tap water
- Best option: Put it back in the socket immediately
- If you can't do that: Store it in cold milk, or have the child hold it in their mouth between their cheek and gums
- Never let it dry out
- Get to a dentist within 20 minutes if possible

The way the tooth is handled in the first few minutes determines whether it can be saved."

3. **Dental management of this case:**

Immediate ED care:

Reimplantation and stabilization:

- Reimplant tooth as described above

- Prepare materials for splinting (or wait for dental consult if arriving soon)
- Keep tooth moist until splinted

Pain management:

- Acetaminophen or ibuprofen (age-appropriate dosing)
- Local anesthesia if needed for manipulation (lidocaine)
- Ice pack to reduce swelling

Medications:

- **Antibiotics:** Amoxicillin 20 mg/kg/day divided three times daily for 7 days
  - Covers oral flora to prevent infection
  - Alternative: Penicillin VK if no amoxicillin available
  - If penicillin allergy: Clindamycin
- **Tetanus:** Check immunization status, update if needed (Tdap if >7 years old)

Splinting (by dentist or oral surgeon):

- Flexible splint to adjacent teeth (usually using wire and composite)
- Splint should be passive (allows slight physiologic movement)
- Leave in place 7-14 days typically
- Rigid splinting can cause ankylosis (tooth fuses to bone—bad outcome)

Dietary instructions:

- Soft diet for 7-14 days
- No biting with front teeth
- Avoid hard, crunchy, or sticky foods
- No contact sports or activities risking reinjury

Oral hygiene:

- Gentle brushing (avoid traumatized area initially)
- Chlorhexidine rinses twice daily
- Keep area clean but be gentle

Emergency dental referral:

- Contact pediatric dentist or oral surgeon immediately
- If after hours, many dental practices have emergency numbers
- Patient needs dental follow-up within 24 hours

Follow-up care (by dentist):

Immediate follow-up (24 hours):

- Assess tooth position and splint

- Radiographs to confirm position
- Adjust splint if needed

Short-term follow-up (weekly for 3-4 weeks):

- Monitor for signs of infection
- Check tooth color (darkening may indicate pulp death)
- Assess for mobility
- Remove splint at appropriate time (usually 7-14 days)

Root canal timing:

- Non-vital teeth (darkening, no response to percussion): Root canal within 2 weeks
- Some dentists start root canal prophylactically in teeth with prolonged dry time
- Timing controversial but generally within 7-14 days if signs of pulp necrosis

Long-term follow-up (months to years):

- Monitor for root resorption (roots gradually disappear—seen on X-ray)
- Watch for ankylosis (tooth fuses to bone, stops erupting as child grows)
- Assess for pulp necrosis development
- May need eventual replacement even if initially successful

Complications to monitor:

Early (days to weeks):

- Infection (swelling, fever, purulent drainage)
- Loss of tooth (falls out again)
- Splint failure

Medium-term (weeks to months):

- Pulp necrosis (tooth darkens, becomes non-vital)
- Root canal infection
- Tooth discoloration

Long-term (months to years):

- External root resorption (tooth root gradually dissolves)
- Internal root resorption (resorption from inside tooth)
- Ankylosis (tooth fuses to bone)
- Arrested tooth development if root not fully formed

4. **Prevention education:**

Provide comprehensive prevention guidance:

For parents and children:

"Now that we're taking care of this injury, let's talk about prevention for the future:

Sports protection:

- Your son should wear a mouthguard for ALL contact sports (baseball, basketball, soccer, hockey, football)
- Custom mouthguards from the dentist work best, but even store-bought ones help
- Mouthguards should be worn during both practices and games
- Replace mouthguards when they show wear or as your son grows

Activity awareness:

- Be cautious during physical play
- Teach proper falling techniques in sports
- Avoid using teeth as tools (opening bottles, tearing packages)
- Never hold objects in mouth during activities

General safety:

- Use seatbelts in cars (prevents facial trauma in crashes)
- Childproof home to prevent falls
- Supervise younger children during play
- Teach children not to run with objects in their mouth

What to do if another dental injury occurs:

For avulsed (knocked out) tooth:

1. Find the tooth
2. Hold by crown, don't touch root
3. Gently rinse if dirty (milk or saline, not tap water)
4. Reimplant immediately if possible, or store in cold milk
5. Get to dentist within 20 minutes

For fractured tooth:

1. Save any broken pieces
2. Rinse mouth with warm water
3. Apply cold compress to reduce swelling
4. See dentist same day

For loosened but not avulsed tooth:

1. Don't wiggle it
2. Soft diet
3. See dentist within 24 hours

Emergency dental kit to keep:

- Dentist's emergency number
- Small container with lid (for storing avulsed tooth)
- Saline solution or milk in small bottle
- Gauze pads
- Cold pack
- Pain reliever (age-appropriate)

Long-term dental care:

- Regular dental checkups every 6 months
- Good oral hygiene
- Fluoride use as recommended
- Address any dental issues promptly

Resources:

- American Academy of Pediatric Dentistry website (has injury guides)
- Your dentist can provide custom mouthguards
- Local sports leagues may have mouthguard programs

The most important thing to remember: Time matters with dental injuries. The faster you act, the better the outcome. Don't hesitate—even if it's after hours, contact an emergency dentist immediately."

Special considerations for this case:

Psychosocial support:

- Child may be traumatized by injury and fearful of treatment
- Use age-appropriate explanations
- Praise cooperation
- Allow parent to comfort and be present
- Consider child life specialist involvement if available

School communication:

- Provide note for school about activity restrictions
- Inform coaches about mouthguard need
- Temporary soft diet may affect lunch choices

Insurance/documentation:

- Dental injuries often covered differently than medical
- May need separate dental insurance claim
- Document thoroughly for insurance purposes
- Sports-related injuries may have different coverage

Follow-up coordination:

- Ensure family has dental appointment scheduled before leaving
- Provide written instructions (family will forget verbal information)
- Give emergency contact numbers
- Schedule medical follow-up if other injuries present

Key learning points from this scenario:

- Time and storage method are critical factors in tooth avulsion survival
- Always reimplant even if conditions aren't ideal—some teeth survive despite prolonged dry time
- Proper handling of avulsed tooth makes difference between saving and losing it
- Education on prevention and emergency management can help families respond better to future injuries
- Coordination between emergency medicine and dentistry is essential for optimal outcomes

This scenario demonstrates the importance of immediate action with dental trauma, proper tooth handling technique, and the value of patient education for both treatment and prevention.

Chapter 9 Summary: Critical Takeaways

You've now completed a comprehensive review of maxillofacial and ocular trauma. These injuries range from minor inconveniences to sight-threatening and life-threatening emergencies. Let's reinforce what matters most for the TCRN exam and clinical practice.

Most Critical Concepts:

1. Airway management in facial fractures:

- Le Fort II and III fractures can compromise airway
- Bilateral mandible fractures destabilize tongue support
- Secure airway early—don't wait for complete obstruction
- Facial instability may make bag-mask ventilation ineffective
- Have surgical airway equipment ready before attempting intubation

2. Vision-threatening emergencies:

- Globe rupture: Never apply pressure, immediate ophthalmology consult
- Retrobulbar hematoma: Requires immediate lateral canthotomy/cantholysis
- Chemical burns: Immediate copious irrigation, don't wait for anything
- Hyphema: Risk of rebleeding days 3-5, monitor IOP
- These injuries require urgent intervention to save vision

3. Time-sensitive dental injuries:

- Avulsed teeth: Best outcomes with reimplantation <20 minutes
- Never touch root, store in milk or saliva if can't reimplant
- Primary teeth: Don't reimplant
- Proper immediate care determines whether tooth survives

4. Fracture recognition patterns:

- Malocclusion indicates mandible or maxilla fracture
- Periorbital ecchymosis with midface trauma suggests Le Fort or orbital fracture
- Infraorbital numbness suggests orbital floor fracture
- CSF rhinorrhea indicates skull base involvement

5. Key assessment maneuvers:

- Midface mobility test differentiates Le Fort types
- Fluorescein staining reveals corneal abrasions
- Halo sign tests for CSF in bloody nasal drainage
- Check extraocular movements and pupil response in orbital trauma

Connecting to Clinical Practice:

Systematic approach to facial trauma:

1. Airway assessment first (especially with midface fractures)
2. Control bleeding
3. Assess vision and eye integrity
4. Examine facial bones systematically
5. Look for CSF leak
6. Check dental occlusion
7. Assess cranial nerve function

Red flags requiring immediate intervention:

- Airway compromise with facial swelling
- Suspected globe rupture
- Retrobulbar hematoma with vision loss
- Chemical eye exposure
- Bilateral mandible fractures
- Le Fort III fractures
- Active uncontrolled epistaxis

Documentation essentials:

- Visual acuity before any intervention (if safe to check)
- Mechanism of injury (especially for penetrating eye injuries)
- Neurovascular status
- Time of tooth avulsion
- Whether CSF leak present

Common Exam Question Patterns:

Watch for questions that:

- Describe malocclusion or facial mobility (testing Le Fort knowledge)
- Present eye injury asking what NOT to do (globe rupture management)
- Give tooth avulsion scenario (test proper handling and reimplantation timing)
- Show periorbital findings (distinguish orbital from other fractures)
- Describe chemical exposure (immediate irrigation)

Building Confidence for Exam Day:

You don't need to memorize every detail about every fracture type. Focus on understanding:

- Which injuries threaten airway, vision, or function
- When immediate intervention is critical
- How to recognize patterns that indicate specific injuries
- What actions can worsen outcomes (pressing on ruptured globe, delaying tooth reimplantation, etc.)

Study Strategies That Work:

Visual learners: Sketch the Le Fort fracture patterns and facial bone anatomy. Draw the layers of the eye and mark where different injuries occur. Visual memory helps with spatial relationships.

Kinesthetic learners: Practice the midface mobility test on yourself (gently). Understand the mechanics of how you'd perform lateral canthotomy. Physical understanding aids recall.

Pattern recognition: When reviewing questions, identify the injury pattern (what constellation of findings points to specific diagnosis). Pattern recognition is faster than working through differential diagnosis step-by-step.

Clinical correlation: When you see facial or eye injuries in practice, consciously apply what you've learned. Real patient encounters cement theoretical knowledge.

Self-Assessment Questions:

Before moving to the next chapter, ask yourself:

- Can I differentiate Le Fort I, II, and III fractures?
- Do I know which eye injuries are true emergencies?
- Can I explain proper tooth avulsion management?
- Do I understand when facial fractures threaten the airway?

If you can answer yes with confidence, you're ready to proceed. If any areas feel uncertain, review those specific sections.

Final Thoughts on Chapter 9:

Maxillofacial and ocular trauma requires balancing multiple concerns: airway, vision, function, and cosmesis. While dramatic in appearance, not all facial injuries are emergencies. However, missing the true emergencies—airway compromise, vision-threatening injuries, time-sensitive dental trauma—can have devastating consequences.

You've learned to identify these critical situations and respond appropriately. This knowledge protects your patients from preventable disability and guides you toward correct prioritization when multiple injuries compete for attention.

Looking Ahead:

You've now completed 9 of the 14 main content chapters. You're building a comprehensive foundation in trauma nursing. Each chapter connects to others—airway management spans multiple injury types, shock recognition applies universally, and systematic assessment remains constant.

As you progress through the remaining chapters, you'll continue developing the clinical judgment and pattern recognition that defines expert trauma nursing. The knowledge you're building isn't just for exam success—it's the foundation of safe, effective trauma care that will serve your patients throughout your career.

Chapter 10: Special Populations

Trauma doesn't discriminate by age, size, or health status, but the way trauma affects different populations varies dramatically. A mechanism that causes minor injuries in a healthy young adult can be catastrophic for a pediatric patient, elderly person, pregnant woman, or bariatric patient. Understanding these physiological differences and adapting your assessment and management accordingly isn't just good nursing—it's lifesaving.

This chapter explores how trauma presents differently across special populations and how to modify your approach for optimal outcomes. You'll learn the unique anatomical and physiological considerations that make each population vulnerable, recognize injury patterns specific to each group, and master the assessment and intervention modifications necessary for safe, effective care.

Pediatric Trauma Considerations

Children are not just small adults. Their unique anatomy, physiology, and injury patterns require specialized knowledge and adapted approaches. Understanding these differences helps you recognize serious injuries that might be subtle in presentation and avoid interventions that could harm rather than help.

Anatomical and Physiological Differences

Cardiovascular system:

Children have remarkable cardiovascular reserve. Their hearts can compensate for blood loss far better than adults by dramatically increasing heart rate and peripheral vasoconstriction. This means a pediatric trauma patient can maintain normal blood pressure despite losing 25-30% of their blood volume.

Here's the critical point: **by the time a child becomes hypotensive, they've already lost significant blood volume and are in severe shock**. A child with tachycardia, cool extremities, and delayed capillary refill but normal blood pressure is in compensated shock and needs aggressive intervention immediately. Don't wait for blood pressure to drop—you'll be too late.

Normal vital signs vary by age:

Infant (0-12 months): HR 100-160, BP 70-90 systolic

Toddler (1-3 years): HR 90-150, BP 80-100 systolic

Preschool (3-6 years): HR 80-140, BP 80-110 systolic

School age (6-12 years): HR 70-120, BP 90-120 systolic

Adolescent (12-18 years): HR 60-100, BP 100-120 systolic

Respiratory system:

Children have higher metabolic rates and oxygen consumption per kilogram than adults. They desaturate faster when apneic and have less respiratory reserve. Their airways are smaller, making even minor swelling or obstruction more significant.

Key differences:

Larger tongue relative to mouth size (easier airway obstruction)

More anterior and cephalad (higher) larynx

Floppy epiglottis that can obstruct view during intubation

Narrowest part of airway is at cricoid ring (not vocal cords like adults)

Smaller functional residual capacity (less oxygen reservoir)

What this means practically: A child can go from adequate oxygenation to critical hypoxia in seconds. Bag-valve-mask ventilation is often more effective than in adults if done properly, but improper technique (too much pressure or volume) easily causes gastric distension and aspiration.

Skeletal system:

Children's bones are more flexible and cartilaginous than adults. They can absorb tremendous force without fracturing, but this means the force gets transmitted to underlying organs. A child can have severe internal injuries with minimal or no external signs.

The flexibility also means:

Greenstick fractures (incomplete fractures) are common

Buckle fractures (compression injuries) occur where adult bones would break completely

Growth plate injuries can affect future bone growth

Rib fractures in children indicate severe force (ribs are very flexible)—if present, suspect serious underlying injury and possible abuse

Thermoregulation:

Children have larger body surface area relative to mass, leading to rapid heat loss. Hypothermia develops quickly and worsens outcomes by impairing coagulation and increasing metabolic demands. Keep the room warm, use warming devices, and warm all fluids.

Psychological factors:

Children may not communicate pain or symptoms clearly. They're frightened by the trauma, the hospital environment, and separation from parents. Anxiety can mimic or mask serious symptoms. When possible, allow parents to stay with the child—it calms the child and improves your assessment accuracy.

Common Pediatric Injury Patterns

Blunt trauma predominates: Motor vehicle crashes (as passengers or pedestrians), falls, bicycle crashes, and abuse account for most pediatric trauma. Penetrating trauma is less common but increasing in some areas.

Head injuries: Children have proportionally larger heads and weaker neck muscles, making head injury the leading cause of death in pediatric trauma. Diffuse axonal injury and cerebral edema are more common than focal mass lesions. Children can develop significant intracranial pressure with smaller hematomas than adults.

Abdominal injuries: Solid organ injuries (spleen, liver, kidneys) are common because children's abdomens are more protuberant and organs less protected by ribs and abdominal musculature. Handlebar injuries classically cause duodenal hematomas or pancreatic injuries in children.

Spinal injuries: Cervical spine injuries in children often occur at higher levels (C1-C3) than in adults (C5-C7) because of larger head size and ligamentous laxity. SCIWORA (Spinal Cord Injury Without Radiographic Abnormality) occurs in children—they can have significant spinal cord injury with normal X-rays and CT scans due to spinal column elasticity.

Pattern injuries: Certain injury patterns raise abuse concerns:

Bruising in non-mobile infants (babies who can't roll or crawl shouldn't have bruises)

Bruising in unusual patterns (handprints, belt marks, loop marks)

Injuries at different healing stages

Fractures inconsistent with stated mechanism

Delay in seeking care

Changing or inconsistent history

Assessment Modifications

Primary survey adaptations:

Airway:

Position carefully—neck flexion or hyperextension can obstruct airway

Use jaw thrust, avoid head tilt if spinal injury possible

Appropriate-sized equipment: Estimate based on length-based tape (Broselow tape) or formula: ETT size = (age in years/4) + 4

Have multiple sizes available—one size smaller and larger

Breathing:

Watch for signs of respiratory distress: nasal flaring, retractions, grunting

Auscultate carefully—transmitted sounds can be misleading

Bag-valve-mask technique critical—proper seal, appropriate volume (just enough to see chest rise)

Circulation:

Recognize shock early—tachycardia, cool extremities, delayed capillary refill, altered mental status BEFORE hypotension

IV access challenging—intraosseous (IO) route is excellent alternative. Don't delay resuscitation with multiple IV attempts. Two failed IV attempts = go to IO

Fluid resuscitation: 20 mL/kg boluses of crystalloid, reassess after each bolus

Blood products: 10 mL/kg packed red blood cells

Disability:

Modified Glasgow Coma Scale for infants/young children (nonverbal components)

AVPU scale useful: Alert, responds to Voice, responds to Pain, Unresponsive

Fontanelle assessment in infants (bulging suggests increased ICP)

Exposure:

Completely undress but prevent hypothermia

Warm room, warm blankets, warming lights

Efficient examination to minimize heat loss

Pain Management

Children feel pain just as much as adults but may not express it the same way. Inadequate pain control is both inhumane and clinically problematic—it increases stress response, worsens outcomes, and makes assessment harder.

Assessment tools:

FLACC scale (Face, Legs, Activity, Cry, Consolability) for non-verbal children

Wong-Baker FACES scale for children who can point

Numeric rating scale for older children and adolescents

Medication considerations:

Weight-based dosing essential

Avoid IM injections when possible (painful, absorption unpredictable)

Intranasal fentanyl excellent for moderate to severe pain

Oral medications when appropriate (acetaminophen, ibuprofen for mild pain)

Never withhold opioids for fear of masking abdominal findings—this outdated practice causes unnecessary suffering

Family-Centered Care

Parents are terrified when their child is injured. They need information, reassurance, and inclusion in care when appropriate.

Communication strategies:

Speak directly to older children when explaining procedures

Use developmentally appropriate language (no medical jargon for young children)

Be honest—children sense deception and it increases anxiety

Allow parents to stay during procedures when possible (research shows this benefits both child and parent)

If parents must leave, assign someone to update them frequently

Family presence during resuscitation: Research supports allowing family presence during resuscitation when:

A staff member is assigned to support them

They're positioned where they can see but not interfere

They're prepared for what they'll witness

They can leave if they choose

Benefits include better family psychological outcomes, increased satisfaction with care, and no interference with medical care.

Child Abuse Recognition

Healthcare providers are mandated reporters. Any suspicion of abuse must be reported to appropriate authorities—Child Protective Services or law enforcement.

Red flags:

Injury inconsistent with developmental stage (baby with "fell off couch" injury but can't roll)

Delay in seeking care

Changing or vague history

History inconsistent between caregivers

Caregiver more concerned about consequences than child's welfare

Pattern injuries (bruises in shape of object)

Multiple injuries at different healing stages

Bruising in unusual locations (ears, neck, genitals, buttocks)

Fractures in non-ambulatory infants

Retinal hemorrhages (suggest shaken baby syndrome)

Your role:

Document objectively—describe what you see, not conclusions ("multiple circular bruises on back" not "cigarette burns")

Use body diagrams to document injury locations

Photograph injuries when possible

Preserve evidence (clothing, if suspicious for assault)

Report suspicions—investigation is not your role, reporting is

Support the child and non-offending family members

Geriatric Trauma Patients

The population is aging, and elderly trauma patients are increasingly common. They present unique challenges: they're more likely to be injured from minor mechanisms, have worse outcomes from similar injuries, and their presentation can be deceptively benign despite serious injury.

Physiological Changes with Aging

Cardiovascular: Aging hearts lose elasticity and compliance. They can't increase heart rate or contractility as effectively during stress. Many elderly patients take beta-blockers or calcium channel blockers that prevent normal tachycardia response to shock.

What this means: **An elderly patient can be in severe shock with a heart rate of 80 bpm** because medications prevent compensatory tachycardia. A "normal" blood pressure of 120/80 may actually represent relative hypotension if their baseline is 160/90. Always ask about baseline vital signs and medications.

Cardiac reserve is limited—elderly hearts can't handle the same fluid loads as younger patients without developing pulmonary edema. Resuscitation requires careful balance: adequate volume to maintain perfusion without causing fluid overload.

Respiratory: Decreased chest wall compliance, reduced lung elasticity, and diminished cough reflex increase pneumonia risk and make ventilatory failure more likely. Elderly patients desaturate more slowly than children but recover more slowly and are less tolerant of hypoxia.

Chronic conditions like COPD or pulmonary fibrosis reduce baseline function. An elderly patient with COPD may normally saturate at 88-92%, so "normal" oxygen saturation of 95% might not indicate adequate reserve.

Neurological: Brain atrophy is normal with aging. This creates space for blood to accumulate subdurally after minor head trauma. An elderly person can have a significant subdural hematoma from a ground-level fall, with symptoms developing gradually over days to weeks.

Cognitive impairment (dementia, Alzheimer's) complicates assessment. Is the confusion from head injury or baseline? Always try to establish baseline mental status from family or medical records.

Renal: Kidney function declines with age. Elderly patients have less ability to concentrate urine, handle sodium loads, or clear medications. They're more susceptible to acute kidney injury from hypoperfusion, contrast dye, or medications.

Chronic kidney disease is common. Know baseline creatinine and GFR—acute changes indicate new injury or inadequate resuscitation.

Musculoskeletal: Osteoporosis means bones fracture from minor trauma. A ground-level fall can cause hip fractures, vertebral compression fractures, or distal radius fractures. Decreased muscle mass and strength increase fall risk and injury severity.

Degenerative spine changes are universal. Elderly patients often have baseline spinal stenosis, making them more vulnerable to spinal cord injury from minor trauma or hyperextension.

Skin and thermoregulation: Thin, fragile skin tears easily and heals slowly. Elderly patients develop hypothermia quickly and are more susceptible to pressure injuries from immobilization.

Common Geriatric Injury Patterns

Falls: The most common mechanism. Even ground-level falls cause serious injuries: hip fractures, subdural hematomas, vertebral compression fractures, and rib fractures.

Risk factors for falls:

- Medications (sedatives, antihypertensives, diuretics)
- Sensory deficits (vision, proprioception)
- Environmental hazards (loose rugs, poor lighting)
- Gait instability
- Cognitive impairment

Motor vehicle crashes: Elderly drivers have higher crash rates per mile driven. Age-related changes in vision, reaction time, and judgment contribute. They're more likely to be injured and less likely to survive similar-severity crashes compared to younger adults.

Pedestrian struck: Elderly pedestrians have slower crossing speeds and may not judge vehicle speeds accurately. They suffer more severe injuries when struck.

Elder abuse: Often overlooked. Signs include unexplained injuries, multiple injuries at different healing stages, poor hygiene, malnutrition, over-sedation, or caregiver preventing private conversation with patient.

Assessment and Management Modifications

History gathering:

Obtain detailed medication list—know which drugs affect vital signs or coagulation

Determine baseline functional status—was patient independent, using walker, bedbound?

Establish baseline mental status from family

Ask about recent illness or changes that might have precipitated the injury

Identify advance directives or healthcare proxies

Vital sign interpretation:

Compare to patient's baseline, not age-based normals

Consider medication effects on heart rate and blood pressure

Lower threshold for concern—"normal" vital signs may not be normal for this patient

Earlier aggressive intervention—don't wait for obvious shock

Anticoagulation considerations: Many elderly patients take warfarin, direct oral anticoagulants (DOACs like apixaban, rivaroxaban), or antiplatelet agents (aspirin, clopidogrel). These dramatically increase bleeding risk and affect management:

Warfarin:

Check INR immediately

Elevated INR with bleeding: Give vitamin K, fresh frozen plasma (FFP), or prothrombin complex concentrate (PCC)

Head injury on warfarin: High suspicion for intracranial bleeding, lower threshold for CT

DOACs:

No readily available reversal for most (except dabigatran—use idarucizumab)

Bleeding management: Stop drug, supportive care, consider PCC

Half-lives vary—know when last dose was taken

Antiplatelet agents:

Increase bleeding risk, especially with head injury

No specific reversal

Consider platelet transfusion for severe bleeding

Increased subdural hematoma risk

Pain management: Start low, go slow with medications. Elderly patients are more sensitive to opioids and sedatives. Smaller doses often provide adequate relief. Monitor closely for respiratory depression.

Non-opioid options (acetaminophen, topical agents, regional blocks) are excellent adjuncts and may reduce opioid requirements.

Fracture management: Early surgical fixation of hip fractures improves outcomes by allowing earlier mobilization, reducing complications. Prolonged bed rest causes pneumonia, pressure injuries, DVT, and deconditioning.

Vertebral compression fractures are often managed conservatively with pain control and bracing, but some benefit from vertebroplasty or kyphoplasty.

Preventing Complications

Pulmonary:

Aggressive pulmonary hygiene (incentive spirometry, early mobilization)

Appropriate DVT prophylaxis

Careful fluid management to avoid overload

Pressure injuries:

Frequent repositioning

Pressure-relieving surfaces

Early mobilization when possible

Excellent skin care

Delirium:

Maintain day-night orientation (lights during day, dark at night)

Glasses and hearing aids in place

Minimize unnecessary medications

Early mobilization

Family presence

Functional decline:

Physical and occupational therapy consultation early

Discharge planning started on admission

Address why fall occurred to prevent recurrence

Pregnancy-Related Trauma

Trauma complicates 6-7% of pregnancies and is the leading cause of maternal death from non-obstetric causes. Managing pregnant trauma patients requires caring for two patients simultaneously while understanding how pregnancy changes physiology and injury patterns.

Physiological Changes in Pregnancy

Cardiovascular: Pregnancy causes dramatic cardiovascular changes that alter trauma presentation:

Blood volume: Increases 40-50% by third trimester. This creates physiologic anemia (dilutional) but provides a protective buffer against blood loss. A pregnant patient can lose 30-35% of blood volume before showing signs of shock—but this comes at the fetus's expense. Maternal vital signs may appear stable while the fetus is severely compromised from inadequate placental perfusion.

Heart rate: Increases 10-20 bpm during pregnancy. Baseline tachycardia is normal, making it harder to recognize shock from heart rate alone.

Blood pressure: Decreases in second trimester (lowest at 24-28 weeks), then rises toward pre-pregnancy levels in third trimester. "Normal" blood pressure may actually be elevated for that patient at that gestational age.

Cardiac output: Increases 30-40%. The heart works harder throughout pregnancy.

Supine hypotension syndrome: After 20 weeks gestation, the gravid uterus compresses the inferior vena cava when patient is supine, reducing venous return and cardiac output. Always tilt patients left lateral or manually displace uterus to the left.

Respiratory:

Minute ventilation increases 50% (breathing more deeply and slightly faster)

Functional residual capacity decreases (diaphragm pushed up by uterus)

Mild respiratory alkalosis is normal (compensatory metabolic acidosis)

Decreased oxygen reserve—desaturates faster if apneic

Gastrointestinal:

Delayed gastric emptying and decreased LES tone—high aspiration risk

Stomach displaced upward—penetrating injuries to upper abdomen more likely to involve stomach

Renal:

GFR increases 50%

Serum creatinine and BUN lower than non-pregnant—"normal" values may indicate renal impairment

Mild hydronephrosis is normal (progesterone effect)

Hematologic:

Hypercoagulable state—increased DVT risk but also increased clotting ability

Fibrinogen doubles—normal values 200-400 mg/dL, pregnancy 400-600 mg/dL

Mild thrombocytopenia common

Mechanisms and Injury Patterns

Blunt trauma (most common):

Motor vehicle crashes account for majority

Domestic violence increases during pregnancy

Falls (balance changes, ligamentous laxity)

Penetrating trauma:

Gunshot and stab wounds

Uterus may protect maternal organs but fetus is vulnerable

In late pregnancy, enlarged uterus fills abdomen—penetrating trauma to abdomen likely hits uterus/fetus

Unique pregnancy-related injuries:

Placental abruption: Partial or complete separation of placenta from uterine wall, most common cause of fetal death from maternal trauma. Occurs in 1-5% of minor trauma, up to 50% of major trauma.

Signs:

Vaginal bleeding (may be absent if blood contained behind placenta)

Abdominal pain and uterine tenderness

Firm, contracting uterus (tetanic contraction)

Fetal distress or demise

Diagnosis: Clinical suspicion, ultrasound (may not show abruption), fetal monitoring shows fetal distress Treatment: Mild cases may observe; severe cases need emergent delivery

Uterine rupture: Uncommon but catastrophic. Risk higher with previous cesarean section.

Signs:

Severe abdominal pain

Palpable fetal parts through abdomen

Loss of fetal heart tones

Maternal shock

Treatment: Emergency cesarean section, hysterectomy often needed

Fetomaternal hemorrhage: Fetal blood enters maternal circulation from trauma. Can cause fetal anemia and sensitization if mother is Rh-negative and fetus Rh-positive.

Diagnosis: Kleihauer-Betke test (detects fetal cells in maternal blood) Treatment: Rh-negative mothers get RhoGAM to prevent sensitization

Direct fetal injury: Skull fractures, intracranial hemorrhage, long bone fractures possible from trauma, especially penetrating or severe blunt trauma.

Assessment Priorities

Primary survey modifications:

Airway:

High aspiration risk—early intubation if needed

Rapid sequence intubation with cricoid pressure

Breathing:

Supplemental oxygen to all pregnant trauma patients (maintain maternal saturation >95% for fetal benefit)

Chest tube placement one to two interspaces higher than normal (diaphragm elevated)

Circulation:

Left lateral tilt or manual left uterine displacement to relieve IVC compression

Aggressive fluid resuscitation—remember, maternal vital signs stable while fetus compromised

Two large-bore IVs above diaphragm (avoid lower extremity IVs—if major bleeding, won't reach heart effectively due to IVC compression)

Disability/Exposure:

Same as non-pregnant

Prevent hypothermia

Secondary survey additions:

Obstetric assessment:

Fundal height (estimates gestational age: fundus at umbilicus = 20 weeks, at xiphoid = 36 weeks)

Fetal heart rate (normal 120-160 bpm)

Uterine tone (soft and non-tender is normal)

Vaginal exam for bleeding, amniotic fluid, or prolapsed cord

Continuous fetal monitoring if viable gestational age (usually >20-24 weeks)

Diagnostic considerations:

All imaging necessary for maternal care should be done—radiation risk to fetus is minimal and maternal death is worse for fetus

Shield abdomen when possible but don't delay necessary imaging

CT with contrast: Generally safe, iodinated contrast doesn't cross placenta significantly

MRI: Safe in pregnancy, no radiation

Management Principles

Mother is the primary patient: Optimal fetal outcome depends on optimal maternal outcome. Resuscitate the mother aggressively. Everything that helps the mother helps the fetus.

Early obstetric consultation: Involve OB early for viable pregnancies. They guide decisions about delivery timing, fetal monitoring, and pregnancy-specific complications.

Fetal monitoring:

Continuous fetal heart rate monitoring for viable gestations

Minimum 4-6 hours for minor trauma, 24-48 hours for significant trauma

Monitoring detects placental abruption and fetal compromise before symptoms obvious

Rh status:

Determine maternal Rh status and antibody screen

Rh-negative mothers with trauma get RhoGAM (unless father known to be Rh-negative or mother already sensitized)

Dose: 300 mcg IM covers 30 mL fetal-maternal hemorrhage

Kleihauer-Betke test determines if larger dose needed

Perimortem cesarean section: If mother in cardiac arrest and fetus viable (usually >24 weeks), perform emergency cesarean section within 4-5 minutes of arrest. This improves outcomes for both mother (relieves IVC compression, improves resuscitation success) and fetus.

Indications:

Maternal cardiac arrest

Viable fetus (>24 weeks)

Failed maternal resuscitation after 4 minutes

Don't delay for obstetric consultation or OR—do it in the ED. Fetal survival depends on delivery within 5 minutes of maternal arrest.

Domestic Violence Screening

Pregnancy is a high-risk time for domestic violence. Screen all pregnant trauma patients privately (without partner present):

Questions:

"Do you feel safe at home?"

"Has anyone hurt you or threatened you?"

"Are you afraid of your partner?"

If positive:

Provide resources (hotline numbers, safe houses)

Document thoroughly

Involve social work

Safety plan before discharge

Bariatric Trauma Patients

Obesity (BMI >30) and morbid obesity (BMI >40) are epidemic. Bariatric patients present unique challenges in trauma care, from assessment difficulties to equipment limitations and increased complication risks.

Physiological Considerations

Cardiovascular:

Increased blood volume and cardiac output to perfuse adipose tissue

Hypertension common—know baseline blood pressure

Cardiomegaly and left ventricular hypertrophy common

Increased risk of arrhythmias

Difficult IV access—may need ultrasound guidance or central access

Respiratory:

- Restrictive lung pattern from chest wall weight and abdominal mass
- Obstructive sleep apnea common
- Obesity hypoventilation syndrome in some patients
- Difficult airway—short neck, redundant pharyngeal tissue
- Desaturate faster when apneic, harder to ventilate
- Higher risk of aspiration

Metabolic:

- Diabetes mellitus common—check glucose, know baseline control
- Dyslipidemia
- Fatty liver disease

Pharmacologic:

- Medication dosing complex—some by total body weight, some by ideal body weight, some by adjusted body weight
- Lipophilic drugs have larger volume of distribution
- Consult pharmacy for appropriate dosing

Assessment Challenges

Physical examination:

- Difficult to palpate pulses, assess jugular venous pressure
- Abdominal exam less reliable—harder to detect tenderness, guarding, or masses
- External landmarks obscured—makes procedures more difficult

Diagnostic imaging:

- Weight limits on CT scanners (usually 350-450 lbs, varies by scanner)
- Image quality may be degraded by body habitus
- Ultrasound difficult—adipose tissue impairs penetration
- May need open MRI if patient doesn't fit in standard scanner

Monitoring:

- Standard blood pressure cuffs inaccurate—need appropriate cuff size (bladder covers 80% of arm circumference)
- Small cuffs read falsely high, large cuffs falsely low
- Pulse oximetry may be difficult to obtain

Equipment and Logistical Issues

Patient handling:

Bariatric stretchers and beds required (standard equipment has 350-500 lb limits)

Ceiling lifts or mechanical lift devices needed for transfers

Extra staff required for repositioning

Specialized bariatric equipment: stretchers (1000+ lb capacity), wheelchairs, walkers, commodes

Radiographic equipment:

Standard table weight limits 350-450 lbs

May need specialized bariatric CT scanner or open MRI

Portable X-rays less penetrating—images may be non-diagnostic

OR considerations:

Specialized OR tables with higher weight limits

Longer instruments for surgery through thick abdominal wall

Positioning challenges

Increased anesthetic risk

Injury and Complication Risks

Injuries:

Seatbelts may not fit properly or be worn—higher mortality in crashes

Difficult to assess for rib fractures, flail chest

Pulmonary contusion harder to diagnose and manage

Abdominal injuries harder to detect clinically

Complications: Bariatric patients have higher rates of:

Pulmonary complications (pneumonia, ARDS, PE)

Cardiovascular complications

Wound complications (infection, dehiscence)

Pressure injuries

DVT and PE (despite higher doses of prophylaxis)

Difficulty with mobilization and rehabilitation

Management Strategies

Airway:

- Anticipate difficult airway—have experienced provider and backup plan
- Video laryngoscopy helpful
- Ramping positioning (stacked blankets or ramp to align external auditory meatus with sternal notch) improves intubation view
- Earlier intubation if respiratory distress—won't improve on own

Breathing:

- Aggressive pulmonary care—incentive spirometry, early mobilization
- CPAP or BiPAP for those with sleep apnea (bring own machine if has one)
- Higher PEEP requirements on ventilator
- Prone positioning very difficult but sometimes necessary for ARDS

Circulation:

- Ultrasound-guided IV access
- Consider intraosseous access if urgent and IV access difficult
- Central venous access for resuscitation if peripheral access fails
- Higher blood volumes—may need more resuscitation fluid

Medications:

- Consult pharmacy for weight-based medication dosing
- Anticoagulation: Higher doses needed for VTE prophylaxis
- Antibiotics: Some dose on total body weight, others adjusted

Imaging:

- Determine weight limits before transport
- Alternative imaging if patient exceeds limits
- Diagnostic peritoneal lavage or laparoscopy alternatives to CT for abdominal trauma

VTE prophylaxis:

- Early chemical prophylaxis with higher doses (e.g., enoxaparin 40 mg BID instead of daily)
- Sequential compression devices
- Early mobilization critical
- Some recommend duplex ultrasound screening

Wound care:

- Meticulous skin care
- Keep skin folds clean and dry
- Pressure injury prevention—turn frequently, specialized surfaces
- Close monitoring for surgical wound complications

Mobility:

- Physical therapy consultation early
- Bariatric equipment for mobilization
- May need multiple staff for transfers
- Creative solutions for patients exceeding equipment limits

Sensitivity and Respect

Bariatric patients often experience stigma and discrimination in healthcare settings. This is unacceptable and harmful.

Respectful care:

- Use neutral, non-judgmental language
- Ensure appropriate equipment available without making patient feel embarrassed
- Maintain dignity during procedures and transfers
- Address weight-related care needs matter-of-factly
- Private discussions about equipment needs
- Never discuss weight unless medically necessary

Trauma in Special Circumstances

Beyond age and size considerations, certain circumstances require specialized knowledge and modifications to standard trauma care.

Patients with Pre-existing Anticoagulation

Already discussed with geriatric patients, but important enough to emphasize:

Assessment:

- Determine which anticoagulant and last dose
- Check INR for warfarin, PT/PTT
- Lower threshold for imaging, especially head CT

Reversal agents:

- Warfarin: Vitamin K (slow), FFP, or PCC (fast)
- Dabigatran: Idarucizumab
- Apixaban, rivaroxaban: PCC, andexanet alfa (if available)
- Heparin: Protamine sulfate

Decision-making:

Balance bleeding risk against thrombotic risk of stopping anticoagulation

Consult hematology or cardiology if unclear

Some patients can't stop anticoagulation (mechanical heart valves)—manage bleeding and consult specialists

Patients with Implanted Devices

Pacemakers and ICDs:

Note location and type

Can be damaged by chest trauma or defibrillation

Change defibrillator pad position if possible to avoid device

Check device function if directly impacted

Cardiology consultation if malfunction suspected

Ventricular assist devices (VADs):

Patient may have no palpable pulse (continuous flow devices)

Special blood pressure cuffs and Doppler required

Controllers must stay connected—alarms mean emergency

Don't do chest compressions unless VAD failure confirmed

Early cardiothoracic surgery consultation

Insulin pumps:

Note location and remove before MRI

May need to disconnect for procedures—know patient's insulin requirements

Replace with IV insulin if disconnected for extended period

Endocrine consultation if complex management

Orthopedic hardware:

Previous joint replacements, plates, screws, rods

May complicate imaging (artifact on CT/MRI)

Can be damaged by new trauma

May affect surgical approach for new injuries

Immunocompromised Patients

Patients with HIV, cancer, organ transplants, or on immunosuppressive medications have unique vulnerabilities.

Infection risk:

Higher rates of post-traumatic infection

More aggressive antibiotic prophylaxis for open wounds

Lower threshold for admission and monitoring

Atypical organisms more common

Wound healing:

- Delayed or impaired healing
- Higher rate of wound complications
- May need different surgical approaches

Medication interactions:

- Immunosuppressants may interact with antibiotics or other medications
- Continue home immunosuppressants when possible to prevent rejection (transplant patients)
- Consult pharmacy and patient's specialists

Transfusion considerations:

- Some immunocompromised patients need CMV-negative or irradiated blood products
- Check patient's medical record or contact their specialist

Patients with Spinal Cord Injury

Trauma patients with pre-existing spinal cord injury require special consideration.

Autonomic dysreflexia: Can occur in patients with injury at T6 or above. Noxious stimulus below injury level causes unopposed sympathetic response.

Signs:

- Sudden severe hypertension (can be life-threatening)
- Bradycardia
- Pounding headache
- Sweating and flushing above injury level
- Pale, cool skin below injury level

Common triggers in trauma: Distended bladder, fecal impaction, pain, fractures

Treatment:

- Sit patient upright if possible
- Remove triggering stimulus (catheterize bladder, remove restrictive clothing)
- Antihypertensive medication if needed
- Monitor closely—can rapidly become hypertensive crisis

Baseline assessment:

- Establish patient's baseline motor and sensory function
- New deficits indicate new injury, not just pre-existing condition
- Ask patient to describe their normal function and any changes

Pressure injury prevention:

- Existing injuries may be present
- High risk for new injuries from immobilization
- Meticulous pressure relief and skin care
- Early mobilization to usual seating system when medically appropriate

Respiratory considerations:

Patients with high cervical injuries may have limited respiratory reserve

Baseline abnormal breathing patterns

Lower threshold for respiratory support

Patients with Intellectual or Developmental Disabilities

Communication:

Speak directly to patient when possible, not just caregivers

Use simple, clear language

Give extra time for processing and response

Visual aids or demonstrations may help

Some patients communicate non-verbally—learn their communication methods

Behavioral responses:

May not understand what's happening—increased anxiety and behavioral responses

Unfamiliar environment and people are frightening

May not cooperate with examination or procedures

Not "being difficult"—expressing fear and confusion in their way

Management strategies:

Caregiver or family presence extremely helpful

Maintain routines when possible

Familiar objects from home can comfort

Quiet, calm environment

Chemical restraints last resort—try behavioral interventions first

Consult patient's usual care team for management strategies

Pain assessment:

May not verbalize pain clearly

Watch for behavioral indicators: agitation, self-injury, changes from baseline

Caregivers can often identify pain behaviors

Use appropriate pain scales (FLACC for non-verbal patients)

Incarcerated Patients

Prisoners and detained individuals have same right to medical care as other patients.

Security considerations:

Correctional officers remain with patient

Restraints may be in place—can be temporarily removed for medical procedures if safe

Keep officers informed of medical plan

Maintain chain of custody for belongings and specimens if required

Medical care:

Provide standard, high-quality care regardless of criminal history

Privacy maintained within security constraints

Treat with same respect as all patients

Document objectively, separate from feelings about alleged crimes

Consent and confidentiality:

Incarcerated patients can consent for themselves unless cognitively impaired

HIPAA still applies—don't share information with correctional staff beyond security needs

Forensic evidence collected if ordered by law enforcement with proper warrant/consent

Homeless Patients

Unique vulnerabilities:

Often have untreated chronic conditions

May delay seeking care

Nutritional deficiencies common

Higher rates of substance use disorders and mental illness

May have experienced previous trauma (PTSD common)

Assessment considerations:

Complete medical history may be unknown

Medication allergies and current medications may be uncertain

Baseline functional status unclear

May minimize symptoms or try to leave AMA to avoid admission

Discharge planning:

Standard discharge instructions may not apply (no home, no phone, no transportation)

Need creative solutions: shelter placement, respite care, connection with social services

Medication regimen must be feasible (can't refrigerate insulin if living outside)

Follow-up appointments need to be accessible

Trauma-informed care:

Many homeless individuals have trauma histories

Build trust, explain all procedures

Maintain dignity and respect

Involve social work early

Connect with community resources

Patients with Substance Use Disorders

Active intoxication:

Alcohol and drugs complicate assessment—is altered mental status from intoxication or head injury?

Assume head injury present until proven otherwise

Some drugs (cocaine, methamphetamine) cause agitation, tachycardia, hypertension mimicking other conditions

Toxicology screen helps but doesn't change trauma management priorities

Withdrawal risk:

Chronic alcohol users at risk for withdrawal seizures and delirium tremens

Timing: Usually begins 6-48 hours after last drink

Prevention: CIWA protocol, benzodiazepines, thiamine, folate, multivitamin

Monitor closely—withdrawal can be life-threatening

Opioid use:

Patients on chronic opioids have tolerance—need higher doses for pain control

Don't withhold appropriate analgesia due to addiction concerns

If on buprenorphine or methadone, continue when possible

Acute withdrawal uncomfortable but not life-threatening (unlike alcohol)

Pain management considerations:

Undertreating pain is unethical regardless of substance use history

Use multimodal analgesia (regional blocks, non-opioids, adjuncts)

Addiction medicine consultation if available

Establish clear, structured pain management plan

Stigma:

Patients with substance use disorders face significant healthcare stigma

Provide non-judgmental, compassionate care

Focus on medical needs, not moral judgments

Offer treatment resources if patient interested

Patients with Mental Illness

Assessment challenges:

Baseline psychiatric symptoms may be present

Differentiate baseline from new trauma-related changes

Contact psychiatric providers for baseline information

Don't assume all behavioral changes are psychiatric—rule out medical causes

Medication management:

Continue psychiatric medications when possible

Abrupt discontinuation causes withdrawal or symptom recurrence

Some psych medications interact with trauma medications

Consult psychiatry or pharmacy for complex regimens

Trauma-specific considerations:

Patients with PTSD may be triggered by trauma care environment

Explain procedures clearly

Offer choices when safe to do so

Minimize restraints (can be re-traumatizing)

Trauma-informed approach: safety, trustworthiness, choice, collaboration

Suicide risk:

Self-inflicted injuries may indicate suicide attempt

Screen for suicidal ideation

Psychiatric consultation for intentional self-harm

Remove means (pills, sharps) and implement safety measures

Continuous observation if suicidal

Chapter 10 Practice Questions (Complete 40 Questions)

Question 1: A 3-year-old child has a heart rate of 140 bpm and blood pressure of 85/50 after blunt trauma. These vital signs indicate:

A) Normal for age
B) Compensated shock
C) Decompensated shock
D) Hypertension

Answer: A

Explanation: Normal heart rate for a toddler (1-3 years) is 90-150 bpm, and normal systolic BP is 80-100. These vital signs are within normal limits for age. Always compare pediatric vital signs to age-appropriate norms, not adult values.

Question 2: When should you suspect compartment syndrome in a pediatric patient with forearm fracture?

A) When pain is controlled with over-the-counter medication
B) When pain is severe with passive finger extension
C) When capillary refill is 2 seconds
D) When the child is sleeping comfortably

Answer: B

Explanation: Severe pain with passive stretching of muscles in the affected compartment is the earliest and most reliable sign of compartment syndrome at any age. Pain with passive finger extension indicates volar compartment syndrome. Don't wait for late signs like absent pulses.

Question 3: A pregnant patient at 28 weeks gestation is hypotensive when supine. The appropriate intervention is:

A) Aggressive fluid boluses
B) Vasopressor administration
C) Left lateral tilt or manual left uterine displacement
D) Head-down position

Answer: C

Explanation: After 20 weeks gestation, the gravid uterus can compress the inferior vena cava when the patient is supine, causing supine hypotension syndrome. Tilting left lateral or manually displacing the uterus to the left relieves this compression and improves venous return.

Question 4: Which finding in a 6-month-old with "fall from couch" history raises concern for abuse?

A) Single bruise on forehead
B) Clavicle fracture
C) Multiple bruises at different healing stages
D) Crying during examination

Answer: C

Explanation: Multiple bruises at different healing stages suggest repeated trauma and raise concern for abuse. Additionally, non-mobile infants shouldn't have multiple bruises from normal activity. Single injuries from plausible mechanisms are more consistent with accidents, but multiple injuries at different stages warrant investigation.

Question 5: An 82-year-old on warfarin with INR of 3.8 has a subdural hematoma. Initial management includes:

A) Observation only
B) Vitamin K administration and possible prothrombin complex concentrate
C) Aspirin therapy
D) Discharge with outpatient follow-up

Answer: B

Explanation: Elevated INR with intracranial bleeding requires immediate reversal. Vitamin K reverses warfarin but takes hours to work. Prothrombin complex concentrate (PCC) provides immediate clotting factors. Fresh frozen plasma is an alternative. Don't delay reversal—intracranial bleeding can expand rapidly.

Question 6: A child's Glasgow Coma Scale score is 8. This indicates:

A) Mild brain injury
B) Moderate brain injury
C) Severe brain injury requiring intubation
D) Normal consciousness

Answer: C

Explanation: GCS ≤8 indicates severe brain injury and is an indication for endotracheal intubation to protect the airway and allow controlled ventilation for ICP management. This applies to both adults and children. GCS 13-15 is mild, 9-12 is moderate, ≤8 is severe.

Question 7: Intraosseous (IO) access in pediatric patients should be used when:

A) First-line for all pediatric trauma
B) After two failed IV attempts or when immediate access needed
C) Only in cardiac arrest
D) Never in children

Answer: B

Explanation: IO access is appropriate after two failed peripheral IV attempts or when immediate vascular access is critical and IV placement will take too long. It provides rapid, reliable access comparable to central venous access. Any medication or fluid that can go IV can go IO.

Question 8: What makes rib fractures in children particularly concerning?

A) They heal slowly
B) They indicate severe force was applied
C) They always require surgery
D) They cause more pain than in adults

Answer: B

Explanation: Children's ribs are very flexible and can absorb tremendous force before fracturing. If ribs do fracture, it indicates severe force was applied, raising concern for significant underlying injuries (pulmonary contusion, solid organ injuries) and possible abuse in young children.

Question 9: A pregnant trauma patient at 32 weeks has vaginal bleeding, abdominal pain, and a firm, tender uterus. This suggests:

A) Normal pregnancy changes
B) Urinary tract infection
C) Placental abruption
D) Preterm labor only

Answer: C

Explanation: Vaginal bleeding, abdominal pain, and firm/tender uterus after trauma are classic signs of placental abruption. This is the most common cause of fetal death from maternal trauma. Continuous fetal monitoring and obstetric consultation are urgent. Severe cases require emergent delivery.

Question 10: The primary goal when managing pregnant trauma patients is:

A) Immediate delivery of the fetus
B) Optimal maternal resuscitation
C) Limiting radiation exposure
D) Fetal monitoring

Answer: B

Explanation: The mother is the primary patient. Optimal fetal outcome depends on optimal maternal outcome. Aggressive maternal resuscitation is the best way to help the fetus. Don't withhold necessary interventions (including radiation) for maternal care due to pregnancy concerns.

Question 11: An elderly patient has "normal" blood pressure of 120/80 after trauma but appears in shock. This may indicate:

A) Anxiety
B) Relative hypotension if baseline BP is normally 160/90
C) Adequate resuscitation
D) Improved condition

Answer: B

Explanation: Many elderly patients have baseline hypertension. A "normal" blood pressure of 120/80 may actually represent relative hypotension and shock in someone whose baseline is 160/90. Always ask about baseline vital signs and compare current values to patient's normal.

Question 12: Pediatric fluid resuscitation for hemorrhagic shock starts with:

A) 10 mL/kg bolus
B) 20 mL/kg bolus
C) 40 mL/kg bolus
D) 1 liter bolus

Answer: B

Explanation: Pediatric fluid resuscitation begins with 20 mL/kg crystalloid boluses, reassessing after each bolus. This is different from adult fixed-volume boluses. Blood products are given at 10 mL/kg. Weight-based dosing is essential in pediatrics—calculate the patient's weight and dose accordingly.

Question 13: A bariatric patient (BMI 48) requires medication dosing:

A) Based on total body weight for all medications
B) Based on ideal body weight for all medications
C) Varies by medication—consult pharmacy
D) Same as non-bariatric patients

Answer: C

Explanation: Medication dosing in bariatric patients is complex. Some medications dose on total body weight, some on ideal body weight, some on adjusted body weight, and some have maximum doses. Always consult pharmacy for appropriate dosing to avoid underdosing (ineffective treatment) or overdosing (toxicity).

Question 14: SCIWORA (Spinal Cord Injury Without Radiographic Abnormality) is most common in:

A) Elderly patients
B) Pediatric patients
C) Pregnant patients
D) Bariatric patients

Answer: B

Explanation: SCIWORA occurs when spinal cord injury exists without visible fracture or abnormality on X-ray or CT. It's most common in children due to spinal column elasticity—the spine can stretch and injure the cord, then return to normal position. MRI may show cord injury when other imaging is normal.

Question 15: An Rh-negative pregnant patient with abdominal trauma requires:

A) No special treatment
B) RhoGAM administration
C) Immediate cesarean section
D) Platelets

Answer: B

Explanation: Rh-negative mothers with trauma should receive RhoGAM (Rh immune globulin) to prevent sensitization if the fetus is Rh-positive. Trauma can cause fetomaternal hemorrhage (fetal blood entering maternal circulation). RhoGAM prevents maternal antibody formation that could affect current or future pregnancies.

Question 16: Which statement about geriatric trauma patients is correct?

A) They have the same outcomes as younger patients with similar injuries
B) They have worse outcomes even with minor injuries
C) They don't need aggressive resuscitation
D) Ground-level falls never cause serious injury

Answer: B

Explanation: Elderly patients have significantly worse outcomes than younger patients with similar injury severity. They have less physiologic reserve, more comorbidities, and higher complication rates. Even minor mechanisms (ground-level falls) cause serious injuries. They require aggressive, appropriate resuscitation.

Question 17: A child is "acting normally" after head trauma. This means:

A) No serious injury is present
B) Safe to discharge home
C) Head injury still possible—children compensate well initially
D) No further assessment needed

Answer: C

Explanation: Children can appear normal initially despite serious head injury due to excellent compensatory mechanisms. They can deteriorate suddenly. "Acting normal" doesn't rule out injury. Maintain appropriate suspicion based on mechanism, and provide clear return precautions to caregivers about warning signs.

Question 18: Perimortem cesarean section in maternal cardiac arrest should be performed:

A) Only in the operating room
B) After 30 minutes of failed resuscitation
C) Within 4-5 minutes of arrest if fetus viable (>24 weeks)
D) Never

Answer: C

Explanation: If maternal resuscitation fails and fetus is viable (typically >24 weeks gestation), perform emergency cesarean section within 4-5 minutes of arrest. This can be done in the ED—don't wait for OR or obstetrics. Benefits both mother (relieves IVC compression) and fetus. Infant survival depends on delivery within 5 minutes of maternal arrest.

Question 19: An elderly patient on a beta-blocker has a heart rate of 78 bpm after trauma. This:

A) Indicates adequate resuscitation
B) Rules out shock
C) May represent inadequate compensation for shock
D) Is always normal for elderly patients

Answer: C

Explanation: Beta-blockers prevent compensatory tachycardia in response to shock. A heart rate of 78 bpm might represent inability to mount appropriate tachycardic response to hypovolemia. Don't rely on heart rate alone to assess shock in patients on beta-blockers or calcium channel blockers. Look at other signs: mentation, skin perfusion, urine output, lactate.

Question 20: A bariatric patient exceeds CT scanner weight limit (450 lbs). Alternative imaging for abdominal trauma includes:

A) No imaging necessary
B) Diagnostic peritoneal lavage or serial exams
C) Ultrasound only
D) Discharge without evaluation

Answer: B

Explanation: When patients exceed imaging equipment limits, alternatives include diagnostic peritoneal lavage (DPL), diagnostic laparoscopy, or very close serial clinical exams with low threshold for surgical exploration. Never discharge without adequate evaluation due to equipment limitations. Some facilities have bariatric CT scanners or open MRI as alternatives.

Question 21: The most important intervention to prevent morbidity in bariatric trauma patients is:

A) Strict bed rest
B) Early mobilization
C) Low-calorie diet
D) Limiting visitors

Answer: B

Explanation: Early mobilization is critical for preventing complications in bariatric patients: pneumonia, DVT, pressure injuries, and deconditioning. Despite logistical challenges with mobility, getting patients up and moving as soon as medically safe significantly improves outcomes.

Question 22: A 5-year-old has a femur fracture with different explanation from each parent. This suggests:

A) Parents are confused
B) Normal in stressful situations
C) Possible child abuse requiring investigation
D) Nothing concerning

Answer: C

Explanation: Inconsistent or changing history between caregivers is a red flag for child abuse. The injury doesn't match the explanations, or caregivers can't agree on what happened. This warrants investigation, thorough documentation, and reporting to child protective services. Healthcare providers are mandated reporters.

Question 23: A patient with pre-existing complete C6 spinal cord injury has blood pressure 200/110 and severe headache. This suggests:

A) Hypertensive emergency from other cause
B) Autonomic dysreflexia
C) Normal for spinal cord injury patients
D) Stroke

Answer: B

Explanation: Sudden severe hypertension with headache in a patient with spinal cord injury at T6 or above indicates autonomic dysreflexia. Common trigger in trauma is bladder distension. Treatment: sit upright, remove trigger (catheterize bladder), give antihypertensives if needed. Can be life-threatening if untreated.

Question 24: Appropriate pain scale for a non-verbal child with developmental disability is:

A) Numeric rating scale
B) Visual analog scale
C) FLACC scale (Face, Legs, Activity, Cry, Consolability)
D) McGill Pain Questionnaire

Answer: C

Explanation: FLACC scale assesses pain in non-verbal patients by observing facial expression, leg position, activity, cry, and consolability. Each scored 0-2, total 0-10. It's appropriate for young children and patients who can't self-report pain due to developmental disabilities, intubation, or altered mental status.

Question 25: A pregnant patient at 35 weeks needs CT scan for abdominal trauma. The appropriate approach is:

A) Refuse CT due to radiation risk
B) Wait until after delivery
C) Perform CT with abdominal shielding if possible
D) Substitute with ultrasound only

Answer: C

Explanation: Don't withhold necessary imaging from pregnant patients. Radiation risk to fetus from single CT is minimal and far less risky than missing maternal injuries. Shield abdomen when possible without compromising image quality. Maternal wellbeing is priority—maternal death is worse for fetus than radiation exposure.

Question 26: Signs of elder abuse include:

A) Single injury consistent with stated mechanism
B) Prompt presentation for care
C) Multiple injuries at different healing stages with vague history
D) Patient accompanied by attentive family

Answer: C

Explanation: Multiple injuries at different healing stages with vague, inconsistent, or changing history suggest abuse. Other red flags: delay in seeking care, caregiver preventing private conversation with patient, injuries inconsistent with mechanism, poor hygiene or malnutrition, over-sedation. Healthcare providers are mandated reporters for elder abuse.

Question 27: A child has tachycardia, cool extremities, delayed capillary refill, and normal blood pressure. This indicates:

A) Normal vital signs
B) Compensated shock requiring immediate intervention
C) Anxiety only
D) Adequate resuscitation

Answer: B

Explanation: Children can maintain normal blood pressure despite 25-30% blood loss through compensatory tachycardia and vasoconstriction. Tachycardia, cool extremities, and delayed capillary refill indicate compensated shock requiring immediate aggressive intervention. By the time blood pressure drops (decompensated shock), significant blood loss has occurred.

Question 28: Fetal heart rate monitoring after maternal trauma should continue for at least:

A) 1 hour for all patients
B) 4-6 hours minimum, longer for significant trauma
C) 30 minutes
D) No monitoring needed if mother stable

Answer: B

Explanation: Continuous fetal heart rate monitoring should be performed for minimum 4-6 hours after minor trauma, 24-48 hours after significant trauma in viable pregnancies (>20-24 weeks). Monitoring detects placental abruption and fetal compromise before symptoms are obvious. Contractions, fetal heart rate decelerations, or other abnormalities warrant extended monitoring and obstetric consultation.

Question 29: A homeless patient needs discharge after minor trauma. Appropriate discharge planning includes:

A) Standard written instructions
B) Collaboration with social work for shelter placement and accessible follow-up
C) No special considerations
D) Prescription for narcotic pain medication

Answer: B

Explanation: Standard discharge instructions don't work for homeless patients (no home for rest/elevation, no phone for follow-up calls, no refrigeration for some medications). Work with social work to arrange shelter, ensure prescriptions are feasible (can't refrigerate insulin if living outside), make follow-up accessible, and connect with community resources. Consider respite care if medical needs require.

Question 30: VTE prophylaxis in bariatric patients often requires:

A) Standard dosing
B) No prophylaxis needed
C) Higher doses than standard patients
D) Only mechanical prophylaxis

Answer: C

Explanation: Bariatric patients need higher doses of chemical VTE prophylaxis due to increased volume of distribution and higher VTE risk. Example: enoxaparin 40 mg twice daily instead of once daily, or 0.5 mg/kg twice daily. Use both chemical and mechanical prophylaxis. Some centers use duplex ultrasound screening. Despite higher doses, bariatric patients still have elevated VTE rates.

Question 31: A 70-year-old with dementia has altered mental status after fall. The appropriate approach is:

A) Assume it's baseline dementia
B) Attribute to dementia without further workup
C) Establish baseline from family and investigate changes
D) No treatment needed

Answer: C

Explanation: Never assume altered mental status is baseline without verification. Establish baseline from family or medical records, then investigate any changes from baseline. Patients with dementia can still have delirium, head injuries, or other acute issues causing mental status changes. Attributing everything to dementia causes missed diagnoses.

Question 32: What is the most common cause of death in pediatric trauma?

A) Abdominal injuries
B) Extremity injuries
C) Head injuries
D) Burn injuries

Answer: C

Explanation: Head injury is the leading cause of death in pediatric trauma. Children's proportionally larger heads, weaker neck muscles, and thinner skulls make them vulnerable. Diffuse axonal injury and cerebral edema are more common than in adults. Even minor mechanisms can cause significant head injury in children.

Question 33: A patient with insulin pump needs CT scan. The appropriate action is:

A) Leave pump in place
B) Remove pump before MRI but can stay for CT
C) Disconnect permanently
D) Give oral diabetes medications instead

Answer: B

Explanation: Insulin pumps must be removed before MRI (magnetic field damages pump) but can stay for CT. If pump is disconnected for extended period, patient may need IV insulin replacement. Document pump settings and location. Coordinate with endocrinology for complex cases. Replace pump and verify function after imaging.

Question 34: A child with handlebar injury to abdomen is at high risk for:

A) Splenic injury
B) Duodenal hematoma or pancreatic injury
C) Kidney laceration
D) Liver injury

Answer: B

Explanation: Handlebar injuries (bicycle or motorcycle) cause direct blow to epigastrium, compressing duodenum and pancreas against spine. Classic injuries are duodenal hematoma, duodenal perforation (often delayed), and pancreatic injury. Elevated amylase/lipase, epigastric tenderness, and mechanism should raise suspicion. Some injuries present with delayed symptoms.

Question 35: Appropriate blood pressure cuff size for bariatric patients requires:

A) Largest cuff available
B) Cuff bladder covering 80% of arm circumference
C) Standard adult cuff
D) Any cuff that fits

Answer: B

Explanation: Blood pressure cuff bladder should cover 80% of arm circumference for accurate measurement. Too small a cuff reads falsely high, too large reads falsely low. Bariatric patients often need thigh cuffs on the arm. Inaccurate cuff size leads to inappropriate treatment decisions.

Question 36: A pregnant patient in third trimester has palpable fetal parts through abdomen and lost fetal heart tones. This suggests:

A) Normal fetal position
B) Uterine rupture
C) Placental abruption
D) Preterm labor

Answer: B

Explanation: Palpable fetal parts through abdomen with loss of fetal heart tones indicates uterine rupture—complete tear in uterine wall with fetus expelled into peritoneal cavity. This is catastrophic for both mother and fetus. Risk higher with previous cesarean section. Requires emergency cesarean/hysterectomy and massive resuscitation.

Question 37: An elderly patient with osteoporosis falls from standing. Appropriate imaging includes:

A) No imaging needed for ground-level fall
B) Targeted imaging based on complaints
C) Low threshold for imaging—minor falls cause significant fractures
D) Observation only

Answer: C

Explanation: Osteoporotic bones fracture from minimal trauma. Ground-level falls in elderly patients can cause hip fractures, vertebral compression fractures, distal radius fractures, and other injuries. Have low threshold for imaging based on mechanism, even if patient seems stable. What's trivial trauma for young adults is serious for elderly with osteoporosis.

Question 38: A child abuse report should be made when:

A) Definitive proof of abuse exists
B) Suspicion of abuse exists
C) Only if caregiver confesses
D) After complete investigation

Answer: B

Explanation: Healthcare providers are mandated reporters who must report suspicion of abuse, not just confirmed abuse. Investigation is the role of child protective services and law enforcement, not healthcare providers. Report any reasonable suspicion—you don't need proof. Failure to report when suspicion exists is a violation of mandatory reporting laws.

Question 39: Developmentally appropriate explanation for a 5-year-old needing IV placement is:

A) "We need to put a small straw in your arm to give you medicine"
B) "This is for intravenous access for fluid resuscitation"
C) No explanation needed
D) Explain only to parents

Answer: A

Explanation: Use simple, age-appropriate language for children. Avoid medical jargon. Concrete, simple terms they understand work best ("small straw" for catheter, "medicine" for fluids). Be honest but gentle. Children understand more than we think and deserve explanations. Speaking directly to children (while including parents) shows respect and reduces anxiety.

Question 40: A patient with VAD (ventricular assist device) in cardiac arrest should receive:

A) Immediate chest compressions
B) Check VAD function before compressions
C) Defibrillation only
D) No resuscitation

Answer: B

Explanation: Patients with continuous-flow VADs may have no palpable pulse normally. Before performing chest compressions, verify VAD failure (check alarms, connections, pump function). If VAD is functioning, compressions aren't needed and may damage device. If VAD has failed, then perform CPR. Early cardiothoracic surgery consultation essential. These are complex patients requiring specialized knowledge.

Clinical Scenarios

Clinical Scenario 1: Pediatric Trauma with Compensated Shock

A 4-year-old boy was struck by a car while crossing the street. He's brought in by ambulance crying and asking for his mother. Initial vitals: HR 158, BP 88/54, RR 32, SpO_2 96% on non-rebreather mask, temperature 36.2°C.

On exam, he's anxious and crying. Skin is pale and cool with capillary refill of 4 seconds. Breath sounds equal bilaterally. Abdomen is mildly distended and diffusely tender without obvious guarding. Pelvis stable. No obvious extremity deformities. GCS 15 (E4, V5, M6).

Weight is estimated at 18 kg using Broselow tape.

Questions:

Is this child in shock? What clinical findings support your assessment?

What are your immediate priorities and interventions?

The nurse obtains IV access and asks how much fluid to give. What is your answer?

After 20 mL/kg crystalloid, vitals are HR 142, BP 92/58. The child is less anxious but abdomen more distended. What do you suspect and what's the next step?

Answers:

Shock assessment: Yes, this child is in compensated shock despite "normal" blood pressure. Supporting findings:

Tachycardia: HR 158 is elevated even for a frightened 4-year-old (normal up to 140 for preschool age)

Cool, pale skin with delayed capillary refill (4 seconds): Indicates peripheral vasoconstriction, the body shunting blood from skin to vital organs

Blood pressure 88/54: While within "normal" range for age (80-110 systolic), it's at the lower end. In context of other findings, this suggests compensated shock

Tachypnea (RR 32): Compensatory response to metabolic acidosis from poor perfusion

Mechanism: Pedestrian struck by car—high-energy mechanism with high likelihood of internal injuries

Distended, tender abdomen: Suggests intra-abdominal bleeding

Critical concept: Children maintain blood pressure through remarkable cardiovascular compensation until 25-30% blood loss. This child is maintaining BP at cost of significant vasoconstriction and tachycardia. He needs immediate intervention before decompensating to hypotensive shock.

Immediate priorities:

Airway/Breathing:

- Continue high-flow oxygen via non-rebreather (already in place)
- Monitor respiratory effort closely—tachypnea may worsen
- Prepare for possible intubation if mental status deteriorates

Circulation:

- Establish two large-bore IVs immediately (or IO if two IV attempts fail)
- Send labs: CBC, type and crossmatch, comprehensive metabolic panel, coagulation studies, lactate
- Begin fluid resuscitation (calculated below)
- Activate pediatric trauma team and massive transfusion protocol
- Keep patient warm (room temperature up, warming lights, warm fluids)

Assessment:

- FAST exam to identify free fluid
- Portable chest and pelvis X-rays
- Continuous monitoring (cardiac monitor, pulse oximetry, blood pressure every 5 minutes)
- Frequent reassessment—pediatric patients can deteriorate rapidly

Family:

- Allow parents to be with child if possible (reduces anxiety for both)
- Assign team member to update parents
- Explain procedures in developmentally appropriate language to child

Definitive care preparation:

- Contact pediatric surgery immediately
- Prepare for possible OR or CT (if stabilizes)
- If FAST positive with ongoing instability, will need emergent laparotomy

Fluid resuscitation calculation:

Weight: 18 kg (from Broselow tape)

Initial bolus: 20 mL/kg of crystalloid (normal saline or lactated Ringer's)

- Calculation: 18 kg × 20 mL/kg = 360 mL
- Give 360 mL crystalloid rapidly (wide open)
- Reassess after completion

Key points:

- Pediatric resuscitation is weight-based, not fixed volumes
- Give boluses, reassess, repeat as needed
- Maximum 60 mL/kg crystalloid before switching to blood products
- If needs blood: 10 mL/kg packed red blood cells (180 mL for this patient)
- Use blood warmer for all products
- O-negative blood if type-specific not available
- Consider massive transfusion protocol if continues requiring resuscitation

Clinical deterioration suggests:

Assessment after fluid bolus:

- HR improved from 158 to 142 (still elevated but better)
- BP improved slightly 88→92 systolic
- Less anxious (improved cerebral perfusion)
- BUT abdomen MORE distended (concerning)

Interpretation: This child has **ongoing intra-abdominal hemorrhage**. The fluid bolus temporarily improved hemodynamics but bleeding continues, causing progressive abdominal distension.

Evidence:

- Partial response to fluid (HR and BP improved but not normalized)
- Increasing abdominal distension despite resuscitation
- Mechanism (high-energy blunt trauma) consistent with solid organ injury

Next steps—URGENT:

Immediate:

- FAST exam NOW (if not already done)—will likely show free fluid
- Continue resuscitation with blood products (don't give more crystalloid)
- Give 10 mL/kg (180 mL) PRBCs immediately
- Activate massive transfusion protocol with pediatric ratios
- Notify OR of impending arrival

Diagnostic decision:

- If FAST positive + hemodynamic instability = direct to OR for exploratory laparotomy
- If stabilizes with blood products = CT to characterize injuries and determine if non-operative management possible
- This child is NOT stable enough for CT—continued distension with partial response to resuscitation = needs surgery

Surgical plan:

Emergent exploratory laparotomy

Likely findings: splenic or liver laceration (most common in pediatric blunt abdominal trauma)

May attempt splenorrhaphy (spleen repair) rather than splenectomy if possible—preserves immune function

Damage control approach if coagulopathic: pack, warm, correct coagulopathy, return for definitive repair

Ongoing management:

Address hypothermia (child already 36.2°C—will worsen with fluids and OR)

Monitor for coagulopathy (dilutional and hypothermic)

Keep parents informed—prepare them that child needs surgery

Pediatric ICU bed arranged for post-op care

Key learning points:

Recognize compensated shock in children before hypotension develops

Weight-based dosing is essential in pediatrics

Partial response to resuscitation with worsening abdominal exam indicates ongoing bleeding

Don't delay surgery in unstable patients—CT is for stable patients only

Pediatric trauma requires specialized knowledge of age-specific norms and responses

---

Clinical Scenario 2: Geriatric Trauma with Anticoagulation

A 78-year-old woman slipped on ice and struck her head on the sidewalk. She was initially alert but is now increasingly confused. EMS reports she was "fine" initially, then became lethargic during transport.

Current vitals: HR 76, BP 164/92, RR 16, SpO2 95% on room air.

Medical history obtained from EMS includes atrial fibrillation (on warfarin), hypertension, diabetes, and osteoporosis. Medications: warfarin 5 mg daily, metoprolol 50 mg BID, lisinopril 20 mg daily, metformin 1000 mg BID.

Examination shows confusion (oriented only to person), 4 cm laceration on right temporal area, no other obvious trauma. Pupils equal and reactive. Right-sided weakness noted with pronator drift. GCS 13 (E3, V4, M6).

Questions:

What is your primary concern and why is anticoagulation significant?

The daughter asks if her mother's blood pressure is "normal." How do you interpret these vital signs?

Labs return with INR 3.2. What are your immediate interventions while awaiting CT results?

CT shows 8 mm acute subdural hematoma with 3 mm midline shift. What is the management plan?

Answers:

Primary concern:

Expanding intracranial hematoma is the primary concern. This patient has:

Classic presentation of evolving intracranial bleeding:

- Initial lucid interval (alert after injury)
- Progressive deterioration (confusion, letharness)
- Focal neurological findings (right-sided weakness)
- Declining GCS (13, indicating moderate brain injury)

Anticoagulation significance:

- Warfarin increases bleeding risk dramatically—even minor head trauma can cause significant intracranial hemorrhage
- INR >3 indicates significant anticoagulation (therapeutic range 2-3 for AFib)
- Subdural hematomas expand more rapidly in anticoagulated patients
- Without reversal, bleeding will continue and patient will deteriorate

Mechanism consideration:

- Ground-level fall in elderly on anticoagulation is HIGH RISK for intracranial bleeding
- Age + anticoagulation + head trauma = very concerning combination
- Brain atrophy (normal aging) creates space for blood to accumulate before symptoms appear

Time-sensitive injury:

- Progressive symptoms indicate ongoing bleeding/mass effect
- Every minute counts—brain can only tolerate so much compression
- Reversal must begin immediately, not after CT confirmation

Vital sign interpretation:

These vital signs are ABNORMAL for this patient despite seeming "normal" by standard:

Blood pressure 164/92:

- Elevated, but need to know her baseline
- Could be her normal (many elderly have baseline hypertension)

OR could represent Cushing's response to increased intracranial pressure (hypertension + bradycardia with irregular respirations)

In context of head injury and declining mental status, concerning for elevated ICP

Heart rate 76:

Seems normal, but she's on metoprolol (beta-blocker)

Beta-blockers prevent compensatory tachycardia

May represent relative bradycardia (unable to mount appropriate response)

In Cushing's triad, would expect bradycardia with hypertension

Respiratory rate 16:

Normal rate, but need to assess pattern and depth

Irregular respirations part of Cushing's triad

Interpretation for daughter: "Your mother's blood pressure is elevated, which combined with her confusion and the fact that she's on a blood thinner, is concerning for bleeding in her brain. Even though her heart rate looks normal, she's on a medication that prevents it from rising even when there's a problem. We're treating this very seriously and getting a CT scan of her brain immediately. We're also going to reverse her blood thinner right now to stop any bleeding."

Action based on vitals:

These suggest possible increased ICP (Cushing's response)

Don't wait for "textbook" Cushing's triad (late finding)

Immediate head CT

Immediate reversal of anticoagulation

Prepare for possible neurosurgical intervention

Immediate interventions for INR 3.2:

DON'T wait for CT results to reverse anticoagulation—clinical picture warrants immediate reversal

Reversal protocol:

Vitamin K (Phytonadione):

Dose: 10 mg IV (slow push over 10-20 minutes to avoid anaphylaxis)

Effect: Takes 12-24 hours to work (too slow for acute emergency)

Purpose: Provides sustained reversal after faster agents wear off

Prothrombin Complex Concentrate (PCC)—PREFERRED:

Dose: 25-50 units/kg IV (approximately 2000-4000 units for 80 kg patient)

- Effect: Immediate reversal (within minutes)
- Contains factors II, VII, IX, X—exactly what warfarin depletes
- Advantages: Small volume, fast, effective
- Give this FIRST

Fresh Frozen Plasma (FFP)—Alternative if PCC unavailable:

- Dose: 15 mL/kg (approximately 4-6 units)
- Effect: 30-60 minutes
- Disadvantages: Large volume (may worsen cerebral edema), slower than PCC, less effective

Tranexamic acid (TXA)—Consider:

- Some protocols include TXA 1 gram IV to prevent hematoma expansion
- Evidence mixed but may help in intracranial hemorrhage

Other immediate interventions:

- Stat head CT (patient should already be there or en route)
- Neurosurgery consultation STAT (call even before CT if high suspicion)
- Elevate head of bed 30 degrees (reduces ICP if increased)
- Avoid hypotension (maintain cerebral perfusion)
- Repeat INR 30 minutes after reversal to confirm
- Serial neurological assessments every 15-30 minutes
- Correct any coagulopathy (platelets if low, check fibrinogen)

Hold warfarin:

- Obviously don't give next dose
- Decision to restart will be made later in consultation with neurosurgery and cardiology
- Balance stroke risk from AFib vs. re-bleed risk

Management plan for subdural hematoma:

CT findings interpretation:

- 8 mm subdural hematoma = significant (generally >5 mm is clinically significant)
- 3 mm midline shift = definite mass effect
- Acute subdural (bright on CT)
- Combined with clinical deterioration = surgical candidate

Immediate management:

Medical optimization:

- Continue anticoagulation reversal (already started)
- Recheck INR—goal <1.5, ideally <1.3 before surgery

Maintain systolic BP 140-160 (adequate cerebral perfusion without worsening bleeding)

Prevent secondary brain injury:

- Avoid hypotension (maintain cerebral perfusion pressure)
- Avoid hypoxia (keep O2 sat >95%)
- Prevent hyperthermia
- Maintain normoglycemia (diabetes management)

Seizure prophylaxis: Consider levetiracetam or phenytoin

Neurosurgical intervention:

Indications for surgery (this patient meets multiple):

- Hematoma >10 mm thickness OR
- Midline shift >5 mm OR
- GCS decline OR
- Progressive neurological deficits

This patient has 8 mm hematoma, 3 mm shift, declining GCS, and focal deficits—clear surgical candidate

Surgical options:

Craniotomy: Most definitive, allows complete evacuation, better outcomes for acute SDH with mass effect

Burr holes: Less invasive but may be inadequate for acute organized clot

Decision by neurosurgeon based on clot characteristics and patient factors

Timing:

Urgent surgery once INR corrected

Don't delay excessively—outcome better with earlier intervention

Balance: need adequate coagulation but can't wait indefinitely while ICP rises

ICU management post-op:

Neurological ICU monitoring

ICP monitoring may be placed

Serial CT scans to assess for re-bleed

Gradual wean from sedation with neuro checks

DVT prophylaxis (mechanical only initially, chemical once bleeding risk reduced)

Early mobilization when appropriate

Rehabilitation planning

Anticoagulation decision:

Complex decision involving neurosurgery, cardiology, patient/family

Timing of restart depends on:

- Bleeding control
- Stroke risk from AFib (CHA2DS2-VASc score)
- Type of hematoma
- Other options (can consider different anticoagulant with better reversibility)

Typically wait at least 7-14 days, sometimes longer

May transition to DOAC (easier to reverse than warfarin) when restarting

Prognosis discussion with family:

Age is adverse factor (elderly have worse outcomes from brain injury)

Anticoagulation worsened bleeding

Surgical intervention and reversal improve outcomes

Recovery may be prolonged

Risk of permanent deficits

Some patients recover well, others have residual disability

Honest, compassionate communication about uncertainty

Key learning points:

Low-threshold for head CT in elderly with any head trauma, especially if anticoagulated

Ground-level falls cause serious injury in elderly

"Normal" vital signs may not be normal—know baseline and medications

Reverse anticoagulation immediately based on clinical suspicion, don't wait for imaging

Subdural hematomas in elderly evolve over hours to days—progressive symptoms warrant urgent intervention

Beta-blockers mask compensatory responses—can't rely on tachycardia to indicate shock

---

Clinical Scenario 3: Pregnancy Trauma with Placental Abruption

A 32-year-old woman at 34 weeks gestation was the restrained driver in a motor vehicle crash (frontal impact, moderate damage). She complains of abdominal pain and contractions. She reports normal pregnancy with no complications.

Vitals: HR 108, BP 118/76, RR 20, SpO2 98% on room air.

Examination shows seatbelt bruising across lower abdomen. Fundal height 32 cm (appropriate for dates). Fetal heart rate 142 bpm on initial check. Uterus feels firm and tender. Vaginal exam shows no obvious bleeding, cervix closed. No other injuries apparent.

Questions:

What pregnancy-specific injury does the clinical picture suggest?

How should this patient be positioned and why?

Fetal monitoring shows late decelerations and decreased variability. What does this indicate and what interventions are needed?

The patient suddenly develops vaginal bleeding with persistent uterine contractions. Fetal heart tones drop to 90 bpm. What has occurred and what is your immediate action?

Answers:

Pregnancy-specific injury suggested:

Placental abruption is highly suspected based on:

Mechanism:

- Motor vehicle crash with frontal impact
- Restrained driver (seatbelt across abdomen)
- Deceleration forces shear placenta from uterine wall
- Occurs in 1-5% minor trauma, up to 50% major trauma

Clinical findings:

- Abdominal pain (placental separation is painful)
- **Firm, tender uterus** (classic finding—tetanic contraction from bleeding behind placenta)
- Contractions (irritable uterus from bleeding)
- Seatbelt bruising across abdomen (direct evidence of force to pregnant abdomen)
- Gestational age 34 weeks (viable fetus at risk)

Key point: Vaginal bleeding may be ABSENT (50% of abruptions)

- Blood can be contained behind placenta (concealed abruption)
- Absence of vaginal bleeding does NOT rule out abruption
- Firm, tender, contracting uterus is the key finding

Differential considerations:

- Uterine contusion (less likely with this degree of tenderness)
- Preterm labor (but wouldn't cause firm, tender uterus)
- Uterine rupture (less likely without prior cesarean, would see more dramatic presentation)

Pathophysiology:

- Deceleration causes placenta to shear from uterine wall
- Bleeding occurs into space between placenta and uterus
- Reduces placental surface area for gas exchange

Fetus becomes hypoxic from decreased oxygen delivery

Can progress from partial to complete abruption

Maternal coagulopathy can develop (DIC) if severe

Patient positioning:

Left lateral tilt or manual left uterine displacement—ESSENTIAL

Rationale:

At 34 weeks, gravid uterus is large enough to compress IVC when supine

IVC compression reduces venous return → decreased cardiac output

This causes supine hypotension syndrome

Maternal hypotension reduces placental perfusion

Fetal distress worsens from decreased maternal cardiac output

In patient with possible abruption (already compromised placental function), any reduction in perfusion is dangerous

How to achieve:

Option 1: Left lateral tilt

Tilt backboard/stretcher 15-30 degrees to left

Or place wedge (rolled towels, foam) under right hip

Keeps patient in semi-supine position for procedures while relieving IVC compression

Option 2: Manual uterine displacement

Staff member manually pushes uterus to patient's left

Effective but requires dedicated person

Useful during procedures when can't tilt (intubation, etc.)

Exception:

If CPR needed, can't tilt—perform manual left uterine displacement during compressions

If patient in arrest >4 minutes with viable fetus, prepare for perimortem C-section

Other positioning considerations:

Spinal precautions if mechanism suggests spinal injury

Can maintain c-spine while tilting entire board

Head of bed can be elevated if respiratory distress (but maintain left tilt)

Monitoring while positioned:

Maternal vital signs

- Continuous fetal heart rate monitoring
- Watch for improvement in both with proper positioning

Fetal heart rate abnormalities indicate:

Late decelerations and decreased variability = FETAL DISTRESS from inadequate placental perfusion

Understanding fetal heart rate patterns:

Normal fetal heart rate:

- Baseline: 110-160 bpm (this fetus 142—initially normal)
- Variability: 6-25 bpm fluctuation (shows intact nervous system)
- Accelerations with movement (reassuring)
- No concerning decelerations

Late decelerations:

- Heart rate decreases AFTER uterine contraction peaks
- Caused by uteroplacental insufficiency
- Indicates fetus not getting adequate oxygen
- Placenta can't meet fetal oxygen demands during contraction
- Very concerning pattern

Decreased variability:

- Loss of normal beat-to-beat variation
- Indicates fetal hypoxia affecting brainstem function
- Combined with late decelerations = severe fetal compromise

In context of suspected abruption:

- Placental separation reduces functional placenta
- Less surface area for maternal-fetal gas exchange
- Fetus becomes progressively hypoxic
- Without intervention, fetal death imminent

Immediate interventions:

Optimize maternal status (improves fetal perfusion):

- Ensure left lateral tilt in place
- **High-flow oxygen** to mother (goal: maternal SpO2 >95%, ideally 100%)
  - Increases maternal PaO2
  - Improves oxygen gradient across placenta
  - Helps hypoxic fetus
- **IV fluid resuscitation:**
  - Two large-bore IVs if not already present

- Crystalloid bolus 500-1000 mL
- Increases maternal blood volume
- Improves uteroplacental perfusion pressure

Correct hypotension aggressively:

- Maternal BP directly affects placental perfusion
- This patient's BP seems "normal" but may be relatively low
- Goal: maintain normal to slightly elevated BP for optimal placental flow

Stop any uterotonics:

- If patient receiving any medications causing contractions, stop immediately
- Contractions worsen placental perfusion

Prepare for delivery:

- Immediate obstetric consultation (should already be involved)
- Notify NICU of impending delivery of 34-week infant in distress
- Notify anesthesia
- Type and crossmatch maternal blood
- Consider tocolytics to stop contractions if not contraindicated (controversial in abruption)

Delivery decision:

- Non-reassuring fetal heart rate pattern = indication for delivery
- Severity determines urgency
- Options:
  - **Emergent C-section** (most likely given fetal distress and abruption)
  - Vaginal delivery if cervix favorable and fetus can tolerate (unlikely in this scenario)

Maternal monitoring:

- Abruption can cause maternal coagulopathy (DIC)
- Check coagulation studies (PT, PTT, fibrinogen, platelets)
- Have blood products available
- Monitor for postpartum hemorrhage risk

Fetal monitoring:

- Continuous monitoring until delivery
- If pattern worsens (persistent bradycardia), move to immediate C-section

Prepare resuscitation equipment for premature infant

Clinical deterioration—vaginal bleeding and fetal bradycardia:

What occurred: Progression to severe or complete placental abruption

New findings:

Vaginal bleeding (previously absent, now present)

Persistent uterine contractions (irritable uterus)

Fetal bradycardia (90 bpm, critical—normal 110-160)

Interpretation:

Abruption progressing from partial to more complete

More placental surface separating from uterus

Blood now tracking down and out (vaginal bleeding)

Fetus severely hypoxic from massive loss of placental function

Fetal heart rate 90 bpm = severe distress, imminent fetal death without delivery

This is a TRUE OBSTETRIC EMERGENCY

Immediate actions—SIMULTANEOUS:

Call overhead code/emergency:

"Obstetric emergency, [location], need OB, anesthesia, NICU stat"

All hands on deck

Notify team:

OB attending and resident to bedside NOW

Anesthesia to bedside NOW

OR to prepare for stat C-section

NICU team to OR/bedside for neonatal resuscitation

Continue maternal resuscitation:

Continue high-flow oxygen

Rapid IV fluid resuscitation

Activate massive transfusion protocol (abruption can cause massive maternal bleeding)

Check coagulation studies stat

Crossmatch 4-6 units PRBCs

Have FFP, platelets, cryoprecipitate available

Prepare for immediate delivery:

Patient to OR immediately (don't wait for labs, imaging, etc.)

If cesarean section can be started within 5 minutes, go to OR

If delay to OR, consider emergency C-section in ED/L&D (decision by OB)

For 34-week fetus with heart rate 90, minutes matter

Set up for emergency C-section:

Prep and drape abdomen

Anesthesia provides fastest safe option (usually general in true emergency)

Surgical instruments ready

Neonatal resuscitation equipment ready and checked

Neonatal team scrubbed and ready

Informed consent:

If time allows: explain emergency to patient, obtain verbal consent

If no time: proceed under emergency doctrine (life-saving intervention when patient can't consent)

Document clearly

Delivery and immediate post-delivery:

Cesarean section:

Rapid delivery of infant

NICU team resuscitates infant (likely needs aggressive resuscitation given distress and prematurity)

Deliver placenta and inspect for completeness

Assess amount of abruption (% of placenta separated)

Maternal management:

Assess for postpartum hemorrhage (high risk with abruption)

Uterotonics (oxytocin, methergine, misoprostol) to contract uterus

Correct coagulopathy if present

Monitor for DIC (can develop hours after delivery)

ICU monitoring if unstable or coagulopathic

Neonatal management:

34-week infant may need respiratory support

NICU admission

Assess for hypoxic injury

Glucose monitoring (premature infants at risk for hypoglycemia)

Family communication:

Update family immediately about mother and baby status

Explain what happened (placental separation, emergency delivery)

Honest about neonatal prognosis (34 weeks generally good prognosis if resuscitated promptly)

Support family through crisis

Key learning points:

- Placental abruption can occur without vaginal bleeding—firm, tender uterus is key finding
- Seatbelt sign in pregnancy raises high suspicion for abruption
- Continuous fetal monitoring essential—fetal distress indicates severity
- Maternal resuscitation improves fetal outcomes (oxygen, fluids, left tilt)
- Non-reassuring fetal heart rate = delivery indication
- Fetal bradycardia in setting of abruption = immediate delivery needed
- Abruption can progress rapidly—vigilant monitoring required
- Mother can appear stable while fetus severely compromised

Clinical Scenario 4: Bariatric Patient with Assessment Challenges

A 52-year-old male (weight 385 lbs, BMI 54) fell down stairs at home. He complains of right leg and chest pain. He has difficulty breathing and can't stand.

Medical history: Morbid obesity, Type 2 diabetes, hypertension, sleep apnea (uses CPAP), previous DVT.

Vitals: HR 104, BP obtained with thigh cuff on arm reads 158/94, RR 26, SpO2 89% on room air.

He's sitting upright on EMS stretcher, appears anxious and in pain. Lower right leg has obvious deformity. You attempt to examine his chest but adipose tissue makes assessment difficult.

Questions:

- What are the immediate airway and breathing concerns specific to this bariatric patient?
- How do you approach the physical examination given body habitus limitations?
- The patient needs imaging but weighs more than your CT scanner limit (450 lbs). What are your options?
- What VTE prophylaxis is appropriate and why is this patient particularly high risk?

Answers:

Airway and breathing concerns specific to bariatric patients:

Current presentation:

- **Hypoxemia (SpO2 89%):** Significantly below normal, indicates inadequate oxygenation
- **Tachypnea (RR 26):** Respiratory distress
- **Chest pain:** Could indicate rib fractures, pulmonary contusion, or cardiac issue
- **Sitting upright:** Patient positioning himself for maximum respiratory effort—lying flat would worsen breathing
- **Anxiety:** May be from hypoxia, pain, or both

Bariatric-specific respiratory concerns:

Baseline respiratory compromise:

- **Restrictive lung disease:** Chest wall weight and abdominal mass compress lungs
- **Reduced functional residual capacity:** Less oxygen reserve
- **Obstructive sleep apnea:** Narrowed upper airway from pharyngeal tissue
- **Obesity hypoventilation syndrome:** Some bariatric patients chronically hypoventilate
- **Patient uses CPAP at home:** Confirms sleep apnea diagnosis

Why hypoxia is particularly concerning:

- Limited respiratory reserve means rapid desaturation
- Harder to ventilate with bag-mask if needed (stiff chest wall)
- Difficult airway if intubation needed (short neck, redundant tissue)
- Positional considerations (supine worsens breathing)

Trauma-specific concerns:

- Fall down stairs can cause rib fractures, pulmonary contusion
- Adipose tissue makes chest wall assessment difficult
- May not appreciate rib fractures or flail chest on exam
- Splinting from pain reduces tidal volume

Critical point: Lower threshold for respiratory failure due to baseline compromise + acute injury

Immediate interventions:

Oxygenation:

- High-flow oxygen via non-rebreather mask immediately
- Goal: $SpO_2 \geq 94\%$ (>92% minimum, but aim higher)
- If doesn't improve with supplemental O_2, consider:
  - Bringing patient's home CPAP (improves oxygenation and he's familiar with it)
  - BiPAP or CPAP in ED
  - Early intubation if worsening

Positioning:

- Keep patient upright (30-45 degrees minimum)
- DON'T lay flat—will worsen respiratory mechanics
- Reverse Trendelenburg if needed for procedures
- Extra pillows/positioning devices

Airway assessment:

Assess for difficult airway features:

- Short neck (obscured by adipose tissue)
- Limited neck mobility

- Mallampati score if possible (predicts intubation difficulty)

Anticipate difficult airway—have backup plan ready:

- Video laryngoscopy
- Bougie
- Supraglottic airway (LMA)
- Surgical airway equipment immediately available

Ramping position if intubation needed:

- Stack blankets/towels to align external auditory meatus with sternal notch
- Improves laryngoscopy view dramatically
- Essential for successful intubation in bariatric patients

Pain management affecting breathing:

- Chest and leg pain causing splinting (shallow breathing)
- Adequate analgesia improves respiratory effort
- Consider regional techniques (rib blocks for chest pain)
- Multimodal approach reduces opioid requirements and respiratory depression risk

Monitoring and early intervention:

- Continuous pulse oximetry
- Capnography if available (monitors ventilation)
- ABG if concerns about adequacy of ventilation (may have baseline hypercapnia)
- **Low threshold for positive pressure ventilation:**
  - BiPAP/CPAP if deteriorating
  - Intubation if failing non-invasive support
  - Don't wait until complete respiratory failure

Critical decision points:

- **Improving with oxygen and positioning:** Continue close monitoring, prepare for intubation if worsens
- **Not improving or worsening:** Strongly consider early intubation while patient still has some reserve, rather than waiting for crisis
- **If intubates:** Anticipate difficult airway, use experienced provider, have backup plans ready
- **Physical examination approach with body habitus limitations:**

General principles:

- **Be thorough despite challenges**—don't assume injuries aren't present just because hard to assess
- **Use all available tools**—imaging, lab work, and clinical judgment together

Serial examinations—repeat frequently as injuries may become apparent over time

Lower threshold for imaging—when exam unreliable, imaging fills gaps

Specific examination strategies:

Chest assessment (current priority given respiratory distress):

Inspection:

Observe chest wall movement for symmetry (may see despite adipose tissue)

Look for bruising, abrasions (may be hidden in skin folds—examine carefully)

Note any paradoxical movement (flail chest)

Respiratory effort—using accessory muscles, retractions

Palpation:

Press firmly to palpate ribs through adipose tissue

Feel for crepitus (rib fractures, subcutaneous emphysema)

Check for chest wall stability

May need deeper palpation than usual—communicate with patient about pressure

Auscultation:

Challenging but still valuable

Breath sounds may be diminished throughout due to body habitus

Compare side to side—asymmetry more important than absolute quality

Listen in multiple locations including axillae and back (if can roll patient)

Pearl: Transmitted sounds can be misleading in bariatric patients—abnormal sounds on one side may transmit to other side

Percussion:

Limited utility (dampened by adipose tissue)

Still attempt—may detect large hemothorax or pneumothorax

Adjunct tools:

Ultrasound (FAST and lung ultrasound):

May be technically challenging but often still possible

Can identify pneumothorax, hemothorax, rib fractures

Lung ultrasound shows lung sliding (rules out pneumothorax)

Imaging essential:

Chest X-ray immediately (portable if patient can't move to radiology)

CT chest if stable enough and within scanner weight limit

Extremity assessment (right leg deformity):

Inspection:

Obvious deformity visible

Look for open wounds, bone protrusion

Color of foot (perfusion)

Palpation:

Neurovascular assessment critical:

Pulses: May be difficult to palpate—use Doppler ultrasound

Dorsalis pedis and posterior tibial arteries

Compare to uninjured side

Sensation: Light touch, can patient feel?

Motor: Can patient wiggle toes, dorsiflex, plantarflex?

Capillary refill: >2 seconds concerning

Temperature: Cool extremity suggests vascular compromise

Compartment assessment:

Palpate leg compartments (may be difficult through adipose tissue)

Most important: Pain assessment

Pain out of proportion to injury?

Pain with passive stretch of muscles?

Progressive pain despite immobilization and analgesia?

Don't rely on pulses—compartment syndrome occurs before pulses lost

Splinting:

Immobilize fracture

Recheck neurovascular status after splinting

Pad bony prominences well (increased pressure injury risk)

Abdominal assessment:

Major challenges:

Large pannus (abdominal apron of adipose tissue) obscures palpation

May need to lift pannus to examine

Maintain patient dignity while being thorough

Approach:

Inspect for bruising, abrasions (check under pannus/folds)

Palpate firmly in all quadrants

Difficult to detect subtle findings

Focus on gross abnormalities: rigidity, severe tenderness, masses

Assess for distension (hard to determine—know patient's baseline if possible)

FAST exam:

Can be technically challenging

Free fluid may be harder to see

Still attempt—often successful despite body habitus

Liberal use of CT:

Physical exam less reliable

CT often necessary to rule out injuries

(Assuming patient within weight limit—see next question)

Documentation:

Document examination challenges encountered

Note what was able to be assessed and what wasn't

Record workarounds used (ultrasound, imaging)

Serial exams documented to show changes over time

Imaging options when patient exceeds CT scanner weight limit:

Problem: Patient weighs 385 lbs, CT scanner limit 450 lbs—he's within limit, BUT:

Need to verify actual scanner limit at your facility

Limits vary: some 350 lbs, some 450 lbs, bariatric scanners 550-700 lbs

Gantry size also matters (patient circumference may exceed opening even if weight acceptable)

For this scenario, assume he exceeds your facility's limit

Alternative diagnostic strategies:

Option 1: Transfer to facility with bariatric scanner

Some centers have CT scanners designed for bariatric patients (higher weight limits, larger gantries)

Considerations:

Is patient stable for transfer?

How far is the facility?

What's the time delay?

Is benefit worth risk of transport?

Best for: Stable patients who need detailed imaging for operative planning

Option 2: Open MRI

Open MRI scanners have no enclosed tube

Often accommodate larger patients

Limitations:

Longer scan times than CT

Not ideal for unstable patients

May not be available emergently

Image quality sometimes inferior to CT

Best for: Stable patients, specific indications (spinal cord imaging)

Option 3: Serial clinical examinations

Close, frequent physical examinations by experienced clinician

Look for developing signs of injury:

Worsening abdominal tenderness

Developing peritonitis

Hemodynamic deterioration

New neurological findings

Requires:

ICU or step-down level monitoring

Experienced examiner

Very low threshold for surgical exploration

Clear documentation of serial findings

Best for: Patients with concerning mechanism but initially stable

Option 4: Diagnostic peritoneal lavage (DPL)

Invasive but definitive for intraperitoneal blood

Insert catheter into peritoneum, instill saline, aspirate and analyze

Positive if:

Gross blood on aspiration

RBC >100,000/mm³

WBC >500/mm³

Bile, bacteria, or food fibers present

Limitations:

Invasive

Doesn't identify specific injuries or retroperitoneal injuries

Doesn't assess chest or extremities

May be technically difficult in bariatric patients (thick abdominal wall)

Best for: Unstable patients when can't get to imaging

Option 5: Diagnostic laparoscopy

Minimally invasive surgical exploration

Can visualize abdominal organs directly

Advantages:

Identifies and sometimes treats injuries

More sensitive than DPL

Can assess diaphragm, anterior peritoneum

Limitations:

Requires OR and anesthesia

Technically challenging in bariatric patients (thick abdominal wall, large liver)

May miss some retroperitoneal or posterior injuries

Difficult airway makes anesthesia higher risk

Best for: Equivocal cases needing definitive assessment

Option 6: Selective conservative management with targeted imaging

Plain radiographs for obvious fractures

Ultrasound for FAST exam (abdominal free fluid, pneumothorax)

Focused MRI if specific concern (spinal cord injury)

Clinical judgment combined with available imaging

Best for: Specific injuries where targeted approach adequate

For this patient's specific injuries:

Leg fracture:

Plain X-rays adequate for diagnosis

Shows fracture pattern, guides treatment

CT not necessary unless complex injury or operative planning

Chest injury:

Portable chest X-ray immediately

May show rib fractures, pneumothorax, hemothorax

Lung ultrasound supplements X-ray findings

If X-ray shows significant injury (pneumothorax, hemothorax), treat accordingly

CT chest helpful for surgical planning but may not be essential for immediate management

Abdominal concerns (mechanism—fell down stairs):

FAST exam first-line

If positive FAST + unstable → OR for exploratory laparotomy

If negative FAST + stable → close serial exams

If equivocal or high suspicion → consider DPL or diagnostic laparoscopy

Transfer for bariatric CT if stable and time permits

Decision-making framework:

How stable is the patient?

What imaging is essential vs. nice-to-have?

What alternatives exist?

What's the risk-benefit of each option?

What does the patient/family prefer?

Documentation:

Clearly document equipment limitations

Explain decision-making process

Justify chosen approach

If outcomes differ from what CT might have shown, demonstrate reasonable clinical judgment was used

VTE prophylaxis in this high-risk bariatric patient:

Why this patient is extremely high risk for VTE:

Multiple risk factors present:

Obesity itself:

BMI 54 (severe/morbid obesity)

Obesity increases VTE risk 2-3 fold

Venous stasis from increased abdominal pressure

Chronic inflammation

Endothelial dysfunction

Trauma:

Any trauma increases VTE risk

Immobilization from leg fracture

Endothelial injury from vascular damage

Hypercoagulable state from stress response

Immobilization:

Can't bear weight on right leg (fracture)

Limited mobility baseline (severe obesity)

Will be bed-bound or severely limited during recovery

Venous stasis from immobility

Previous VTE history:

Most important risk factor for future VTE

Indicates underlying hypercoagulability

Once had DVT, lifetime increased risk

Other factors:

Age 52 (risk increases with age)

Diabetes (increased VTE risk)

Likely prolonged hospitalization

VTE risk without prophylaxis: VERY HIGH (>40%)

Appropriate prophylaxis—MULTIMODAL approach:

Chemical prophylaxis:

Standard dosing INADEQUATE—need higher doses:

Enoxaparin (preferred):

Standard dose: 40 mg SC daily

Bariatric dose: 40 mg SC twice daily OR 0.5 mg/kg SC twice daily

For 385 lbs (175 kg): 0.5 mg/kg × 175 kg = 87.5 mg, round to 90 mg divided as 45 mg twice daily

Alternative: Some protocols use 30 mg SC three times daily

Heparin:

5,000 units SC three times daily (higher frequency than standard BID)

Less predictable absorption in bariatric patients

Fondaparinux:

Weight-based dosing

5 mg SC daily for 50-100 kg

7.5 mg SC daily for >100 kg

10 mg SC daily for some bariatric patients

Timing:

Start within 24 hours of admission unless contraindicated

Earlier is better

- Balance bleeding risk from trauma vs. VTE risk (VTE risk usually higher)

Duration:

- Throughout hospitalization minimum
- Extended prophylaxis (28 days) for high-risk patients
- Until fully mobile

Mechanical prophylaxis:

Sequential compression devices (SCDs):

- Apply to both legs (or uninjured leg if bilateral not possible)
- Keep on except during physical therapy/ambulation
- Ensure proper fit—bariatric-sized devices may be needed

Graduated compression stockings:

- If appropriate size available
- Often standard sizes don't fit bariatric patients
- Don't force undersized stockings—can cause injury

Both chemical AND mechanical together:

- Multimodal approach superior to either alone
- Mechanical provides additional benefit beyond chemical alone

Early mobilization:

- **Single most important intervention**
- Get patient up as soon as medically safe
- Physical therapy consultation immediately
- Even chair sitting better than bed rest
- Non-weight-bearing on injured leg but can still mobilize with assistive devices

Monitoring and surveillance:

Clinical monitoring:

- Daily assessment for DVT signs (leg swelling, pain, warmth)
- Pulmonary embolism symptoms (chest pain, dyspnea, hypoxia)
- Bleeding complications from anticoagulation

Consider duplex ultrasound screening:

- Some centers screen high-risk patients
- Baseline and weekly ultrasounds
- Can detect asymptomatic DVT before PE develops
- Controversial—not universally recommended but reasonable in this patient

IVC filter consideration:

- If contraindication to chemical prophylaxis AND very high risk
- Retrievable filter preferred
- This patient has history of DVT—some would consider filter

Usually reserve for patients who can't receive anticoagulation

Special considerations:

Medication dosing complexity:

- Consult pharmacy for appropriate dosing
- Anti-Xa levels can be checked to verify adequacy (goal 0.2-0.5 for prophylaxis)
- Renal function monitoring (adjust doses if renal impairment)

Long-term anticoagulation:

- Patient has prior DVT—may need therapeutic anticoagulation, not just prophylaxis
- Contact patient's usual physician
- May already be on chronic anticoagulation
- Coordinate with hematology if complex

Balancing risks:

- Trauma patients have bleeding risk
- This patient's VTE risk very high
- Generally, benefits of prophylaxis outweigh bleeding risk
- Individualize based on specific injuries
- If intracranial bleeding: delay chemical prophylaxis, use mechanical only initially

Patient/family education:

- Explain VTE risk and importance of prophylaxis
- Encourage mobilization and leg exercises
- Report warning signs immediately (leg swelling, chest pain, dyspnea)
- Compliance with SCDs important

Documentation:

- VTE risk assessment documented
- Prophylaxis regimen clearly ordered
- Contraindications noted if any
- Rationale for chosen approach

Expected outcomes with appropriate prophylaxis:

- VTE risk reduced from >40% to ~5-10%
- Early mobilization further reduces risk
- Multimodal approach provides best protection
- Vigilant monitoring allows early detection if VTE occurs despite prophylaxis

Key learning points from this scenario:

- Bariatric patients have unique physiological challenges affecting all aspects of trauma care
- Assessment is more difficult—use all available tools and serial examinations
- Equipment limitations require creative solutions—never let equipment dictate care
- VTE risk is dramatically elevated—aggressive multimodal prophylaxis essential

Early mobilization benefits multiple outcomes (pulmonary, VTE, pressure injuries, deconditioning)

Medication dosing requires careful calculation and pharmacy consultation

Respectful, dignified care is essential—bariatric patients face healthcare stigma and discrimination

Chapter 10: Special Populations - Summary and Key Takeaways

You've completed a comprehensive exploration of how trauma care differs across special populations. Let's consolidate the critical concepts that will serve you on the TCRN exam and in clinical practice.

Pediatric Trauma: Essential Concepts

Physiological differences matter:

- Children compensate remarkably—maintain BP until 25-30% blood loss
- **Hypotension is a late, ominous sign in children**—act on tachycardia, cool skin, delayed capillary refill
- Larger heads, flexible skeletons—serious internal injuries with minimal external signs
- Hypothermia develops rapidly—keep warm

Assessment modifications:

- Age-appropriate vital signs—compare to normal for age, not adult values
- Weight-based interventions: 20 mL/kg fluid boluses, 10 mL/kg blood
- IO access after two IV attempts—don't delay resuscitation
- Modified GCS or AVPU for young children

Injury patterns:

- Head injury leading cause of death
- Flexible ribs—if fractured, indicates severe force
- SCIWORA possible—spinal cord injury with normal imaging
- Handlebar injuries cause duodenal/pancreatic trauma

Child abuse recognition:

- Injuries inconsistent with developmental stage or history
- Multiple injuries at different healing stages
- Delay in seeking care, changing history
- Pattern injuries (bruising in shapes, locations)
- **Healthcare providers are mandated reporters**—report suspicion, not just proof

Family-centered care:

- Include parents when safe and appropriate
- Developmentally appropriate communication
- Honest but gentle explanations

Family presence during resuscitation benefits child and family

Geriatric Trauma: Critical Considerations

Physiological changes with aging:

Limited cardiovascular reserve—can't increase HR or BP effectively

Medications (beta-blockers) mask compensatory responses

"Normal" vital signs may represent shock in elderly patient

Brain atrophy allows subdural hematomas from minor trauma

Assessment priorities:

Establish baseline—compare current findings to patient's normal

Ask about home medications, especially anticoagulants

Lower threshold for imaging and intervention

Ground-level falls cause serious injuries in elderly

Anticoagulation management:

High index of suspicion for bleeding in anticoagulated patients

Immediate reversal for intracranial hemorrhage:

Warfarin: Vitamin K + PCC or FFP

DOACs: Specific reversals when available, PCC otherwise

Don't wait for CT to reverse if high clinical suspicion

Complications prevention:

Pulmonary: Aggressive pulmonary hygiene, early mobilization

Pressure injuries: Frequent repositioning, pressure relief

Delirium: Orientation, glasses/hearing aids, minimize medications

Functional decline: Early PT/OT, discharge planning

Pain management:

Start low, go slow

More sensitive to opioids and sedatives

Multimodal approach reduces opioid requirements

Pregnancy Trauma: Dual Patient Care

Physiological changes:

- Blood volume increased 40-50%—can lose significant volume before signs
- Maternal vital signs may be stable while fetus severely compromised
- Supine hypotension after 20 weeks—always left lateral tilt or manual uterine displacement
- Hypercoagulable state—increased DVT risk

Unique pregnancy injuries:

- **Placental abruption:** Most common cause of fetal death
  - Vaginal bleeding may be absent
  - Firm, tender, contracting uterus
  - Continuous fetal monitoring detects fetal distress
- **Uterine rupture:** Catastrophic, presents with severe pain, palpable fetal parts
- **Fetomaternal hemorrhage:** Rh-negative mothers need RhoGAM

Management principles:

- **Mother is primary patient**—optimal maternal resuscitation is best fetal care
- Don't withhold necessary interventions (including radiation) due to pregnancy
- Continuous fetal monitoring for viable pregnancies (>20-24 weeks)
- Early obstetric consultation
- Perimortem C-section within 4-5 minutes if maternal arrest with viable fetus

Fetal monitoring interpretation:

- Late decelerations = uteroplacental insufficiency
- Decreased variability = fetal hypoxia
- Non-reassuring patterns = delivery indication

Bariatric Trauma: Special Challenges

Assessment difficulties:

- Physical exam less reliable—difficult palpation
- Vital signs challenging—need appropriate cuff size
- Lower threshold for imaging when exam limited
- Use ultrasound, serial exams when CT unavailable

Respiratory concerns:

- Baseline restrictive lung disease, reduced reserve
- Difficult airway if intubation needed
- Keep upright positioning when possible

Early mobilization critical

Equipment limitations:

Weight limits on CT scanners, OR tables, beds

Alternative strategies: Transfer to bariatric center, DPL, diagnostic laparoscopy, serial exams

Never let equipment dictate inadequate care

VTE prophylaxis:

Extremely high risk (obesity + trauma + immobility)

Higher doses needed: Enoxaparin 40 mg BID or weight-based dosing

Multimodal: Chemical + mechanical + early mobilization

Consider screening ultrasounds in very high-risk patients

Medication dosing:

Complex—some by total weight, some by ideal weight

Always consult pharmacy

Monitor drug levels when available

Respectful care:

Bariatric patients face healthcare stigma

Provide dignified, non-judgmental care

Ensure appropriate equipment available without embarrassment

Special Circumstances: Key Points

Immunocompromised patients:

Higher infection risk—aggressive prophylaxis

May need special blood products (CMV-negative, irradiated)

Continue immunosuppressants when possible (transplant patients)

Spinal cord injury patients:

Autonomic dysreflexia: Severe hypertension from noxious stimulus below injury level

Establish baseline function—new deficits indicate new injury

High pressure injury risk

Patients with developmental disabilities:

Communicate directly with patient when possible

Caregiver presence extremely helpful

Behavioral pain indicators when can't verbalize

Allow extra time and patience

Substance use disorders:

Intoxication complicates assessment—assume head injury until proven otherwise

Withdrawal risk—especially alcohol (can be life-threatening) Appropriate pain management regardless of substance use history	Non-judgmental care, offer treatment resources

TCRN Exam Success Strategies

Recognizing special population questions: Watch for questions that:	**Key phrases that signal special population considerations:**
Specify patient age, weight, or pregnancy status Mention pre-existing conditions or medications Describe "normal" findings that should concern you in special populations Test whether you know age-appropriate norms or modifications	"Ground-level fall in 80-year-old" → Serious injury possible, anticoagulation concern "Seatbelt sign in pregnant patient" → Placental abruption risk "Child compensating well" → May be in shock despite normal BP "BMI >40" → Equipment limitations, dosing considerations, VTE risk
Common question patterns:	**Integration with other chapters:**
Pediatric shock: Will patient have "normal" BP? (Yes, until decompensated) Geriatric vital signs: Are these truly normal? (Need baseline) Pregnancy positioning: What's essential? (Left lateral tilt) Bariatric dosing: How to calculate? (Varies by drug, consult pharmacy)	Shock recognition applies differently across populations (Chapter 3) Airway management modified for pediatric, bariatric (Chapter 3) Injury patterns vary (abdominal Chapter 5, orthopedic Chapter 6) Pain management considerations throughout

Building Clinical Judgment

Success with special populations requires:

Knowing the norms for each population

Recognizing when "normal" isn't normal for that patient

Modifying your approach based on unique physiology

Anticipating complications specific to each population

Acting earlier and more aggressively when reserve is limited

Practice application: When you encounter exam questions about special populations:

Identify which special population (age, pregnancy, obesity, comorbidity)

Consider how physiology differs from "standard" adult

Interpret findings in context of that population

Choose interventions appropriate for that patient

Anticipate population-specific complications

Self-Assessment

Before moving forward, ensure you can answer:

How does shock present differently in children vs. adults?

Why can't I rely on heart rate in elderly patients on beta-blockers?

What makes placental abruption the most common cause of fetal death in maternal trauma?

How do I calculate appropriate medication doses in bariatric patients?

When am I mandated to report suspected abuse?

If any areas feel uncertain, review those sections. Understanding special populations is essential for recognizing when standard approaches need modification.

Your Progress

Congratulations! You've completed Chapter 10 and mastered how trauma care adapts across diverse populations. This knowledge ensures you provide safe, effective care to every patient regardless of age, size, or special circumstances.

Chapter 11: Psychosocial Aspects and Professional Issues

Trauma nursing extends far beyond managing physical injuries. The psychological and emotional dimensions of trauma care—for patients, families, and healthcare providers—are equally critical to understand and address. This chapter explores the human side of trauma nursing: supporting patients and families through crisis, managing the emotional weight of traumatic death, collecting evidence while maintaining compassionate care, recognizing violence and abuse, and protecting yourself from the cumulative toll of trauma work.

These aren't peripheral topics—they're central to competent trauma nursing. Understanding crisis intervention prevents psychological harm. Knowing how to support families during resuscitation improves outcomes and satisfaction. Proper evidence collection can help prosecute perpetrators and protect future victims. Recognizing abuse can save lives. And maintaining your own wellbeing ensures you can continue providing excellent care without burning out.

The TCRN exam tests these concepts because they're essential to trauma nursing practice. More importantly, mastering these skills makes you a more complete, effective, and resilient trauma nurse.

Crisis Intervention

Every trauma patient experiences crisis—a disruption of their psychological equilibrium caused by a traumatic event that overwhelms their usual coping mechanisms. As a trauma nurse, you're often the first healthcare provider to interact with patients and families in crisis. How you respond in those initial moments can significantly influence their psychological recovery.

Understanding Crisis Response

Crisis isn't just about the injury severity—it's about the person's perception of threat and their ability to cope. A minor injury can create major psychological crisis if the person perceives it as life-threatening or if it triggers past trauma. Conversely, some people with severe injuries remain psychologically stable because they have effective coping mechanisms or strong support systems.

Crisis unfolds in predictable phases:

Impact phase: The immediate aftermath of trauma. The person may be in shock, disbelief, or denial. They might seem calm or detached—this doesn't mean they're fine. Shock is a protective mechanism that allows the brain to process overwhelming information gradually.

Common responses: "This isn't happening," "I'm fine," apparent calm despite severe injury, emotional numbness, difficulty processing information.

Recoil phase: Reality begins setting in, usually within hours. Emotional responses emerge—fear, anger, grief, guilt, anxiety. The person starts comprehending what happened and what it means for their life.

Common responses: Crying, panic, anger outbursts, repetitive questions, withdrawal, inability to make decisions.

Recovery phase: The person begins adapting to their new reality. They start problem-solving and using coping mechanisms. This phase can take days to months depending on injury severity and individual factors.

Not everyone follows this linear path. Some people cycle through phases multiple times. Others get stuck in one phase. Understanding these patterns helps you provide appropriate support at each stage.

Crisis Intervention Principles

Effective crisis intervention in trauma settings follows specific principles designed to provide immediate psychological stabilization.

1. Safety first—physical and psychological

Before addressing emotional needs, ensure physical safety. You can't provide crisis intervention to someone actively bleeding or struggling to breathe. Once physical stabilization begins, shift attention to psychological safety.

Psychological safety means the person feels protected from immediate threats and believes their physical needs are being addressed. Simple statements establish this: "You're in the hospital now. We're taking care of your injuries. You're safe here."

2. Provide clear, honest information

Uncertainty amplifies anxiety. People in crisis desperately need information to regain a sense of control. Provide clear, honest updates about what's happening, what you're doing, and what comes next.

What this looks like in practice:

"I'm starting an IV line now to give you fluids and pain medication"

"The doctor is examining your X-rays to determine if surgery is needed"

"We're waiting for the CT scanner to be available. It should be about 15 minutes"

Avoid medical jargon: "We need to rule out a pneumothorax" means nothing to most people. Instead: "We're checking to make sure your lung isn't collapsed."

Be honest about uncertainty: If you don't know something, say so, but add what you're doing to find out: "I don't know yet if you'll need surgery. The trauma surgeon will examine you shortly and explain the plan."

3. Allow emotional expression

People in crisis need to express emotions. Crying, anger, fear—these are normal responses to abnormal situations. Don't minimize or suppress emotions with statements like "You need to calm down" or "Everything will be fine."

Instead, validate their feelings:

"I can see this is very frightening for you"

"It's completely normal to feel scared right now"

"You've been through something terrible. These feelings make sense"

Create space for expression: Sometimes people need permission to fall apart. "It's okay to cry. You've been through a lot." Other times they need permission to delay processing: "You don't have to talk about what happened right now. We're focused on your medical care."

4. Support coping mechanisms

Everyone has ways of managing stress. Some people need to talk through events repeatedly. Others need silence to process internally. Some want family present; others want to be alone initially. When possible, support the person's preferred coping style.

Assess coping by asking:

"What helps you when you're stressed or scared?"

"Would you like someone with you, or would you prefer some quiet time?"

"How can I best support you right now?"

Respect healthy coping mechanisms even if they're not what you'd choose. If someone wants to pray, facilitate that. If they need to call a specific family member, help them do so. If they find music calming, provide earbuds.

Recognize maladaptive coping: Some responses hinder recovery or safety. If someone wants to leave against medical advice or refuses necessary treatment due to fear or denial, intervene appropriately while still showing respect and empathy.

5. Mobilize resources

No one should face crisis alone. Help connect people with support systems and resources.

Immediate resources:

Family and friends (help with phone calls, facilitate visits)

Chaplain or spiritual care provider

Social workers

Language interpreters if needed

Patient advocates

Long-term resources:

Mental health referrals for trauma counseling

Support groups (survivors of specific injuries, trauma survivors generally)

Community resources (housing assistance, disability services, victim advocacy)

Financial counseling if injury impacts employment

Don't wait for people to ask: Many don't know what resources exist or feel uncomfortable requesting help. Proactively offer: "Would you like to speak with a counselor who specializes in helping people who've experienced trauma?" or "Our social worker can help you navigate insurance and disability questions when you're ready."

Special Populations in Crisis

Different groups experience and express crisis differently. Culturally competent crisis intervention recognizes these variations.

Children: Experience crisis through a developmental lens. Young children may not understand death, disability, or permanence of injury. They may be more concerned about separation from parents than their injuries.

Approach:

Use age-appropriate language

Provide honest but simple explanations

Allow parents/caregivers to stay when possible

Offer comfort items (stuffed animals, blankets)

Don't assume stoicism means coping—children often suppress emotions to avoid burdening adults

Elderly patients: May have experienced previous trauma or loss, influencing current crisis response. Sensory impairments may complicate communication. Concern about loss of independence often dominates psychological response.

Approach:

Speak clearly, face them when talking (for lip reading)

Address them directly, not through family (unless cognitive impairment present)

Acknowledge concerns about independence honestly

Respect their life experience and coping strategies

Cultural considerations: Culture profoundly influences crisis expression and coping. In some cultures, stoic acceptance is valued; in others, loud emotional expression is expected and healthy. Some cultures prefer family-centered decision making; others prioritize individual autonomy.

Approach:

Ask about cultural or religious practices that might help

Use professional interpreters, not family members (for accuracy and to avoid burdening family with medical information)

Learn about common cultural responses in your community

Never assume—ask individuals about their preferences and needs

Patients with mental illness: Pre-existing mental health conditions can complicate crisis response. Anxiety disorders may amplify fear responses. Depression may impair coping. PTSD from previous trauma may be triggered.

Approach:

Ask about pre-existing mental health conditions and current medications

Recognize that crisis may exacerbate underlying conditions

Involve psychiatric consultation early if needed

Don't attribute all distress to mental illness—their fear and upset are valid responses to trauma

Trauma-Informed Care

This approach recognizes that many trauma patients have histories of previous trauma—abuse, violence, combat, disasters, or other traumatic experiences. Current trauma can trigger past trauma, complicating psychological response.

Principles of trauma-informed care:

1. Safety: Create physical and emotional safety. Explain procedures before doing them. Ask permission when possible. Respect personal space.

2. Trustworthiness and transparency: Be honest and consistent. Follow through on commitments. Explain reasoning behind decisions.

3. Peer support: Connect patients with others who've experienced similar trauma when appropriate.

4. Collaboration: Involve patients in decisions about their care when possible. This restores a sense of control lost during trauma.

5. Empowerment: Focus on strengths and resilience, not just problems. Recognize that survival itself demonstrates strength.

Red flags for trauma history:

Extreme distress with routine procedures

Dissociation (seeming "checked out" or detached from reality)

Hypervigilance or startle responses

Panic with loss of control

Requests that providers be specific gender

Response: Don't probe trauma history during acute care—that's not the time. Instead, modify your approach to maximize safety and control. "I need to examine your abdomen. Would you like the door closed for privacy?" or "I'm going to touch your shoulder now to help position you."

Family Presence During Resuscitation

Should family members be present during resuscitation of their loved one? This question once had a universal "no" answer in healthcare. Research and evolving practice now demonstrate that family presence, when properly supported, benefits families and doesn't harm resuscitation efforts.

Evidence Supporting Family Presence

Multiple studies across emergency and critical care settings show consistent findings:

Benefits for families:

Reduced anxiety and depression in bereavement

Fewer symptoms of post-traumatic stress

Better acceptance of death when it occurs

Feeling they did everything possible for their loved one

No increase in litigation

No harm to resuscitation:

No interference with medical care in vast majority of cases

No increase in performance anxiety for providers once they adjust to practice

Family members rarely need to be removed from the room

Patient perspective: While we can't ask patients in cardiac arrest, survivors report wanting family present. In one study of patients who survived, 94% wanted family present during future resuscitation.

Implementing Family Presence

Family presence during resuscitation requires thoughtful implementation, not simply opening doors and walking away.

Key elements of successful family presence programs:

1. Designated family facilitator

This person—often a nurse, social worker, or chaplain not directly involved in resuscitation—stays with family members, explaining what's happening, providing support, and assessing their response.

Facilitator responsibilities:

Prepare family for what they'll see and hear

Escort them to appropriate location in room (usually foot of bed or against wall where they can see but aren't in the way)

Provide ongoing explanation of procedures in lay terms

Assess family coping and intervene if distress escalates

Remove family if they interfere with care (rare)

Support family if they choose to leave

Provide bereavement support if patient dies

2. Clear team communication

The resuscitation team needs to know family is present and agree to their presence. Team leader makes final decision, but staff input matters.

Before bringing family in: "The patient's wife is here. She's asking to be present during resuscitation. Are we comfortable with family presence?" Address concerns: "I'll stay with her and explain what's happening. If she interferes, I'll remove her immediately."

3. Preparation and boundaries

Prepare family before entering:

"Your husband is very sick. The team is doing everything possible to help him"

"You'll see a lot of medical equipment and many people working quickly"

"You'll hear us giving loud, direct commands—that's normal in resuscitation"

"There will be blood and bodily fluids. This can be upsetting to watch"

"If you feel faint or need to leave, tell me immediately"

"You can speak to him, but please don't touch him or interfere with the team"

Set clear boundaries:

- Where family can stand
- That they may need to step back if procedures require more space
- That they'll need to leave if they interfere with care
- That they can leave anytime—no one will judge them

4. Ongoing support and explanation

During resuscitation, the facilitator provides:

- Simple explanations: "They're giving medications through the IV to help his heart" or "The breathing tube helps get oxygen to his lungs"
- Reassurance about what's normal: "The chest compressions look violent, but they're necessary to circulate blood"
- Support for their presence: "He can probably hear your voice. You can tell him you're here"
- Permission to express emotion: "This is very difficult to watch. It's okay to cry"

5. Decision-making support

If resuscitation reaches a point where decisions must be made (continuing efforts, terminating resuscitation), family presence allows real-time participation in decisions.

This requires:

- Clear explanation of medical situation
- Honest prognosis
- Exploration of patient's known wishes
- Support for whatever decision is made

When Family Presence May Not Be Appropriate

While research supports family presence in most situations, some circumstances warrant careful consideration:

Patient factors:

- Patient previously expressed not wanting family present
- Injuries are extremely graphic (massive trauma, severe burns, dismemberment)

Patient is minor and parents are extremely distressed (may need to focus on parental support before bringing them in)

Family factors:

Extreme combative or violent behavior

Severe intoxication

History of interfering with medical care

Extremely young children (though age alone shouldn't exclude—some mature teens handle presence well)

Situational factors:

Space is extremely limited (though this is rarely absolute contraindication)

Security concerns

Multiple casualties with insufficient facilitators

These aren't absolute contraindications—they're factors requiring individual assessment and sometimes creative solutions (video link if room too small, allowing presence for brief periods with frequent check-ins if distress is high).

Cultural and Religious Considerations

Some cultures and religions have specific practices around dying that influence family presence preferences.

Be aware of:

Cultures that emphasize communal death rituals (may want extended family present)

Religious practices requiring specific prayers or rituals (provide space and time when possible)

Beliefs about communication with dying or deceased (some believe hearing is last sense to go, some practice specific words or prayers)

Gender considerations (some religions restrict who can touch body)

Ask about needs: "Are there cultural or religious practices that are important for you during this time?" and "How can we support your family's traditions while providing medical care?"

Supporting Staff with Family Presence

Team members who aren't comfortable with family presence need support, not judgment.

Common concerns:

Performance anxiety (feeling watched)

Worry about family seeing procedures (especially invasive ones)

Fear of lawsuits

Concern about protecting family from traumatic images

Address concerns through:

Education about research supporting family presence

Debriefing after family presence experiences

Acknowledging that discomfort decreases with experience

Respecting provider boundaries while encouraging growth

Remember: The goal isn't forcing everyone to love family presence—it's creating systems where family presence can occur safely when appropriate, with proper support for everyone involved.

End-of-Life Care in Trauma

Death in trauma is often sudden, unexpected, and occurs in people not "supposed" to die—young people, previously healthy individuals, parents of small children. This creates unique challenges for end-of-life care.

Recognizing Futility and Terminating Resuscitation

One of trauma care's most difficult decisions is recognizing when resuscitation is futile and death is inevitable. Unlike chronic illness where dying is often a gradual process, trauma death can require active decision to stop trying.

Indications that death is inevitable:

Injuries incompatible with life (massive head trauma, decapitation, hemicorporectomy)

Prolonged pulseless cardiac arrest without reversible cause

Asystole despite appropriate ACLS and trauma resuscitation

Exsanguination from non-survivable vascular injury

Decision-making process:

Team leader assesses situation

Considers: duration of resuscitation, rhythm, reversible causes addressed, overall injury pattern, age and comorbidities

Announces decision to team: "We've exhausted our interventions. The injuries are not survivable. I'm calling the resuscitation at [time]."

Ensures everyone has opportunity to voice concerns before final decision

After termination:

Document time of death

Ensure family notification process begins

Provide team debriefing opportunity

Complete required documentation

Breaking Bad News

Telling someone their loved one has died is one of healthcare's most difficult conversations. In trauma, families often have no preparation—their person was fine hours ago.

The SPIKES protocol provides structure for death notification:

S - Setting:

Private location, sitting down

Bring family together if multiple members present

Have tissues available

Turn off pagers/phones if possible

Bring support person (chaplain, social worker)

P - Perception: Assess what family knows before speaking: "What have you been told so far about your husband's condition?" This prevents shocking them with death announcement before they even know there was serious injury.

I - Invitation: Determine how much information they want: "Would you like me to explain everything that happened?" Some want detailed medical information; others need just essential facts.

K - Knowledge: Deliver the news clearly and compassionately.

Use the "D" word—avoid euphemisms:

"I'm so sorry to tell you that your son has died" (clear)

"He didn't make it" (ambiguous—didn't make what?)

"He passed" (vague, softens to point of confusion)

Be direct but compassionate: "I'm very sorry. Despite everything we did, your mother's injuries were too severe. She died a few minutes ago."

Pause. Let them absorb this. Don't fill silence with medical details yet.

E - Empathy: Acknowledge their pain:

"I'm so very sorry"

"I can't imagine how difficult this is"

"This is devastating news"

Allow emotions: Crying, anger, denial, shock—all are normal. Sit with them. Don't rush. Physical presence matters more than words.

S - Strategy and Summary: After initial shock passes (minutes to hours), address practical needs:

"Would you like to see him?"

"Is there anyone we can call for you?"

"The chaplain/social worker can help with arrangements when you're ready"

"Do you have questions about what happened?"

Special situations:

Sudden unexpected death: "Your daughter was in a car accident. She had very severe injuries. Despite immediate surgery and everything we could do, she didn't survive. I'm so sorry."

Death after prolonged resuscitation: "We worked on your husband for over an hour, trying everything possible. His injuries were too severe. He died at 3:47."

Multiple casualties with some deaths: Prioritize information about immediate family first, then others. "Your son sustained injuries but is stable. I need to tell you about your husband..." Don't make them wait in uncertainty about both.

Viewing the Body

Most families want to see their loved one after death. This helps make death real and allows goodbye. Prepare them and the body.

Prepare the body:

Clean visible blood from face and hands

Cover devastating injuries (sheet over lower body if legs amputated)

Remove unnecessary equipment (keep if helps tell story: "The breathing tube was helping him breathe")

Make room look peaceful (dim lights slightly, remove bloody linens, organize equipment)

Position body naturally (arms at sides, eyes closed if possible)

Prepare the family: "Your wife is in the room. I want to prepare you for what you'll see. She'll look like she's sleeping, but she's very pale because her heart is no longer circulating blood. She still has an IV and breathing tube—we can remove those if you'd like, or leave them if you want to see everything we did. There's a bandage over her chest from surgery. You can touch her and speak to her. Take as much time as you need."

Support during viewing:

Stay nearby but give privacy

Allow rituals (prayers, anointing, specific cultural practices)

Offer keepsakes (lock of hair, handprints, wedding ring)

Allow children to see body if parents consent and child is prepared

Don't rush them—grieving has no timeline

Organ and Tissue Donation

Trauma creates many potential organ donors—young, previously healthy individuals with devastating neurological injuries or death from other causes. Facilitating donation honors the deceased and saves lives.

When to consider donation:

Neurological death (brain death)

Cardiac death (in some protocols)

Age and medical suitability vary by organ/tissue

Process:

Refer all potential donors to organ procurement organization (OPO)—they assess suitability

Don't approach family yourself about donation unless specifically trained

OPO representatives are specially trained in donation discussions

Separation of roles (clinical team focuses on care, OPO team discusses donation) reduces family pressure

Supporting families considering donation:

Provide time and space for decision

Clarify that donation doesn't delay funeral or disfigure body

Acknowledge difficulty of decision during devastating time

Support whatever decision they make

If family declines: "I understand. This is an incredibly personal decision, and there's no right or wrong answer."

If family agrees: "Your generosity will save lives. The donation team will take excellent care of [name]."

Cultural and Religious Considerations in Death

Death practices vary enormously across cultures and religions. Providing culturally competent end-of-life care requires knowledge and humility.

Be aware of:

Autopsy: Some religions prohibit (Jewish, Muslim traditions may object unless legally required)

Body handling: Some traditions require specific gender handle body, specific washing rituals, no embalming

Timing: Some require burial within 24 hours (Jewish, Muslim)

Mourning practices: Varies from quiet private grieving to loud communal wailing

Viewing practices: Some want family present at death, others restrict who can see body

Approach: "Are there cultural or religious practices that are important for your family as we care for [name] after death?" Facilitate when possible, explain limitations honestly when necessary.

Forensic Evidence Collection

Trauma often results from crime—assault, domestic violence, sexual assault, shootings, stabbings. As a trauma nurse, you have dual responsibilities: providing medical care and preserving evidence that may be crucial for prosecution.

Understanding Chain of Custody

Evidence is only useful in court if chain of custody is maintained—documented proof that evidence has been properly collected, labeled, stored, and transferred without contamination or tampering.

Chain of custody requires:

Proper collection by trained personnel

Detailed documentation of what was collected, when, and by whom

Secure storage

Documented transfer between individuals

Continuous documentation until evidence reaches crime lab or court

Your role: You're often the first link in the chain. Improper collection or documentation can render evidence inadmissible, potentially allowing perpetrators to escape prosecution.

General Principles of Evidence Collection

1. **Safety first** Medical care always takes priority over evidence. Don't delay life-saving interventions to collect evidence. However, with minor adjustments, you can often preserve evidence while providing care.

2. **Minimize contamination**

Wear gloves (new gloves for each evidence item)

Don't shake clothing or linens (dislodges trace evidence)

Place each item in separate paper bag (plastic bags trap moisture, degrading biological evidence)

Don't clean wounds until photographed if possible (debris may be evidence)

3. **Document thoroughly**

Photograph injuries (with and without measurement scale)

Document exact quotes from patient about assault

Note time, date, your name on all evidence labels

Describe rather than interpret: "3 cm linear abrasion on left cheek" not "slap mark"

4. **Maintain chain of custody**

Label everything immediately

Never leave evidence unattended

Document every transfer

Secure evidence in locked area until law enforcement retrieval

Clothing as Evidence

Clothing often contains crucial evidence—blood spatter patterns, gunshot residue, DNA from perpetrator, fibers, trace evidence.

Proper clothing collection:

If patient is stable and conscious:

Explain: "Your clothing may contain evidence. We need to collect it for police. We'll give you hospital gown."

Provide privacy

Have patient undress themselves if able (preserves trace evidence better than staff removing)

If staff must remove clothing: Cut along seams when possible (preserves bullet holes, stab marks, tear patterns)

If patient is unstable:

Cut clothing off as needed for medical access

Preserve when possible: cut around holes/tears, not through them

Save all pieces

Handling clothing:

Place each item in separate paper bag

Don't shake out or unfold excessively

If wet with blood: Air dry before bagging if possible (prevents mold)

Label bag with patient name, date, time, your name, contents

Document on evidence log

Special considerations:

Underwear in sexual assault (contains crucial DNA evidence)

Shoes (blood spatter patterns, trace evidence)

Jewelry (may have blood, tissue, or perpetrator's DNA if victim fought back)

Wound Documentation

Injuries tell a story. Proper documentation helps investigators and prosecutors understand what happened.

Photography:

Photograph all injuries

Take overall photo showing body region

Take close-up with measurement scale

Include patient identifier in photo (wristband in frame)

Photograph from multiple angles if needed

Document camera settings and photographer name

Written documentation:

Exact location (use anatomical terms and measurements from landmarks)

Size (length, width, depth if applicable)

Shape and characteristics (linear, circular, irregular, patterned)

Color (red, purple, brown, yellow—indicates age of injury)

Associated findings (swelling, abraded edges, surrounding bruising)

Examples:

"3 cm x 1.5 cm oval purple bruise on right lateral cheek, 2 cm below lateral canthus of eye"

"4 cm linear abrasion on left forearm, mid-forearm level, anterior surface, parallel to long axis of arm"

What NOT to do:

Don't interpret: "Bruise consistent with punch" or "defensive wounds" (that's for investigators)

Don't offer opinions about mechanism

Don't state whether you believe patient's account

Just describe what you see objectively

Projectiles and Foreign Objects

Bullets, knife tips, glass fragments, and other objects removed from wounds are crucial evidence.

Collection:

Remove with instruments (never fingers)

Don't clean or rinse

Place in appropriate container (small plastic container for bullets, larger for knives)

Don't use metal instruments on bullets if avoidable (can create marks confused with rifling)

Label container immediately

Maintain chain of custody

Never throw away foreign objects removed from trauma patients without checking if evidence

Bullets specifically:

Document caliber if known (surgeons may know from extraction)

Preserve any tissue or bone fragments attached (don't clean)

Note location where found in body

Sexual Assault Evidence Collection

Sexual assault evidence collection requires specialized training. Many facilities have Sexual Assault Nurse Examiners (SANEs) who perform these exams.

If SANE not available and you must collect:

Use jurisdiction's sexual assault evidence kit (SAEK)

Follow kit instructions exactly

Maintain patient's autonomy (they can refuse any part of exam)

Document consent for evidence collection separate from medical consent

Collect within 72 hours of assault ideally (DNA degrades over time)

Don't have patient shower or void before collection if possible

Evidence collected:

Clothing (especially underwear)

Swabs from body areas where contact occurred

Fingernail scrapings (if patient scratched perpetrator)

Hair combings (if perpetrator left hair)

Oral swabs (if oral contact)

Photos of all injuries

Blood for DNA reference sample

Support during collection:

Explain each step before doing it

Allow advocate to be present if patient wishes

Proceed at patient's pace

Stop if patient wants to stop

Maintain trauma-informed approach (patient has already experienced violation; don't compound it with invasive exam that feels violating)

Testifying in Court

Evidence you collect may lead to you testifying. Understanding this possibility influences how you document.

If called to testify:

Review medical records thoroughly before court date

Stick to facts, not interpretations

Answer only the question asked

Say "I don't know" or "I don't recall" if you don't—don't guess

Remain professional regardless of attorney tactics

Remember you're advocating for truth, not prosecution or defense

Documentation habits that help in court:

Write legibly

Be thorough but concise

Use objective language

Document exact quotes (especially patient's description of assault)

Note patient's demeanor (crying, flat affect, shaking)

Avoid medical jargon in narrative sections

Legal and Ethical Considerations

Mandatory reporting: Most jurisdictions require healthcare providers report certain injuries:

Suspected child abuse

Suspected elder abuse

Injuries from firearms (some states)

Sexual assault (some states)

Know your state's requirements. Failure to report can result in criminal charges and license sanctions.

Patient consent: In most jurisdictions, you don't need patient consent to report mandatory reportable conditions. For evidence collection beyond what's needed for medical care (like photography), consent practices vary by jurisdiction. Know your facility's policy.

Confidentiality: Evidence collection and mandatory reporting don't override all confidentiality. Information should only be shared with appropriate law enforcement, not discussed with unauthorized individuals.

Violence and Abuse Recognition

Trauma from interpersonal violence presents uniquely. Recognizing abuse patterns, understanding barriers to disclosure, and responding appropriately can literally save lives.

Types of Violence and Abuse

Intimate partner violence (IPV): Physical, sexual, emotional, or economic abuse by current or former intimate partner. Affects all demographics but disproportionately impacts women.

Child abuse: Physical abuse, sexual abuse, neglect, emotional abuse. May be from parents, caregivers, or others with access to child.

Elder abuse: Physical abuse, neglect, financial exploitation, emotional abuse. Often by family caregivers.

Human trafficking: Modern slavery involving forced labor or commercial sexual exploitation. Victims may present with injuries from abuse or occupational hazards.

Red Flags for Violence and Abuse

Injury patterns suspicious for abuse:

Physical abuse indicators:

- Injuries in various stages of healing (suggests repeated trauma)
- Injuries in protected areas (inner arms, inner thighs, torso, genitals)
- Pattern injuries (hand prints, loop marks from cords, implement shapes)
- Injuries inconsistent with stated mechanism
- Delay in seeking care
- Multiple ED visits for injuries

Specific patterns:

- **IPV:** Strangulation marks (petechiae on face, neck bruising), defensive wounds (forearm bruises from blocking), head/face/neck injuries (common targets)
- **Child abuse:** Bucket-handle fractures (from shaking), burns in glove/stocking distribution (from submersion), retinal hemorrhages (from shaking), bruises shaped like objects

Elder abuse: Malnutrition/dehydration in dependent elder, pressure ulcers suggesting neglect, bruising on arms (from grabbing), fractures

Behavioral indicators:

Partner answers all questions, doesn't leave patient alone with staff

Patient minimizes injuries or makes excuses

Fearfulness, especially of specific person

Reluctance to make eye contact

Depression, anxiety, PTSD symptoms

Substance abuse (often coping mechanism)

Inconsistent history between patient and others

Patient's story doesn't match injuries

Environmental indicators:

Child living conditions dangerous or neglected

Elder with unexplained financial problems (suggests exploitation)

Evidence of substance abuse in household

Isolation (abusers isolate victims from support systems)

Screening for Violence and Abuse

Universal screening—asking all patients about violence—identifies more victims than screening only "suspicious" cases.

When to screen:

Routine part of trauma assessment

Private setting (never screen with potential abuser present)

Non-judgmental tone

For patients with cognitive impairment or language barriers, use trained interpreters

Screening questions:

IPV screening:

"Do you feel safe at home?"

"Has anyone at home hurt you or threatened you?"

"Are you in a relationship where you've been physically hurt or threatened?"

Child abuse screening (ask caregivers):

"How did this injury occur?" (assess plausibility)

"Who was supervising when this happened?"

"Has your child had injuries like this before?"

Elder abuse screening:

"Has anyone hurt you or touched you without your consent?"

"Has anyone taken your money or belongings without permission?"

"Are you afraid of anyone?"

Human trafficking indicators:

Does patient have identification documents?

Can they leave their residence/job freely?

Are they living and working in same location?

Do they owe money to employer?

Signs of physical abuse or deprivation

If patient discloses abuse:

Believe them: "I believe you, and I'm glad you told me"

Validate feelings: "You don't deserve to be hurt. This isn't your fault"

Ensure immediate safety: "Are you safe to go home today?"

Document disclosure in patient's own words: "Patient states 'My husband punched me in the face three times yesterday'"

Provide resources without pressure: "Would you like to speak with an advocate who helps people in situations like yours?"

Respect autonomy: "I can't make you leave, but I want you to know there are options and people who can help"

If patient denies abuse but you suspect it:

Don't pressure or accuse

Provide information anyway: "Here's a card with the domestic violence hotline number. You can call anytime, even just to talk"

Document your concerns objectively: "Multiple bruises in various stages of healing, inconsistent with stated mechanism"

Offer follow-up: "I'd like to see you back here in a week to check on your injuries"

Safety Planning

For patients who acknowledge abuse but aren't ready to leave the situation, safety planning can reduce harm.

Components of safety planning:

Immediate safety:

Identify safe room in house (with exit and without weapons)

Keep phone accessible for calling 911

Create code word to signal danger to trusted friend/family

Pack essential items (ID, medications, money, keys) and hide or store with trusted person

Know where to go in emergency (shelter address, trusted friend's home)

Financial safety:

Open separate bank account if possible

Save money gradually if safe to do so

Document financial abuse (save statements showing accounts emptied, etc.)

Legal safety:

Know how to obtain protective order

Document abuse (photos of injuries, copies of threatening texts/emails)

Keep important documents accessible (birth certificates, social security cards, lease/deed)

Emotional safety:

Connect with support groups or counseling

Maintain contact with supportive friends/family

Recognize abuse patterns and triggers

Provide written safety plan discretely: Abusers often monitor victims closely. Offer to store safety plan information in medical record or give resources disguised as general health information.

Mandatory Reporting

Understanding your legal obligations protects vulnerable populations and protects you legally.

Child abuse reporting:

Mandatory in all states for healthcare providers

Report if you suspect abuse, not just if you're certain

Immunity from liability for good-faith reports

Failure to report can result in criminal charges and license sanctions

Don't need parent/guardian permission to report

Child protective services investigates, not you

What triggers mandatory reporting:

Physical injuries suggesting abuse

Sexual abuse or suspicion thereof

Neglect (inadequate food, shelter, medical care, supervision)

Emotional abuse (in some jurisdictions)

Elder abuse reporting:

Mandatory in most states for healthcare providers

Similar standards as child abuse (suspicion, not certainty)

Report to Adult Protective Services

Capacity issues complicate (competent adults can refuse intervention)

Intimate partner violence reporting:

Not universally mandatory

Some states require reporting injuries from weapons or specific severity

Know your state's requirements

Even where not mandatory, provide resources

How to make reports:

Call designated agency (Child Protective Services, Adult Protective Services)

Provide patient information, nature of concerns, basis for suspicion

Follow up with written report if required

Document in medical record that report was made

Notify patient when appropriate (exceptions for child abuse when parent is abuser)

Supporting Victims of Violence

Beyond legal requirements, your response to violence victims impacts their healing and safety.

Immediate support:

Provide medical care for injuries

Assess immediate safety

Offer crisis intervention

Connect with advocates (domestic violence, sexual assault, child protection)

Provide resources regardless of whether patient plans to use them

Long-term considerations:

- Understand leaving abusive relationships is complex and dangerous (most dangerous time is when victim attempts to leave)
- Don't judge if patient returns to abuser or refuses to leave
- Maintain connection: "I'm here if you need help in the future"
- Document thoroughly (medical records may be crucial in future legal proceedings)

Vicarious trauma warning: Caring for violence victims takes emotional toll. Use debriefing, peer support, and your own counseling resources when needed. This work affects you—acknowledge and address that.

Compassion Fatigue and Self-Care

Trauma nursing extracts a price. Witnessing suffering daily, making life-and-death decisions, and absorbing others' trauma creates cumulative stress that can lead to compassion fatigue, burnout, and secondary traumatic stress. Understanding these risks and actively protecting your wellbeing isn't selfish—it's essential for sustaining your ability to care for others.

Understanding Compassion Fatigue

Compassion fatigue is the emotional and physical exhaustion that results from prolonged exposure to others' suffering, particularly in caregiving professions. Unlike burnout (which results from workplace stress generally), compassion fatigue specifically relates to empathic engagement with suffering.

How compassion fatigue develops:

When you care for trauma patients, your natural empathy means you absorb some of their emotional pain. This is what allows you to provide compassionate care. But repeated exposure without adequate recovery creates an accumulation of secondary trauma.

Think of it like a sponge absorbing water. Initially, the sponge has capacity. But if you keep exposing it to water without wringing it out, it becomes saturated and can't absorb anymore. Worse, the prolonged wetness degrades the sponge itself.

Symptoms of compassion fatigue:

Physical symptoms:

- Exhaustion not relieved by sleep
- Frequent illness (immune system suppression from chronic stress)
- Headaches, GI problems, muscle tension
- Sleep disturbances (difficulty falling asleep, nightmares, waking frequently)

Emotional symptoms:

- Emotional numbness or detachment
- Feeling overwhelmed by others' suffering

Difficulty separating work from personal life

Reduced empathy (feeling less for patients than you used to)

Intrusive thoughts about patients or traumatic cases

Anxiety, depression, irritability

Feeling like your work doesn't matter

Behavioral symptoms:

Avoidance (calling in sick, avoiding difficult patients, not volunteering for trauma activations)

Isolation from colleagues, friends, family

Increased use of alcohol or other substances to cope

Decreased work performance

Difficulty making decisions

Cynicism about work or patients

Cognitive symptoms:

Difficulty concentrating

Confusion or disorientation

Decreased attention to detail

Negative self-image or self-doubt

Questioning your career choice

Risk Factors for Compassion Fatigue

Some factors increase vulnerability to compassion fatigue:

Personal factors:

High empathy levels (your greatest strength becomes a vulnerability)

Personal trauma history (caring for trauma patients triggers your own unresolved trauma)

Poor boundaries between work and personal life

Perfectionism (setting unrealistic standards for yourself)

Being early in career (less developed coping mechanisms)

Being highly experienced (cumulative exposure effect)

Work environment factors:

High patient acuity and volume

Frequent exposure to dying patients, especially children

Lack of control over work conditions

Insufficient staffing

Lack of organizational support

No debriefing or processing opportunities after difficult cases

Culture that views self-care as weakness

Specific trauma types that increase risk:

Pediatric trauma (especially abuse)

Cases involving colleagues or their family members	Prolonged resuscitations that fail
Mass casualty incidents	Violent trauma (particularly when ongoing threat exists)
Cases that trigger personal experiences	

Burnout vs. Compassion Fatigue vs. Secondary Traumatic Stress

These terms are related but distinct:

Burnout:

Results from chronic workplace stress

Develops gradually over time

Characterized by exhaustion, cynicism, reduced efficacy

Related to work conditions more than specific emotional toll

Example: Feeling exhausted and frustrated by mandatory overtime, understaffing, administrative burden

Compassion fatigue:

Results specifically from empathic engagement with suffering

Can develop gradually or suddenly

Characterized by reduced capacity for empathy and compassion

Related to the emotional cost of caring

Example: Finding yourself feeling nothing when a patient cries, where you used to feel deeply moved

Secondary traumatic stress (STS):

Results from indirect exposure to trauma through caring for trauma victims

Can develop suddenly after particularly traumatic case

Mirrors symptoms of PTSD (intrusive thoughts, avoidance, hyperarousal, negative mood)

Related to absorbing patients' traumatic experiences

Example: Having nightmares about a pediatric trauma patient's injuries, avoiding caring for similar patients

These often co-occur. A nurse might experience burnout from understaffing, compassion fatigue from constant exposure to suffering, and secondary traumatic stress from particularly horrific cases—all simultaneously.

Prevention Strategies

Preventing compassion fatigue requires intentional, ongoing effort. It doesn't happen accidentally.

Self-awareness:

Regular self-assessment is crucial. Ask yourself monthly:

- How's my energy level compared to three months ago?
- Am I sleeping well?
- Do I still feel moved by patients' stories?
- Am I isolating from friends and family?
- Have I noticed changes in my health, mood, or behavior?
- Am I using alcohol or other substances more?

Early recognition allows early intervention. Don't wait until you're completely depleted to act.

Boundaries:

Professional boundaries protect both you and patients:

Physical boundaries:

- Take scheduled breaks (actually leave the unit)
- Use your vacation time
- Don't routinely stay late or come early
- Turn off work notifications when off-duty

Emotional boundaries:

- Recognize you can care deeply without taking on patients' emotions as your own
- Practice empathy without absorption: "I understand your pain" rather than "I feel your pain as my own"
- Accept that you can't fix everything
- Differentiate between compassion (caring about their suffering) and codependence (making their suffering your responsibility to eliminate)

Cognitive boundaries:

- Leave work thoughts at work when possible
- Don't ruminate about cases during personal time
- Practice thought-stopping techniques when work thoughts intrude

Setting boundaries isn't callousness—it's sustainability. You can't help others if you're depleted.

Work-life balance:

Actively cultivate life outside work:

Relationships:

- Maintain relationships with non-healthcare friends
- Spend quality time with family
- Join groups unrelated to medicine
- Protect relationship time (no work talk during family dinner)

Hobbies and interests:

- Engage in activities you enjoy
- Learn new skills unrelated to nursing
- Create (art, music, writing, gardening)
- Move (exercise, dance, sports)

Rest:

- Prioritize sleep (7-9 hours)
- Practice relaxation techniques
- Allow downtime without productivity goals
- Disconnect from technology regularly

Meaning and purpose:

- Remember why you chose trauma nursing
- Reflect on positive patient outcomes
- Connect your work to larger values
- Celebrate small victories

Workplace strategies:

Advocate for organizational support:

Debriefing after critical events:

- Formal debriefing process after mass casualties, pediatric deaths, colleague injuries
- Informal check-ins after difficult shifts
- Normalize discussing emotional impact
- Led by trained facilitators when possible

Adequate staffing:

- Appropriate nurse-patient ratios
- Adequate support staff
- Manageable schedules with sufficient time off

Professional development:

- Continuing education opportunities
- Career advancement pathways
- Recognition programs
- Mentorship programs (both being mentored and mentoring)

Peer support programs:

- Structured peer support teams
- Access to confidential counseling
- Employee assistance programs
- Resilience training

Team cohesion:

Strong team relationships are protective:

- Support colleagues during difficult cases
- Share coping strategies
- Socialize outside work occasionally
- Acknowledge each other's contributions
- Address conflicts directly and professionally
- Celebrate successes together

Personal resilience practices:

Mindfulness and stress reduction:

- Meditation or deep breathing exercises
- Yoga or tai chi
- Progressive muscle relaxation
- Guided imagery
- Mindfulness apps (Headspace, Calm, Insight Timer)

Physical health:

- Regular exercise (cardiovascular, strength, flexibility)
- Nutritious eating
- Adequate hydration
- Limit caffeine and alcohol
- Regular health checkups

Psychological support:

- Regular therapy or counseling (don't wait until crisis)
- Support groups for healthcare workers
- Spiritual practices if meaningful to you
- Journaling or expressive writing

Professional help when needed:

Know when to seek help:

- Symptoms persist despite self-care efforts
- Functioning impairment (work performance declining, relationship problems)
- Substance use increasing
- Suicidal thoughts
- Inability to stop thinking about work
- Physical symptoms worsening

Resources available:

- Employee assistance programs (free, confidential counseling)
- Private therapists (especially those specializing in healthcare workers)
- Psychiatry if medication might help
- Crisis lines if immediate support needed

Seeking help is strength, not weakness. You wouldn't hesitate to treat a physical injury. Mental health deserves the same respect.

Organizational Responsibility

While individual self-care is crucial, organizations must create environments that support staff wellbeing.

Leadership responsibilities:

- Acknowledge emotional toll of trauma work
- Provide adequate resources for self-care
- Create culture where seeking help is normalized
- Ensure adequate staffing
- Offer flexible scheduling when possible
- Provide professional development opportunities
- Recognize and reward excellent care
- Implement evidence-based resilience programs

Red flags of toxic organizational culture:

- "Suck it up" mentality
- Stigma around mental health
- Expectation of constant availability
- No time for breaks
- Chronic understaffing treated as normal
- No debriefing after critical events
- Emotional reactions dismissed or mocked

If your organization lacks support: Consider advocating for change through proper channels, connecting with colleagues to request resources collectively, or ultimately recognizing when a work environment is unsustainable for your health.

Self-Compassion

You likely excel at showing compassion to patients. Now practice it toward yourself.

Self-compassion involves:

Self-kindness: Treat yourself with the same understanding you'd offer a struggling colleague. When you make mistakes or feel depleted, respond with kindness rather than harsh self-criticism.

Common humanity: Recognize that struggle, imperfection, and compassion fatigue are part of the human experience, not personal failings. Every trauma nurse faces these challenges.

Mindfulness: Acknowledge difficult emotions without over-identifying with them. "I'm experiencing sadness about that patient's death" rather than "I'm a failure because I couldn't save them."

Practical self-compassion:

Notice your inner dialogue. Is it harsh? Would you speak that way to a friend?

When self-critical thoughts arise, pause and reframe: "I'm doing my best in difficult circumstances"

Acknowledge your limits: "I can't save everyone, and that's not a personal failure"

Celebrate what you do accomplish: "I provided comfort even when cure wasn't possible"

Forgive yourself for being human

Building Sustainable Practice

Longevity in trauma nursing requires intentional sustainability planning.

Early career:

- Develop healthy coping mechanisms now
- Build support networks
- Learn to set boundaries
- Seek mentorship from resilient senior nurses
- Start self-care practices before you feel you need them

Mid-career:

- Reassess regularly (are current strategies working?)
- Be willing to adjust work arrangements (unit, shift, hours)
- Consider developing expertise that provides variety (education, management, specialty roles)
- Mentor newer nurses (teaching reinforces meaning)

Late career:

- Recognize changing capacity (what was sustainable at 25 may not be at 55)
- Consider transitional roles (case management, education, quality improvement)
- Share wisdom with next generation
- Plan for retirement transition (identity beyond "trauma nurse")

Throughout career:

- Take sabbaticals or extended breaks when needed
- Pursue additional education or certifications for variety
- Participate in professional organizations
- Engage in research or quality improvement
- Remember that changing roles or leaving trauma nursing doesn't equal failure—it means recognizing your needs

Chapter 11 Practice Questions

Question 1: During crisis intervention, the most important initial step is:

A) Providing detailed medical explanations
B) Ensuring physical and psychological safety
C) Contacting family members
D) Administering sedation

Answer: B

Explanation: The foundation of crisis intervention is establishing safety—both physical (treating life-threatening injuries) and psychological (helping the person feel protected and cared for). Only after safety is established can other interventions be effective.

Question 2: Which statement demonstrates appropriate crisis intervention communication?

A) "You need to calm down so we can help you"
B) "Everything will be fine, don't worry"
C) "I can see this is very frightening for you. You're safe here, and we're taking care of your injuries"
D) "Other patients have it much worse"

Answer: C

Explanation: Effective crisis communication validates emotions, provides reassurance about safety, and gives clear information about what's happening. It doesn't minimize feelings, make promises about outcomes, or compare suffering.

Question 3: Research on family presence during resuscitation shows:

A) It increases provider anxiety and medical errors
B) Families always interfere with resuscitation efforts
C) It reduces family anxiety and PTSD symptoms without harming resuscitation
D) It should never be permitted due to legal risks

Answer: C

Explanation: Multiple studies demonstrate that family presence during resuscitation, when properly supported, reduces family members' anxiety, depression, and PTSD symptoms without interfering with medical care or increasing litigation.

Question 4: The primary role of a family facilitator during resuscitation is to:

A) Perform CPR
B) Make medical decisions for the team
C) Explain procedures to family and provide emotional support
D) Keep family members out of the room

Answer: C

Explanation: The family facilitator stays with family members during resuscitation, explaining what's happening in understandable terms, providing emotional support, assessing coping, and intervening if family becomes disruptive (which is rare).

Question 5: When delivering news of a patient's death, you should:

A) Use euphemisms like "passed away" or "didn't make it"
B) State clearly "I'm sorry, your loved one has died"
C) Provide all medical details before mentioning death
D) Have the family guess the outcome

Answer: B

Explanation: Clear, direct language using the word "died" prevents confusion and ambiguity. Euphemisms can be misunderstood. Compassionate directness is most effective: deliver the news clearly, then pause and allow the family to process before providing details.

Question 6: Proper chain of custody for forensic evidence requires:

A) Storing all evidence together in one bag
B) Documenting who collected, handled, and transferred each item
C) Cleaning evidence before packaging
D) Giving evidence directly to family

Answer: B

Explanation: Chain of custody requires meticulous documentation of everyone who handled evidence from collection to court. This proves evidence wasn't tampered with or contaminated, making it admissible in legal proceedings.

Question 7: When collecting clothing as evidence, you should:

A) Cut through bullet holes or tears
B) Place all items in one plastic bag
C) Place each item in a separate paper bag
D) Wash blood-soaked items first

Answer: C

Explanation: Each clothing item goes in a separate paper bag (plastic traps moisture, degrading biological evidence). Cut around, not through, holes or tears to preserve evidence. Never clean items—this destroys evidence.

Question 8: Which injury pattern suggests possible intimate partner violence?

A) Single injury to extremity
B) Multiple injuries in various stages of healing
C) Sports-related fracture
D) Recent surgical scar

Answer: B

Explanation: Multiple injuries in different healing stages suggest repeated trauma over time, a classic pattern in intimate partner violence. Single injuries or those consistent with stated mechanisms are less suspicious.

Question 9: Universal screening for intimate partner violence means:

A) Only screening patients with suspicious injuries
B) Screening all patients in private settings with non-judgmental approach
C) Screening only women
D) Screening only when partner is present

Answer: B

Explanation: Universal screening involves asking all patients about violence in a private, non-judgmental setting. This identifies more victims than screening only "suspicious" cases. Never screen with potential abuser present.

Question 10: If a patient discloses abuse but isn't ready to leave, you should:

A) Force them to leave for their safety
B) Refuse to provide resources until they commit to leaving
C) Provide safety planning and resources while respecting their autonomy
D) Report them to police immediately

Answer: C

Explanation: Respect patient autonomy while providing resources and safety planning. Leaving is most dangerous time in abusive relationships. Forcing someone to leave can increase danger and damage trust. Provide information and support, allowing them to make decisions about their safety.

Question 11: Mandatory reporting of child abuse requires:

A) Certainty that abuse occurred
B) Only suspicion of abuse
C) Parent's permission
D) Proof beyond reasonable doubt

Answer: B

Explanation: Healthcare providers must report suspected child abuse, not just confirmed cases. The threshold is reasonable suspicion, not certainty. Reporters have legal immunity for good-faith reports. Investigation is the responsibility of child protective services, not healthcare providers.

Question 12: Compassion fatigue is characterized by:

A) Increased empathy for patients
B) Reduced capacity for compassion due to prolonged exposure to suffering
C) Occasional tiredness after long shifts
D) Excitement about work

Answer: B

Explanation: Compassion fatigue is the progressive decrease in empathy and compassion resulting from prolonged exposure to others' suffering. It's distinct from normal tiredness—it's a fundamental change in your ability to connect emotionally with patients' pain.

Question 13: Which is an early warning sign of compassion fatigue?

A) Feeling energized by challenging cases
B) Emotional numbness or detachment from patients
C) Enthusiasm for professional development
D) Strong support network

Answer: B

Explanation: Emotional numbness and detachment are early warning signs. Other signs include difficulty separating work from personal life, reduced empathy, intrusive thoughts about cases, and feeling overwhelmed by others' suffering.

Question 14: The difference between burnout and compassion fatigue is:

A) There is no difference
B) Burnout relates to workplace stress generally; compassion fatigue specifically relates to empathic engagement with suffering
C) Compassion fatigue only affects new nurses
D) Burnout is more serious than compassion fatigue

Answer: B

Explanation: Burnout results from chronic workplace stress (understaffing, administrative burden, lack of control). Compassion fatigue specifically results from the emotional cost of empathically engaging with suffering patients. Both are serious, and nurses can experience both simultaneously.

Question 15: An effective strategy for preventing compassion fatigue is:

A) Avoiding all emotional connection with patients
B) Working extra shifts to prove dedication
C) Setting healthy boundaries and maintaining work-life balance
D) Ignoring symptoms until they resolve spontaneously

Answer: C

Explanation: Healthy boundaries and work-life balance are essential prevention strategies. This doesn't mean eliminating empathy—it means caring about patients' suffering without absorbing it as your own, and maintaining a life outside work that provides meaning and restoration.

Question 16: When preparing family to view a deceased loved one, you should:

A) Provide no preparation—they need to see for themselves
B) Describe what they'll see, including medical equipment and changed appearance
C) Only allow viewing if body looks "normal"
D) Require viewing even if family refuses

Answer: B

Explanation: Prepare family by describing what they'll see: changed appearance (pallor, medical equipment still present if not removed, injuries covered with dressings). This preparation prevents additional shock and allows informed decision about viewing.

Question 17: Trauma-informed care includes:

A) Asking detailed questions about all past traumas
B) Creating safety, transparency, and empowerment while recognizing impact of past trauma
C) Treating all patients as if they have PTSD
D) Avoiding all procedures that might cause distress

Answer: B

Explanation: Trauma-informed care recognizes that many patients have trauma histories and modifies approach to maximize safety and control without probing details of past trauma during acute care. It emphasizes safety, transparency, choice, and empowerment.

Question 18: Secondary traumatic stress differs from compassion fatigue in that it:

A) Only affects family members
B) Mirrors PTSD symptoms from indirect trauma exposure
C) Is less serious
D) Only occurs after single events

Answer: B

Explanation: Secondary traumatic stress involves PTSD-like symptoms (intrusive thoughts, avoidance, hyperarousal) from indirect exposure to trauma through caring for trauma victims. It can develop suddenly after particularly horrific cases, while compassion fatigue typically develops gradually.

Question 19: Which action best supports a colleague showing signs of compassion fatigue?

A) Telling them to toughen up
B) Reporting them to management for incompetence
C) Expressing concern privately and suggesting they access support resources
D) Ignoring the signs—it's not your business

Answer: C

Explanation: Express concern privately and supportively, suggesting resources like employee assistance programs or counseling. Create safe space for them to acknowledge struggles. Compassion fatigue isn't weakness or incompetence—it's an occupational hazard requiring support.

Question 20: Proper evidence documentation requires:

A) Interpreting what injuries mean
B) Objective description of what you observe
C) Only photographing obvious injuries
D) Sharing details with unauthorized persons

Answer: B

Explanation: Document objectively—describe exactly what you see without interpretation. "3 cm purple bruise on left cheek" not "bruise consistent with punch." Interpretation is for investigators. Photograph all injuries, document measurements and locations precisely.

Question 21: If a patient refuses to leave an abusive situation, the appropriate response is:

A) Document that they refused and stop providing resources
B) Threaten to call police
C) Respect their decision while providing resources and information for when they're ready
D) Force them to go to a shelter

Answer: C

Explanation: Respect autonomy while ensuring they have resources. Leaving is complex and dangerous—most dangerous time is when victim attempts to leave. Provide domestic violence hotline number, safety planning information, and support regardless of their decision about leaving.

Question 22: Self-compassion in preventing compassion fatigue means:

A) Ignoring your own needs
B) Treating yourself with the same kindness you'd show a struggling colleague
C) Never acknowledging mistakes
D) Working without breaks to prove dedication

Answer: B

Explanation: Self-compassion involves treating yourself kindly, recognizing that struggle is part of the human experience, and acknowledging difficult emotions without harsh self-judgment. It's essential for sustaining compassion for others while protecting your own wellbeing.

Question 23: When should debriefing occur after a critical event?

A) Never—it shows weakness
B) Only if requested by staff
C) Routinely after mass casualties, pediatric deaths, or colleague injuries
D) Only for new staff

Answer: C

Explanation: Formal debriefing should occur routinely after particularly traumatic events (mass casualties, pediatric deaths, deaths of colleagues or their family members). This normalizes discussing emotional impact and provides opportunity for processing, which can prevent compassion fatigue and secondary traumatic stress.

Question 24: The purpose of organ donation discussion is to:

A) Pressure families to donate
B) Provide opportunity for families to honor wishes and help others
C) Only occur if patient carried donor card
D) Reduce hospital costs

Answer: B

Explanation: Organ donation discussion provides families opportunity to honor patient wishes and help others through donation. Approach with sensitivity, never pressure, and separate clinical team (focused on care) from organ procurement organization team (focused on donation discussion).

Question 25: Cultural competence in end-of-life care requires:

A) Treating all patients identically
B) Assuming cultural practices based on appearance
C) Asking about individual cultural or religious practices important to the family
D) Imposing your own beliefs

Answer: C

Explanation: Cultural competence means asking about individual preferences rather than assuming based on perceived ethnicity or religion. "Are there cultural or religious practices important for your family as we care for your loved one?" allows families to guide culturally appropriate care.

Clinical Scenarios

Clinical Scenario 1: Crisis Intervention with Multiple Trauma

A 28-year-old woman arrives after a motor vehicle crash. She sustained multiple injuries including femur fracture, pneumothorax, and facial lacerations. She's conscious and in severe pain, crying and repeatedly asking "Am I going to die? Where's my daughter? Was anyone else hurt?"

Her vital signs are stabilizing after initial resuscitation, but she remains extremely anxious and agitated despite pain medication. The social worker reports her daughter (age 3) is being treated in pediatrics with minor injuries. Her husband was driving and died at the scene.

Questions:

How do you address her immediate psychological crisis while managing medical care?

Should you tell her about her husband's death now, or wait until she's more stable?

How do you address her concerns about her daughter?

What resources should be mobilized to support her?

Answers:

Addressing immediate psychological crisis:

Establish safety first (already underway with medical stabilization): The foundation of crisis intervention is physical safety. Her injuries are being addressed, which is essential before psychological needs can be met. Continue medical care while simultaneously addressing psychological crisis.

Provide clear, honest information about HER status: "I know this is terrifying. You've been in a serious accident and you have some significant injuries—a broken leg, some damage to your lung, and cuts on your face. We're treating all of these. You're getting stronger. You're not going to die."

Be specific and concrete: Her question "Am I going to die?" needs clear answer. Vague reassurance ("You'll be fine") doesn't reduce anxiety. Specific information does: "Your vital signs are stable. Your lung is re-expanding with the chest tube. The orthopedic surgeon will repair your leg. These are serious injuries, but you're going to survive this."

Validate her emotions: "It's completely normal to feel scared right now. You've been through something terrible. These feelings make sense."

Address immediate control: "I can't make everything okay right now, but I can tell you exactly what we're doing to help you" then provide clear explanation of each intervention and what happens next.

Use therapeutic presence: Maintain calm demeanor, speak clearly and slowly, make appropriate eye contact, stay physically present rather than appearing rushed.

Timing of death notification:

This requires careful judgment. **Consider:**

Against immediate disclosure:

- She's in acute crisis with multiple injuries
- She's already maximally stressed
- Her cognitive processing may be impaired by pain, medications, trauma response
- Adding grief to current crisis could overwhelm coping

For immediate disclosure (with support):

- She's repeatedly asking about others
- Delaying creates more distress from uncertainty
- She may learn from others (staff conversations, family, her daughter mentioning daddy)
- Finding out you knew and didn't tell damages trust
- She has right to know

Best approach—provide truth with maximum support:

"You asked if anyone else was hurt. I need to tell you something very difficult. Your daughter is being treated in pediatrics. She has minor injuries and is going to be okay. Your husband was also in the accident. His injuries were very severe. Despite everything the team did, he didn't survive. I'm so sorry."

Then:

- **Stop talking**. Let her process. Silence is okay.
- **Stay present**. Don't leave her alone with this news.
- **Validate emotions**: "This is devastating" (don't minimize: "He's in a better place")
- **Assess safety**: Does grief overwhelm her to point of self-harm risk? Unlikely in this scenario, but assess.
- **Mobilize support**: "The chaplain is here. Our social worker will help with anything you need. Your family is on their way."

Provide information gradually: Don't overwhelm with details. Answer questions as she asks. "What happened?" "There was a collision. The trauma team worked on him, but his injuries were too severe."

Addressing concerns about daughter:

Provide specific, concrete information: "Your daughter is in our pediatric unit. She has a small cut on her forehead that needed a few stitches and a bruised arm. She's scared and asking for you, but she's medically stable. Our pediatric team is taking excellent care of her."

Address her need to see daughter: "I know you need to see her. Right now, we need to stabilize your injuries first—your lung and your leg. As soon as it's medically safe, we'll arrange for you to see her or for someone to bring her picture or video to you."

Creative solutions for mother-daughter reunion:

Video call immediately (pediatrics nurse holds tablet)

Bring recent photo of daughter to mother

Have pediatric team send reassuring message

Once mother stabilized, brief bedside visit with daughter

Reassure about daughter's care: "She's with our best pediatric nurses. They're keeping her comfortable and safe. Family members can be with her. We'll reunite you as soon as medically possible."

Resources to mobilize:

Immediate:

Chaplain for spiritual/emotional support

Social worker for practical assistance (funeral arrangements, childcare, insurance)

Grief counselor

Family liaison to coordinate communication

Ongoing:

Trauma counseling (addressing both physical trauma and sudden loss)

Survivor guilt counseling (common when loved one dies in same accident)

Parenting support (helping daughter process father's death while mother recovers)

Financial counseling (loss of spouse's income)

Support groups (traumatic loss, widow support)

Key takeaway: Crisis intervention requires simultaneous management of physical injuries and psychological needs. Truth delivered with support is better than delayed disclosure. Mobilize comprehensive resources early.

Clinical Scenario 2: Family Presence During Failed Resuscitation

A 16-year-old male arrives in traumatic arrest after gunshot wound to chest. Resuscitation efforts are underway. His mother arrives, hysterical, demanding to see her son. The attending physician says "absolutely not" while the trauma nurse believes family presence should be offered.

After 45 minutes of resuscitation with no response, the team leader is considering terminating efforts. The mother is still in the waiting room, unaware of how critical the situation is.

Questions:

How should the disagreement about family presence be handled in the moment?

If family presence is permitted, how should mother be prepared?

How should resuscitation termination be handled with mother present?

What support does mother need after her son's death?

Answers:

Handling staff disagreement:

Immediate resolution: Team leader makes final decision, but respectfully: "Dr. Smith, I understand your concerns about family presence. Our hospital policy supports family presence when properly facilitated. I'm comfortable proceeding if you are. If not, I'll note your objection in the record, but I believe this is in the family's best interest."

If physician refuses: "I respect your decision as team leader. I'll ensure the family receives frequent updates and we'll bring them in immediately after we stop if efforts are unsuccessful."

Later—address systemically: This isn't personal conflict; it's policy/practice disagreement requiring team education and clear institutional guidelines.

Preparing mother (if permitted):

Assign dedicated facilitator: Don't bring family in unsupported.

Prepare before entering: "Your son is critically injured. The team is doing everything medically possible. I need to prepare you for what you'll see: many people working quickly, medical equipment, blood, your son receiving CPR. It will be very difficult to watch. You can leave anytime. You won't interfere with care, but you can be present and speak to him."

Set boundaries: Where to stand, don't touch patient, facilitator will explain what's happening, may need to step back for procedures.

During resuscitation: Facilitator provides ongoing explanation: "They're doing chest compressions to circulate blood manually. The medications through IV support his heart. They're trying everything."

Termination with family present:

Team leader addresses team first: "We've exhausted our interventions. The injury is not survivable. Unless anyone has additional suggestions, I'm going to call it."

Brief pause for team input, then: "Time of death is 19:47. I'm very sorry."

Address family directly: "Mrs. Johnson, we've done everything medically possible. The injury to your son's heart was too severe. Despite all our efforts, he's died. I'm so very sorry."

Immediate actions:

- Stop CPR gently (not abruptly)
- Leave one nurse with family
- Give family time with body
- Don't rush to remove equipment
- Facilitator stays to support

Support after death:

Immediate:

- Offer viewing (prepare body—clean face, cover wounds, remove excess equipment)
- Provide private space
- Allow cultural/religious rituals
- Offer keepsakes (if appropriate—maybe not with violent death of teen)

Short-term:

- Chaplain support
- Social work for funeral arrangements
- Information about violent crime victim compensation
- Contact information for grief counseling
- Adolescent death support groups

Consider:

- This is violent death—police investigation involved
- Adolescent death creates unique grief

Sudden traumatic loss has different grief trajectory than anticipated death	Mother may have survivor guilt, complicated grief

Key takeaway: Family presence during resuscitation requires preparation, support, and clear communication. Staff training reduces resistance. Witnessing resuscitation efforts can help families accept death when it occurs.

Clinical Scenario 3: Recognizing and Responding to Intimate Partner Violence

A 32-year-old woman presents with facial bruising, wrist fractures, and back pain after "falling down stairs." Her husband accompanies her, answering all questions. She makes minimal eye contact, appears anxious, and flinches when husband touches her arm.

When you finally get her alone (husband went to move the car), she admits: "He pushed me. This isn't the first time. But I can't leave—we have three kids, I don't work, I have nowhere to go. Please don't say anything. He'll know I told you."

Questions:

What about this presentation suggested intimate partner violence before disclosure?

How do you document the injuries and disclosure?

What is your legal obligation regarding reporting?

What resources do you provide when patient refuses to leave?

Answers:

Red flags that suggested IPV:

Injury pattern: Facial injuries common in IPV (intimate areas targeted). Bilateral wrist fractures unusual in falls (defensive injuries from blocking blows).

Mechanism inconsistency: "Falling down stairs" doesn't typically cause bilateral wrist fractures and facial injuries together.

Behavior: Partner answering all questions, not leaving patient alone, patient's anxiety and flinching suggest fear.

Clinical cues: Minimizing injuries, avoiding eye contact, appearing fearful—all suggest abuse history.

Documentation:

Objective injury description:

"Multiple purple/brown bruises on face: 3cm on right cheek, 2cm on left forehead, 4cm on jaw"

"Bilateral wrist fractures confirmed on X-ray"

"Tenderness over lumbar spine"

Document disclosure in patient's exact words:

"Patient states: 'My husband pushed me down. This has happened before. I'm scared to leave because we have three children and I don't have income or a place to go.'"

Behavioral observations:

"Patient appeared anxious, flinching when husband approached"

"Patient only disclosed abuse when alone with nurse"

Avoid interpretation: Don't write "injuries consistent with abuse" or "patient is a victim of domestic violence"—describe facts.

Photograph injuries: With consent, using measurement scale.

Legal obligations:

Know your jurisdiction: IPV reporting requirements vary by state.

Most states: Adult IPV is NOT mandatory reporting (unlike child/elder abuse). Patient autonomy is respected unless specific circumstances require reporting (some states mandate reporting injuries from weapons).

This case: Likely no mandatory reporting obligation. However, provide resources and safety planning.

If children are at risk: May trigger mandatory child abuse reporting if evidence suggests children are being abused or exposed to domestic violence that endangers them. Assess: "Are the children safe? Has he hurt them or do they witness the violence?"

Resources when patient refuses to leave:

Respect autonomy: "I can't force you to leave. I'm worried about your safety, but I respect that you need to make this decision. I want you to have information and resources for when you're ready."

Provide resources discretely:

Domestic violence hotline number (written inside discharge papers or prescription bottle)

Safety planning information

Women's shelter locations

Legal advocacy information

Safety planning:

Identify safe room with exit

Keep phone accessible

Pack essential items and hide or give to friend

Create code word for help

Know where to go in emergency

Medical documentation: "Your medical records can document the abuse. If you ever need evidence for court, these records will be available."

Follow-up: "I'd like to see you back in one week to check your wrist casts. That gives you another opportunity to talk if things change."

Validate feelings: "Leaving is the most dangerous time. You're making the decision that feels safest right now. You know your situation better than anyone."

Key takeaway: Recognize IPV patterns, document thoroughly, provide resources while respecting autonomy, understand reporting requirements, and maintain non-judgmental support.

Chapter 11 Key Takeaways

Crisis Intervention Essentials:

Safety first (physical then psychological)

Provide clear, honest information

Validate emotions without minimizing

Support existing coping mechanisms

Mobilize resources proactively

Family Presence Best Practices:

Benefits families without harming care

Requires designated facilitator

Prepare family for what they'll see

Explain procedures in lay terms

Support through resuscitation and death

End-of-Life Care:

Use clear language: "died" not euphemisms

Prepare family before viewing body

Respect cultural/religious practices

Support organ donation discussions

Provide comprehensive grief resources

Forensic Evidence:

Medical care always takes priority

Maintain chain of custody

Document objectively, not interpretatively

Separate items in paper bags

Preserve evidence even during emergencies

Violence Recognition:

Screen universally, not just suspicious cases

Know injury patterns suggesting abuse

Understand mandatory reporting laws

Provide resources regardless of patient decisions

Document thoroughly for potential legal use

Compassion Fatigue Prevention:

Recognize early warning signs

Set healthy professional boundaries

Maintain work-life balance

Access support resources proactively

Practice self-compassion

Professional Resilience:

Trauma nursing takes emotional toll

Self-care isn't selfish—it's essential

Seek help when needed

Support colleagues experiencing distress

Advocate for organizational support systems

Connecting to Practice

These concepts aren't theoretical—they're daily realities in trauma nursing:

Every trauma activation involves crisis intervention as you calm terrified patients.

Family presence decisions happen during every resuscitation—will you support or resist it?

Death notifications are inevitable in trauma nursing—your delivery impacts families' grief trajectory.

Evidence collection occurs with every assault victim—your documentation may determine justice.

Abuse victims present regularly—your response may save lives.

Your own wellbeing determines career sustainability—neglect it at your peril.

Master these psychosocial skills alongside clinical skills. Technical excellence without human connection is incomplete nursing. Compassionate care without self-preservation is unsustainable practice.

The TCRN exam tests these concepts because they're fundamental to trauma nursing competence. More importantly, mastering them makes you a complete, effective, and resilient trauma nurse.

Study Tips for Chapter 11:

Crisis intervention: Remember the order—safety, information, validation, coping support, resources

Family presence: Know the research supports it and the facilitator role is key

Evidence: Chain of custody and objective documentation are critical

Abuse: Recognize patterns, know reporting laws, respect autonomy while providing resources

Compassion fatigue: Identify early signs and prevention strategies

Common Exam Patterns:

Scenarios testing appropriate crisis communication

Questions about family presence benefits and implementation

Evidence collection procedures and documentation

Identifying abuse patterns and appropriate responses

Recognizing compassion fatigue symptoms and interventions

Chapter 12: Trauma Systems and Quality Improvement

Understanding how trauma systems work and how they continuously improve is essential for TCRN certification. This chapter moves beyond bedside care to explore the infrastructure that supports optimal trauma outcomes. You'll learn about trauma center designation, how patients are triaged and transferred, how systems measure and improve performance, injury prevention strategies, and disaster response.

These concepts are critical because trauma care doesn't happen in isolation. Even excellent individual nursing care achieves better outcomes within a well-organized trauma system. Understanding these system-level concepts helps you appreciate your role within the larger trauma network and prepares you for leadership opportunities in trauma nursing.

Trauma System Organization

A trauma system is an organized, coordinated effort by a defined geographic region to deliver optimal care to injured patients. Rather than individual hospitals working independently, trauma systems create networks where each facility plays a specific role based on its capabilities.

Levels of Trauma Centers

The American College of Surgeons (ACS) Committee on Trauma designates trauma centers based on resources, capabilities, and commitment to trauma care. Understanding these levels helps you know when patients need transfer versus local management.

Level I Trauma Center (Regional Resource)

These are tertiary care facilities providing the highest level of trauma care. Requirements include:

24/7 immediate availability of surgeons in general surgery, orthopedics, neurosurgery, and other specialties

In-house surgical and anesthesia teams around the clock

Advanced imaging (CT, angiography, interventional radiology) immediately available

Comprehensive critical care capabilities

Trauma research program

Injury prevention and outreach programs

Leadership in trauma education and system development

Annual volume requirements (typically 1,200+ trauma admissions or 240+ with ISS >15)

Clinical implication: Level I centers can manage any injury, no matter how severe. They serve as referral centers for complex cases and provide consultation to lower-level centers.

Level II Trauma Center (Community Trauma Center)

These facilities provide definitive trauma care but may not have all subspecialty services immediately available. Requirements include:

24/7 general surgery coverage

Subspecialty availability (may be on-call rather than in-house)

Most surgical capabilities of Level I but potentially without some highly specialized services

Transfer agreements with Level I centers for cases exceeding their capabilities

Trauma quality improvement program

Clinical implication: Level II centers handle most trauma effectively and transfer only highly complex cases (e.g., severe traumatic brain injury needing neurosurgical expertise not available).

Level III Trauma Center (Rural/Community Hospital)

These facilities provide prompt assessment, resuscitation, emergency operations, and stabilization before transfer if needed. Requirements include:

24/7 emergency physician coverage

General surgery coverage (may be on-call)

Transfer agreements with higher-level centers

Trauma quality improvement program

Limited resources compared to Level I/II but adequate for initial stabilization

Clinical implication: Level III centers focus on rapid stabilization and appropriate transfer. They're critical in rural areas where travel to higher-level centers takes hours.

Level IV and V Trauma Centers (Rural/Remote)

These facilities provide advanced trauma life support before transfer:

- 24/7 physician or advanced practice provider coverage
- Basic resuscitation capabilities
- Transfer agreements
- May be sole healthcare facility in remote areas

Clinical implication: These centers save lives by providing immediate stabilization in areas where the nearest Level I/II center is hours away.

Trauma System Components

Effective trauma systems include coordinated components working together:

Pre-hospital care: EMS providers trained in trauma triage and stabilization, with protocols directing patients to appropriate facilities based on injury severity and transport time.

Trauma center network: Mix of trauma center levels providing appropriate care based on injury and geography, with clear transfer protocols between facilities.

Rehabilitation facilities: Specialized trauma rehabilitation centers for patients requiring extended recovery support.

Data systems: Regional trauma registries collecting outcome data to drive system improvement.

Quality oversight: Regional trauma councils or state agencies monitoring system performance and ensuring standards are met.

Public health integration: Injury prevention programs, violence intervention, and community outreach coordinated across the system.

Inclusive vs. Exclusive Systems

Inclusive systems incorporate all interested facilities willing to meet designation criteria. This approach maximizes access, particularly in rural areas, but requires strong coordination and transfer protocols.

Exclusive systems limit the number of designated trauma centers, theoretically concentrating experience and expertise. However, this may reduce geographic access in some areas.

Most states use inclusive systems, recognizing that broader participation improves overall access while transfer protocols ensure appropriate care levels.

Triage Principles

Trauma triage determines which patients need trauma center care and which level of trauma center is appropriate. Effective triage balances sensitivity (not missing seriously injured patients) with specificity (not over-triaging minimally injured patients).

Field Triage Decision Scheme

The CDC Field Triage Decision Scheme provides a systematic approach to pre-hospital trauma triage using four steps evaluated sequentially.

Step 1: Physiologic criteria (highest priority)

Any of these findings mandate transport to trauma center:

- Glasgow Coma Scale ≤13
- Systolic blood pressure <90 mmHg
- Respiratory rate <10 or >29 breaths/min (or need for ventilatory support)
- Respiratory distress (including in the elderly)

These vital sign abnormalities indicate physiologic compromise requiring trauma center resources regardless of mechanism.

Step 2: Anatomic criteria

Specific injury patterns warrant trauma center care:

- Penetrating injuries to head, neck, torso, or extremities proximal to elbow/knee
- Chest wall instability or deformity (flail chest)
- Two or more proximal long-bone fractures
- Crushed, degloved, mangled, or pulseless extremity
- Amputation proximal to wrist or ankle
- Pelvic fractures
- Open or depressed skull fracture
- Paralysis

These injuries, even in stable patients, often require specialized surgical or critical care.

Step 3: Mechanism of injury criteria

High-energy mechanisms suggest significant force transmission and potential for serious injury:

Falls >20 feet (one story = 10 feet)

High-risk auto crash (intrusion, ejection, death of another occupant, vehicle telemetry data if available)

Auto vs. pedestrian/bicyclist thrown or run over, or impact >20 mph

Motorcycle crash >20 mph

Mechanism alone doesn't mandate trauma center transport if Steps 1-2 are negative, but warrants careful evaluation and consideration of trauma center transport.

Step 4: Special patient or system considerations

Patient or system factors may warrant trauma center transport:

Age >55 years (elderly patients have higher mortality at same injury severity)

Age <15 years (pediatric patients benefit from pediatric trauma expertise)

Pregnancy >20 weeks

Anticoagulation or bleeding disorders

Burns (specific burn criteria determine burn center vs. trauma center)

Time-sensitive extremity injury (vascular compromise, compartment syndrome risk)

End-stage renal disease requiring dialysis

EMS provider judgment

These factors modify risk assessment and may prompt trauma center transport even without other criteria.

Undertriage vs. Overtriage

Undertriage occurs when seriously injured patients are transported to non-trauma centers. This delays definitive care and worsens outcomes. Acceptable undertriage rate is <5%.

Overtriage occurs when minimally injured patients are transported to trauma centers. This uses resources for patients who don't need them but is accepted to minimize undertriage. Acceptable overtriage rate is 25-35%.

The system accepts higher overtriage to ensure seriously injured patients reliably reach trauma centers. Think of it as a safety margin—we're willing to bring four patients with minor injuries to the trauma center to ensure we don't miss the one with serious injuries.

Interfacility Triage

When patients present to non-trauma centers, nurses and physicians must recognize who needs transfer. Transfer criteria include:

Injuries exceeding facility capabilities:

Need for surgical subspecialties not available (neurosurgery, thoracic surgery, pediatric surgery)

Need for interventional radiology or other advanced procedures

Anticipated ICU stay when no ICU beds available

Pediatric trauma at adult-only facility

Physiologic instability:

Persistent shock despite resuscitation

Deteriorating neurological status

Respiratory failure

Resource limitations:

Blood product availability insufficient for massive transfusion

Monitoring capabilities inadequate

Rehabilitation services not available

Transfer Protocols

Effective transfer protocols ensure smooth, safe transitions of care between facilities. Understanding these protocols helps you anticipate transfer needs early and prepare appropriately.

When to Transfer

Transfer decisions balance patient needs with facility capabilities. General principles:

Immediate transfer (during resuscitation):

- Life-threatening injuries clearly exceeding facility capabilities (e.g., ruptured thoracic aorta at non-surgical facility)
- Rapidly deteriorating patients needing immediate specialized intervention

Urgent transfer (after stabilization):

- Serious injuries requiring surgery or interventions not available locally
- Stable patients with injuries that will definitely need higher-level care

Non-urgent transfer:

- Injuries requiring rehabilitation services not available locally
- Need for specialized long-term care

Transfer Process

Effective transfers follow structured processes:

1. Early identification and communication

- Recognize transfer need during initial assessment
- Contact accepting facility early (don't wait until patient "ready")
- Discuss case with accepting physician (often trauma surgeon or intensivist)
- Obtain acceptance and bed assignment

2. Stabilization before transfer

- Secure airway if needed (intubate unstable patients before transport)
- Control hemorrhage
- Establish adequate IV access
- Immobilize spine and fractures
- Insert chest tubes if pneumothorax/hemothorax

Decompress stomach with NGT

Insert Foley catheter for monitoring

Optimize hemodynamics (but don't delay transfer to "fully" resuscitate)

3. Documentation and communication

Complete transfer records including all interventions, medications, fluids given

Copies of all labs, imaging, and diagnostic studies

Transfer form with mechanism, injuries, treatment, and ongoing needs

Direct nurse-to-nurse report

Family communication about transfer and location

4. Mode of transport selection

Ground ambulance:

Most transfers

Distance <50 miles typically

Stable patients

Less costly

Helicopter (air medical):

Distance 50-150 miles (beyond this, fixed-wing may be better)

Time-critical patients (severe TBI, major hemorrhage)

Difficult ground access (rural, congested traffic)

Weather and patient condition permitting (turbulence problematic for some patients)

Fixed-wing aircraft:

Distance >150 miles

Inter-state transfers

More stable flight than helicopter

Requires airports/landing sites at both ends

5. Personnel and equipment

Appropriate skill level for patient acuity (critical care transport team for unstable patients)

Adequate equipment including monitors, oxygen, medications, IV pumps

Blood products if ongoing resuscitation needs

Common Transfer Pitfalls

Delayed recognition of transfer need: Identify early, even if patient initially appears stable. Some injuries declare transfer need early (severe TBI, major vascular injury), while others become apparent over hours (worsening pulmonary contusion, evolving abdominal injuries).

Inadequate stabilization: Don't send unstable airway—intubate before transfer. Secure all lines and tubes. Immobilize all fractures.

Incomplete communication: Receiving facility must know exactly what they're getting—injury details, interventions performed, ongoing issues, and what patient needs.

Documentation gaps: Send complete records. Missing information delays care at receiving facility.

Family considerations: Keep family informed. Provide directions to receiving facility. Some family members may want to accompany patient (policies vary).

Performance Improvement

Trauma performance improvement (PI) is the systematic review of trauma care to identify opportunities for improvement and implement changes that enhance outcomes. This isn't about blame—it's about learning and improving.

Trauma Registry

The trauma registry is the foundation of performance improvement, collecting detailed data on every trauma patient.

Data elements include:

- Demographics and pre-injury factors
- Injury circumstances and mechanism
- Physiologic data (vital signs, GCS)
- Anatomic injuries (coded using Abbreviated Injury Scale)
- Procedures and interventions
- Complications
- Outcomes (mortality, length of stay, discharge disposition, functional status)
- Times (injury to arrival, arrival to intervention, etc.)

This data enables:

- Benchmarking against national standards
- Identifying trends and patterns
- Evaluating specific interventions
- Research on injury patterns and outcomes

PI Process

1. Case identification

Cases are flagged for review based on filters:

- All deaths

Unexpected outcomes (mortality when predicted survival, or survival when predicted death)

Complications (infections, returns to OR, readmissions)

Process deviations (delays to intervention, missed injuries)

High-risk injuries (severe TBI, major vascular injuries)

2. Multidisciplinary review

Trauma PI committee (surgeons, nurses, EMS, anesthesia, radiology, others) reviews cases using structured format:

What happened? (facts of the case)

What went well? (acknowledge good care)

What could be improved? (identify opportunities)

What changes should we make? (action items)

The environment is non-punitive and focused on learning. Individual errors are addressed through separate channels; PI identifies system issues.

3. Preventability determination

For deaths and major complications, the committee considers preventability:

Preventable: Clearly avoidable with different care

Potentially preventable: Might have been avoided with optimal care

Non-preventable: Unavoidable regardless of care provided

This classification is challenging and somewhat subjective, but it focuses improvement efforts where they can make the most difference.

4. Action plans

Identified issues lead to concrete action plans:

Protocol modifications (e.g., earlier activation of massive transfusion protocol)

Education initiatives (e.g., nursing education on compartment syndrome recognition)

Equipment changes (e.g., adding ultrasound machines to resuscitation bays)

Policy revisions (e.g., changing consultation triggers)

5. Loop closure

After implementing changes, the PI process monitors whether improvements occurred. Did the change reduce complications? Improve times to intervention? This "closes the loop" and ensures changes actually work.

Key Performance Indicators

Trauma systems track specific metrics:

Process measures:

- Time from arrival to CT scan for severe TBI
- Time to operative hemorrhage control
- Massive transfusion protocol activation times
- Compliance with evidence-based interventions (DVT prophylaxis, TBI management guidelines)

Outcome measures:

- Risk-adjusted mortality (comparing actual to predicted mortality)
- Complication rates (infections, VTE, pressure injuries)
- Unexpected returns to OR
- Length of stay

System measures:

- Transfer patterns and times
- Undertriage and overtriage rates
- Scene times and transport intervals

These metrics allow tracking trends over time and benchmarking against other facilities.

Nurse Role in PI

Trauma nurses are critical to performance improvement:

Data collection: Accurate documentation in medical records feeds the trauma registry. Missing or inaccurate data undermines PI efforts.

Case identification: Bedside nurses often first recognize complications or issues warranting PI review. Reporting these cases ensures they're reviewed.

Committee participation: Nurse representatives provide frontline perspective on what actually happens during patient care and where system breakdowns occur.

Implementation: Nurses implement many PI-driven changes. Their feedback on practicality and barriers is essential for successful change.

Injury Prevention

The most effective trauma intervention is preventing injury from occurring. Trauma centers have responsibility for injury prevention in their communities.

Levels of Prevention

Primary prevention: Preventing injury before it occurs

Examples: Seatbelt laws, helmet laws, graduated driver licensing for teens, pool fencing

Secondary prevention: Reducing injury severity when incidents occur

Examples: Airbags, crumple zones in vehicles, breakaway bases on baseball fields, energy-absorbing playground surfaces

Tertiary prevention: Preventing complications and disability after injury occurs

This is what hospitals do—preventing infection, VTE, secondary brain injury, etc.

Trauma centers focus on primary and secondary prevention to reduce injury incidence and severity in their communities.

Haddon Matrix

The Haddon Matrix is a framework for analyzing injury prevention opportunities by examining factors before, during, and after injury across human, agent/vehicle, and environment dimensions.

For motor vehicle crashes:

Pre-event (preventing crash):

Human: Driver education, DUI enforcement, graduated licensing

Agent: Anti-lock brakes, electronic stability control

Environment: Road design, lighting, signage

Event (reducing injury during crash):

Human: Seatbelt use, proper child restraints

Agent: Airbags, crumple zones, safety glass

Environment: Guardrails, breakaway signs, median barriers

Post-event (reducing consequences):

Human: First aid training, bystander CPR

Agent: Automatic crash notification, vehicle design allowing rescue access

Environment: Rapid EMS response, trauma system

This framework helps identify multiple intervention points for any injury type.

Common Injury Prevention Programs

Pediatric injury prevention:

- Car seat safety checks and education
- Bike helmet distribution and fitting
- Safe sleep campaigns (preventing suffocation)
- Poison prevention
- Burn prevention (safe hot water temperatures, working smoke detectors)

Violence prevention:

- Hospital-based violence intervention programs (working with assault victims to interrupt cycles of retaliation)
- Safe firearm storage education
- Dating violence prevention
- Suicide prevention screening

Fall prevention:

- Elderly fall prevention (home safety assessments, exercise programs)
- Workplace fall prevention
- Playground safety

Alcohol/substance related injury:

- DUI prevention programs
- Alcohol screening and brief intervention
- Safe ride programs

Implementing Prevention Programs

Effective programs follow evidence-based approaches:

1. **Assess community needs:** What injuries are most common? What populations are at highest risk? Local trauma registry data guides priorities.

2. **Identify evidence-based interventions:** Use proven strategies rather than creating new, untested programs.

3. **Engage stakeholders:** Partner with community organizations, schools, law enforcement, public health agencies. Prevention requires broad collaboration.

4. **Implement systematically:** Pilot test, refine, then expand successful programs.

5. **Evaluate impact:** Track program reach and measure injury reduction. Modify based on results.

Nurse Role in Prevention

Trauma nurses contribute to prevention through:

Bedside prevention counseling: Every trauma admission is a "teachable moment." Discussing injury circumstances and prevention strategies with patients and families can change future behavior.

Community engagement: Participating in car seat checks, helmet fittings, fall prevention education, and other community events.

Advocacy: Supporting evidence-based prevention policies (seatbelt laws, helmet laws, graduated driver licensing, etc.).

Disaster Preparedness

Mass casualty incidents (MCIs) and disasters require systems to care for more patients than usual capacity while maintaining acceptable care quality. Trauma systems and trauma centers play central roles in disaster response.

Types of Disasters

Natural disasters: Earthquakes, hurricanes, tornadoes, floods, wildfires—create surges of injured patients and may disrupt hospital operations.

Technological disasters: Building collapses, transportation crashes, industrial accidents, hazardous material exposures.

Intentional events: Terrorist attacks, active shooter incidents, bombings—require coordination with law enforcement and may involve ongoing threats.

Pandemics: Different challenge—prolonged surge rather than acute spike, with infectious patients requiring isolation rather than traditional trauma care.

Disaster Response Framework

Incident Command System (ICS): Standardized organizational structure used across all disaster responses. Key features:

Unity of command: Each person reports to one supervisor

Span of control: Supervisors manage 3-7 people

Modular organization: Structure expands/contracts based on incident needs

Common terminology: Standardized titles and communication

Hospital incident command includes:

Incident Commander: Overall authority

Operations Section: Direct patient care

Planning Section: Resource tracking, situation updates

Logistics Section: Supplies, equipment, staffing

Finance Section: Cost tracking, procurement

Hospital Disaster Response

1. Activation

Disasters are activated when patient surge exceeds or threatens to exceed normal capacity. Activation triggers:

Notification of all hospital staff

Incident command structure activation

Opening of alternate care areas

Suspension of non-urgent procedures

Cancellation of non-urgent admissions and surgeries

2. Decontamination (if hazmat involved)

Contaminated patients must be decontaminated before entering hospital:

External decontamination area

Remove clothing (removes 80-90% of contamination)

Thorough water wash

Don clean gown before entering facility

Decontamination protects staff and prevents hospital contamination that would require evacuation.

3. Triage

Disaster triage differs from routine triage—the goal shifts from optimal care for each individual to doing the most good for the most people.

START triage (Simple Triage and Rapid Treatment):

Used in field or at hospital entry to quickly categorize patients:

Immediate (Red): Life-threatening injuries requiring urgent intervention to survive

Can't walk, breathing, perfusion compromised, or altered mental status after positioning airway

Examples: Airway compromise, severe bleeding, shock, decreased consciousness

Delayed (Yellow): Serious injuries that can wait hours for treatment

Stable patients with significant injuries

Examples: Most fractures, stable chest injuries, lacerations

Minor (Green): "Walking wounded" with minor injuries

Can walk and have minor injuries

Examples: Sprains, minor lacerations, bruises

Expectant (Black): Injuries incompatible with survival given available resources

Not deceased, but injuries so severe that survival unlikely even with aggressive care

Resources directed to salvageable patients

Examples: Massive head trauma, cardiac arrest in disaster setting

This triage is rapid (30-60 seconds per patient) and focuses on physiologic status, not specific injuries.

4. Treatment areas

Patients are directed to areas based on triage category:

Immediate → Trauma bays, OR

Delayed → ED treatment areas, holding areas

Minor → Designated minor treatment area (often outside main ED)

Expectant → Separated area with comfort care

5. Staffing

Callback of off-duty staff

Reassignment from non-essential areas

Just-in-time training for staff assigned to unfamiliar roles

Shift in nurse-to-patient ratios (accept higher ratios temporarily)

6. Supplies and equipment

Activation of disaster supply caches

Conservation measures (extend use of disposables, use alternatives to preferred supplies)

Requesting mutual aid from other facilities if needed

7. Communication

Regular situation updates to all staff

Coordination with EMS, other hospitals, public health

Public information management (hospital spokesperson handles media)

Family reunification center separate from clinical areas

Nurse Role in Disasters

Pre-disaster preparation:

Participate in disaster drills and exercises

Maintain competency in HAZMAT decontamination if assigned

Know your role in hospital incident command

Keep personal emergency plan current (ensure you can get to hospital and family is cared for)

During disaster response:

Follow incident command structure

Accept assignment to unfamiliar roles with flexibility

Adapt standards of care appropriately (disaster standards accept doing the most good for most people)

Document concisely (may use abbreviated documentation during surge)

Maintain situational awareness and report concerns up chain of command

Post-disaster recovery:

Participate in after-action reviews to identify lessons learned

Recognize signs of stress and seek support (disasters are traumatic for responders too)

Support improvement of disaster plans based on experience

Ethical Considerations

Disasters create ethical challenges:

Resource allocation: When resources are insufficient, who gets them? Guidelines suggest:

Treat most salvageable first

Avoid futile care

Reconsider resource allocation as situation evolves

Crisis standards of care: Disasters may require accepting care that's less than usual standards. This is ethically acceptable when:

Resources are genuinely insufficient

Modifications are necessary to maximize population benefit

Usual standards will be restored as soon as possible

Staff duty to respond: Healthcare workers have ethical duty to respond to disasters, but this is balanced against personal safety and family obligations. Clarify expectations in advance through disaster planning.

Chapter 12 Practice Questions

Question 1: What is the primary difference between Level I and Level II trauma centers?

A) Level II centers cannot perform surgery
B) Level I centers have broader research and education requirements
C) Level II centers only stabilize and transfer
D) Level I centers only accept the most severe cases

Answer: B

Explanation: Level I and II centers both provide definitive surgical care for most trauma. The main distinction is that Level I centers have additional requirements for research programs, education/outreach, and system leadership roles. Both levels can manage severe trauma, but Level I serves as regional resource.

Question 2: According to CDC field triage guidelines, which vital sign alone mandates transport to a trauma center?

A) Heart rate 110 bpm
B) Respiratory rate 25 breaths/min
C) Systolic blood pressure 85 mmHg
D) SpO2 94%

Answer: C

Explanation: Systolic BP <90 mmHg is a Step 1 physiologic criterion requiring trauma center transport. While RR 25 is concerning, the threshold is <10 or >29. HR 110 and SpO2 94% don't meet specific triage criteria alone but warrant careful evaluation.

Question 3: The acceptable undertriage rate in trauma systems is:

A) <5%
B) <15%
C) 25-35%
D) <50%

Answer: A

Explanation: Undertriage (seriously injured patients not going to trauma centers) should be <5% because it directly impacts survival. Systems accept 25-35% overtriage to keep undertriage low, recognizing that bringing some minor injuries to trauma centers is acceptable to ensure severe injuries reliably reach appropriate care.

Question 4: Which patient requires immediate interfacility transfer?

A) Stable patient with isolated femur fracture at hospital with orthopedic surgery
B) Patient with severe TBI at hospital without neurosurgery
C) Patient with minor head injury and normal CT
D) Elderly patient with rib fractures but stable vital signs

Answer: B

Explanation: Severe TBI requires neurosurgical capability for potential intervention (ICP monitoring, evacuation of hematoma). If neurosurgery isn't available and patient has severe TBI, transfer is essential. The other scenarios may not require immediate transfer if the facility can provide appropriate care.

Question 5: What is the primary purpose of the trauma registry?

A) Billing and reimbursement
B) Performance improvement and outcomes tracking
C) Staff scheduling
D) Legal documentation

Answer: B

Explanation: The trauma registry's primary purpose is collecting data for performance improvement, benchmarking, research, and tracking outcomes. While data may support other functions, the core purpose is improving trauma care through systematic data analysis.

Question 6: In START triage, a patient who can walk is categorized as:

A) Immediate (Red)
B) Delayed (Yellow)
C) Minor (Green)
D) Expectant (Black)

Answer: C

Explanation: In START triage, patients who can walk are automatically categorized as Minor (Green) regardless of other factors. The ability to walk indicates adequate perfusion and mental status sufficient to ambulate. These "walking wounded" are directed to minor treatment areas during mass casualty incidents.

Question 7: The Incident Command System (ICS) is characterized by:

A) Multiple people reporting to several supervisors
B) Unity of command with each person having one supervisor
C) Flat organizational structure
D) No defined chain of command

Answer: B

Explanation: Unity of command is a fundamental ICS principle—each person reports to one supervisor. This prevents conflicting directions and maintains clear accountability. Span of control (supervisors managing 3-7 people) and modular organization are other key ICS features.

Question 8: Which represents primary injury prevention?

A) Airbags in vehicles
B) Rapid EMS response
C) Helmet laws
D) DVT prophylaxis in trauma patients

Answer: C

Explanation: Primary prevention prevents injury before it occurs—helmet laws reduce likelihood of head injuries. Airbags are secondary prevention (reducing injury when crashes occur). EMS response and DVT prophylaxis are tertiary prevention (reducing complications after injury occurs).

Question 9: A preventable death in trauma PI is defined as:

A) Any death that occurred
B) Death that was clearly avoidable with different care
C) Death in a patient with severe injuries
D) Death that occurred outside the hospital

Answer: B

Explanation: Preventable deaths are those clearly avoidable with appropriate care. This is distinguished from "potentially preventable" (might have been avoided) and "non-preventable" (unavoidable regardless of care). This classification focuses improvement efforts on cases where different care could have changed outcomes.

Question 10: What mode of transport is most appropriate for a critically ill trauma patient being transferred 120 miles?

A) Ground ambulance
B) Private vehicle
C) Helicopter
D) Fixed-wing aircraft

Answer: C

Explanation: Helicopter transport is optimal for distances 50-150 miles, particularly for critically ill patients where time is essential. Ground is typically used <50 miles, fixed-wing >150 miles. Weather and patient condition must also be considered.

Question 11: The Haddon Matrix analyzes injury prevention across:

A) Time phases and factors
B) Only the human element
C) Just the post-injury period
D) Environmental factors exclusively

Answer: A

Explanation: The Haddon Matrix examines pre-event, event, and post-event time phases across human, agent/vehicle, and environmental factors. This comprehensive framework identifies multiple intervention points for preventing injuries and reducing their severity.

Question 12: Which statement about disaster triage is correct?

A) Focus on optimal care for each individual
B) Goal is doing the most good for the most people
C) Same as routine emergency triage
D) Expectant category means deceased

Answer: B

Explanation: Disaster triage shifts the goal from optimal individual care to maximizing population benefit—doing the most good for the most people. This differs from routine triage where resources allow optimal care for all. Expectant patients are not deceased but have injuries unlikely to survive given available resources.

Question 13: Performance improvement in trauma is best described as:

A) Punitive process for errors
B) Systematic review to identify improvement opportunities
C) Only for cases with bad outcomes
D) Annual review of mortality data

Answer: B

Explanation: Trauma PI is systematic, non-punitive review identifying improvement opportunities. It examines deaths, complications, unexpected outcomes, and process issues to drive system improvements. It's about learning and improving, not blame. Individual errors are addressed separately.

Question 14: Which factor indicates a patient should be transported to a trauma center based on mechanism alone?

A) Minor fender-bender
B) Fall from standing height
C) Fall from 25 feet
D) Low-speed motorcycle crash

Answer: C

Explanation: Falls >20 feet (one story = 10 feet) are high-energy mechanisms warranting trauma center consideration even without obvious injuries. The significant force transmission suggests potential for serious injuries that may not be immediately apparent.

Question 15: Hospital disaster plans should include:

A) Only medical staff roles
B) Decontamination procedures for hazmat incidents
C) Plans for treating unlimited numbers of patients
D) Normal staffing ratios maintained

Answer: B

Explanation: Disaster plans must address decontamination for hazmat incidents to protect staff and facility. Plans include all staff roles (not just medical), acknowledge capacity limits (can't treat unlimited patients), and accept modified staffing ratios during surge.

Question 16: The trauma quality improvement committee should include:

A) Only trauma surgeons
B) Multidisciplinary representatives
C) Only nursing staff
D) Hospital administrators exclusively

Answer: B

Explanation: Effective trauma PI requires multidisciplinary participation including surgeons, nurses, EMS, radiology, respiratory therapy, and others. Different perspectives identify issues that single disciplines might miss, and collaborative problem-solving produces better solutions.

Question 17: Which represents an acceptable action during disaster response?

A) Refusing all unfamiliar assignments
B) Maintaining usual nurse-to-patient ratios
C) Accepting higher patient loads temporarily
D) Providing care only to immediate category patients

Answer: C

Explanation: Disaster response requires accepting modified standards including higher nurse-to-patient ratios. Refusing unfamiliar assignments impedes response. Usual ratios can't be maintained during surge. All triage categories receive appropriate care based on available resources.

Question 18: Trauma center verification by the American College of Surgeons occurs:

A) Monthly
B) Annually
C) Every 3 years
D) Only when problems occur

Answer: C

Explanation: ACS verifies trauma centers every 3 years through site visits evaluating compliance with standards. This regular review ensures centers maintain required capabilities and commitment to trauma care. Facilities must demonstrate ongoing performance between visits.

Question 19: What is the primary advantage of inclusive trauma systems?

A) Limits number of trauma centers
B) Concentrates all trauma at one facility
C) Maximizes geographic access to trauma care
D) Reduces coordination requirements

Answer: C

Explanation: Inclusive systems incorporate all facilities meeting criteria, maximizing geographic access especially in rural areas. While this requires more coordination through transfer protocols, it ensures patients can reach appropriate care regardless of location.

Question 20: Crisis standards of care during disasters are ethically acceptable when:

A) Resources are genuinely insufficient to provide usual care
B) Staff prefer working under relaxed standards
C) The hospital wants to save money
D) Only minor modifications are needed

Answer: A

Explanation: Crisis standards of care are ethically justified only when resources are truly insufficient to maintain usual standards and modifications maximize population benefit. This isn't about convenience or cost savings—it's a necessary response to genuine resource limitations during disasters.

Question 21: Which data element is NOT typically part of trauma registry collection?

A) Injury Severity Score
B) Patient's favorite color
C) Mechanism of injury
D) Discharge disposition

Answer: B

Explanation: Trauma registries collect clinically relevant data including injury severity, mechanism, interventions, complications, and outcomes. Non-clinical information like favorite color isn't relevant to performance improvement or outcomes analysis.

Question 22: The primary goal of injury prevention programs at trauma centers is:

A) Generating revenue
B) Meeting regulatory requirements
C) Reducing injury incidence and severity in the community
D) Providing jobs for staff

Answer: C

Explanation: The fundamental purpose of injury prevention is reducing the burden of injury in the community. While programs may satisfy requirements and employ staff, the core mission is preventing injuries before they occur and reducing severity when they do.

Question 23: In the Field Triage Decision Scheme, which step has the highest priority?

A) Mechanism of injury
B) Physiologic criteria
C) Special considerations
D) Anatomic criteria

Answer: B

Explanation: Physiologic criteria (Step 1) have highest priority because vital sign abnormalities indicate current physiologic compromise requiring immediate trauma center resources. The scheme is sequential—if Step 1 criteria are met, transport to trauma center regardless of other factors.

Question 24: Loop closure in performance improvement refers to:

A) Closing cases without review
B) Monitoring whether implemented changes actually improved outcomes
C) Ending the PI program
D) Completing documentation

Answer: B

Explanation: Loop closure means monitoring whether changes made based on PI findings actually produced improvements. This "closes the loop" by confirming interventions worked or identifying need for further modification. Without this step, you don't know if changes were effective.

Question 25: Which patient would be categorized as "Immediate" (Red) in START triage?

A) Walking patient with arm laceration
B) Breathing patient with weak radial pulse
C) Patient with respiratory rate of 8
D) Deceased patient

Answer: C

Explanation: Respiratory rate <10 or >29 (after positioning airway) categorizes patients as Immediate—they need urgent intervention to survive. Walking patients are Minor (Green). Weak pulse alone (if patient breathing) may be Immediate, but RR 8 definitively meets Immediate criteria. Deceased patients are in a separate category.

Question 26: Transfer of a trauma patient should include:

A) Only basic demographic information
B) Comprehensive communication including mechanism, injuries, interventions, and ongoing needs
C) Just the diagnosis
D) No documentation if verbal report given

Answer: B

Explanation: Effective transfers require comprehensive information: mechanism of injury, all identified injuries, interventions performed, medications given, fluids administered, ongoing issues, and anticipated needs. Incomplete information delays care at the receiving facility.

Question 27: Which represents a process measure in trauma performance improvement?

A) Overall mortality rate
B) Time from arrival to CT scan for severe TBI
C) Patient satisfaction scores
D) Hospital revenue from trauma

Answer: B

Explanation: Process measures track how care is delivered—time to interventions, protocol compliance, etc. Time to CT for severe TBI is a process measure. Mortality is an outcome measure. Satisfaction and revenue aren't clinical performance indicators.

Question 28: The Expectant category in disaster triage means:

A) Patient has already died
B) Patient has injuries incompatible with survival given available resources
C) Patient will definitely survive
D) Patient should be treated first

Answer: B

Explanation: Expectant patients are alive but have injuries so severe that survival is unlikely even with aggressive care given current resource limitations. Resources are directed to more salvageable patients. This isn't the same as deceased—these patients receive comfort care.

Question 29: Which factor would justify helicopter transport over ground ambulance?

A) Distance of 15 miles with stable patient
B) Distance of 80 miles with time-critical severe TBI
C) Any fracture
D) Patient preference alone

Answer: B

Explanation: Helicopter transport is indicated for time-critical patients when distance is 50-150 miles, when ground access is difficult, or when time savings would significantly impact outcome. Severe TBI at 80 miles fits these criteria. Short distances or non-critical patients don't justify helicopter cost and risk.

Question 30: Trauma nurses contribute to performance improvement by:

A) Only collecting data
B) Accurate documentation, case identification, and implementing changes
C) Attending meetings only
D) Working independently without system involvement

Answer: B

Explanation: Nurses contribute throughout the PI cycle: accurate documentation feeds the registry, bedside recognition identifies cases needing review, participation in PI committees provides frontline perspective, and nurses implement many PI-driven changes. PI is a team effort requiring multidisciplinary engagement.

Clinical Scenarios

Clinical Scenario 1: Field Triage Decision

Scenario: You're the charge nurse when EMS calls for medical control. They're at a motor vehicle crash with a 42-year-old male. The patient was unrestrained driver in frontal impact at highway speed. Airbag deployed. Patient is alert and oriented, complaining of chest and abdominal pain. Vitals: HR 88, BP 124/76, RR 18, GCS 15. Physical exam shows seatbelt bruising across chest and abdomen. No obvious deformities.

EMS asks whether to transport to the local community hospital (Level III, 5 minutes away) or the regional trauma center (Level I, 35 minutes away).

Questions & Answers:

What triage criteria apply to this patient?

Step 1 (Physiologic): Negative—vital signs are normal, GCS 15
Step 2 (Anatomic): No definite anatomic criteria met based on prehospital assessment
Step 3 (Mechanism): Positive—high-speed frontal crash (highway speed), airbag deployment indicates significant force, unrestrained increases injury risk
Step 4 (Special considerations): Age 42 (not elderly), no mentioned comorbidities

The mechanism alone (Step 3) indicates trauma center consideration. Additionally, seatbelt sign across chest/abdomen is highly associated with internal injuries that may not be immediately apparent.

What is your recommendation?

Transport to Level I trauma center despite normal vital signs and longer transport time. Rationale: High-energy mechanism, seatbelt sign suggesting occult injuries (possible hollow viscus or solid organ injury), and the need for CT imaging and potential surgical capabilities that Level III may lack. The 30-minute additional transport time is justified given injury risk. Seatbelt sign requires close observation and often delayed presentation of injuries—Level I center provides comprehensive evaluation and monitoring.

Key teaching point: Normal vital signs don't rule out serious injury, especially with high-energy mechanisms and concerning physical findings like seatbelt sign. Appropriate triage prevents undertriage of occult injuries.

Clinical Scenario 2: Performance Improvement Case Review

Scenario: Your trauma PI committee is reviewing a case: 68-year-old male fell from 12-foot ladder. Initial ED assessment showed GCS 15, complaint of hip pain, HR 92, BP 148/86. Pelvis X-ray showed displaced femoral neck fracture. Patient admitted to orthopedics. Twelve hours later, patient became confused and hypoxic. Chest CT showed bilateral pulmonary emboli. Despite treatment, patient died three days later.

Questions & Answers:

What aspects of this case warrant PI review?

Unexpected death in patient with initially stable presentation

Development of major complication (PE) that may have been preventable

Geriatric patient with fall from height (high-risk mechanism for elderly)

Question of appropriate triage (fall from 12 feet meets trauma center criteria)

Timing and adequacy of VTE prophylaxis

Recognition and response to clinical change

What preventability determination might the committee consider?

Potentially preventable. While elderly patients with hip fractures have high PE risk, the committee would examine:

Was VTE prophylaxis initiated appropriately and timely?

Were there contraindications that delayed prophylaxis?

Was the patient mobilized appropriately?

Were early warning signs of deterioration missed?

Should patient have had trauma service consultation given mechanism and age?

What system improvements might emerge from this review?

Protocol revision: Automatic trauma consult for falls >10 feet in patients >65 years

Earlier VTE prophylaxis initiation (within 24 hours if no contraindications)

Enhanced monitoring protocols for geriatric trauma patients

Education on recognizing early signs of PE

Possible implementation of risk assessment tool for VTE in trauma patients

Key teaching point: PI isn't about blame—it's about identifying system improvements that prevent similar outcomes. This case might reveal gaps in geriatric trauma protocols or VTE prevention that, once addressed, improve care for future patients.

Clinical Scenario 3: Disaster Response

Scenario: A commuter train derailment occurs 2 miles from your Level II trauma center at 8 AM. Initial reports indicate 200+ passengers with multiple casualties. Your hospital activates disaster plan. Within 30 minutes, 15 patients arrive simultaneously, with more expected. You're assigned to the triage area.

Patients arriving include:

Patient A: Ambulatory, minor lacerations on arms, complaining of back pain

Patient B: On stretcher, respiratory rate 32, weak radial pulse, confused, bleeding from scalp laceration

Patient C: On stretcher, not breathing despite airway repositioning

Patient D: Moaning, obvious femur fracture, strong radial pulse, follows commands

Patient E: Chest pain, respiratory rate 22, strong pulses, alert and oriented

Questions & Answers:

How would you triage these patients using START?

Patient A: GREEN (Minor)—can walk despite back pain and lacerations

Patient B: RED (Immediate)—RR >29, altered mental status, compromised perfusion (weak pulse)

Patient C: BLACK (Expectant/Deceased)—not breathing after airway positioning (in disaster, CPR isn't performed due to resource limitations)

Patient D: YELLOW (Delayed)—significant injury but stable vital signs, follows commands

Patient E: YELLOW (Delayed)—stable vital signs, alert, chest pain concerning but not immediately life-threatening

Where should each patient be directed?

Patient A → Minor treatment area (likely outside main ED)

Patient B → Resuscitation bay for immediate intervention

Patient C → Designated area with comfort measures (separate from treatment areas)

Patient D → Delayed treatment area for fracture stabilization when resources available

Patient E → Delayed area for cardiac workup and monitoring

What challenges might you face, and how would you address them?

Resource limitations: Accept modified standards—higher nurse-to-patient ratios, abbreviated documentation

Emotional stress: Focus on doing most good for most people; recognize that some patients won't receive usual care

Communication: Use incident command structure; provide regular updates to all staff

Family concerns: Direct families to reunification area separate from clinical spaces

Ongoing arrivals: Continuously reassess and potentially re-triage as situation evolves

Key teaching point: Disaster triage requires shifting mindset from individual optimization to population benefit. This is ethically appropriate when resources are genuinely insufficient. Staff must understand that providing less-than-usual care to some patients allows saving more lives overall.

Key Takeaways - Chapter 12

You've completed the final content chapter of your TCRN preparation. Understanding trauma systems, quality improvement, and disaster response completes your knowledge of how excellent trauma care is organized, measured, and continuously improved.

Critical Concepts to Remember:

Trauma Systems:

Different trauma center levels serve specific roles based on capabilities

Transfer protocols ensure patients receive appropriate care level

Inclusive systems maximize access while maintaining quality through coordination

Triage Principles:

CDC Field Triage uses four sequential steps with physiologic criteria having highest priority

Systems accept overtriage to minimize undertriage (most good for most people)

Mechanism matters—high-energy mechanisms warrant trauma center evaluation even with normal vital signs

Performance Improvement:

PI is non-punitive, systematic review identifying improvement opportunities

Loop closure confirms changes actually worked

Multidisciplinary participation essential for comprehensive review and effective solutions

Injury Prevention:

Most effective trauma intervention is preventing injury before it occurs

Haddon Matrix identifies multiple intervention points

Every trauma admission is a teachable moment for prevention education

Disaster Preparedness:

START triage rapidly categorizes patients during mass casualty incidents

Disaster standards accept modified care to maximize population benefit

Incident Command System provides structure for coordinated response

Connecting to Clinical Practice:

The concepts in this chapter explain the "why" behind many processes you encounter:

Why certain patients are transferred even when your facility could technically manage them

Why every case is reviewed in PI meetings regardless of outcome

Why protocols emphasize specific timeframes and interventions

How your documentation contributes to system-wide improvement

Your Role in the Trauma System:

You're not just a bedside nurse—you're part of an integrated system working to optimize trauma outcomes. Your contributions matter:

Accurate triage ensures patients reach appropriate care

Thorough documentation feeds performance improvement

Recognition of transfer needs prevents delays

Participation in prevention programs reduces future injuries

Disaster preparedness keeps you ready for surge events

Exam Preparation Tips:

Questions on this content often test understanding of:

When to transfer patients (matching capabilities to needs)

Triage criteria and decision-making

Performance improvement processes and terminology

Disaster triage categories and ethical considerations

Remember the underlying principles:

Right patient, right resources, right time

Most good for most people (disaster context)

Continuous improvement benefits all patients

Prevention is the ultimate goal

Final Thoughts:

Trauma nursing exists within a complex system designed to deliver optimal outcomes. Understanding this system makes you a more effective advocate for your patients and a more valuable team member. Whether you're deciding if a patient needs transfer, participating in PI review, or responding to a disaster, you're contributing to a system that saves lives every day.

As you move toward the practice exams, remember that TCRN certification validates not just your clinical knowledge but your understanding of how excellent trauma care is organized, delivered, measured, and improved. You now have the comprehensive foundation you need to succeed on exam day and excel in your trauma nursing career.

Congratulations on completing the core content chapters! Your systematic preparation has equipped you with the knowledge and understanding needed for TCRN certification. As you move into practice exams, remember: you're not just memorizing facts—you're demonstrating the expertise that defines excellent trauma nursing.

TCRN QUESTION-ANSWERING STRATEGY

Systematic Approach for Exam Success

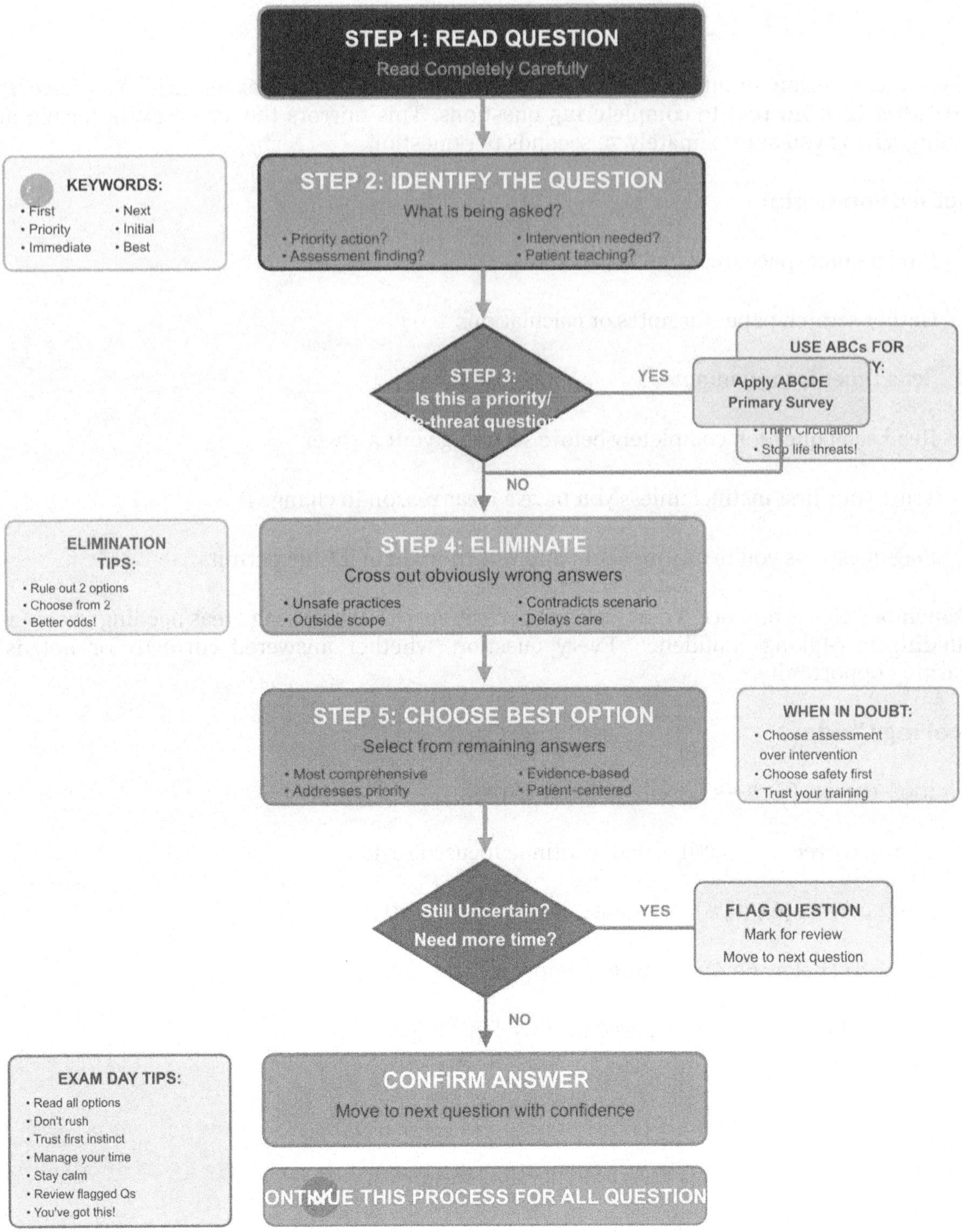

Practice Exam 1

Instructions

This practice exam simulates the actual TCRN certification exam experience. You have **150 minutes (2.5 hours)** to complete 125 questions. This mirrors the actual exam format and timing, giving you approximately 72 seconds per question.

Before you begin:

Find a quiet space free from distractions

Gather scratch paper for notes or calculations

Set a timer for 150 minutes

Read each question completely before selecting your answer

Trust your first instinct unless you have a clear reason to change it

Flag questions you're unsure about and return to them if time permits

Remember, this is practice. Your goal isn't perfection—it's identifying areas needing review and building test-taking confidence. Every question, whether answered correctly or not, is a learning opportunity.

Scoring Guide:

106+ correct (85%+): Excellent, likely to pass

94-105 correct (75-84%): Good, continue focused review

81-93 correct (65-74%): Adequate, needs targeted study

Below 81 (Below 65%): Requires comprehensive review

Take a deep breath. You've prepared for this. Let's begin.

Practice Exam 1 - Questions

Question 1: A patient arrives with Glasgow Coma Scale of 7 after head trauma. What is the priority intervention?

A) Obtain CT scan immediately
B) Endotracheal intubation
C) Administer mannitol
D) Hyperventilate to PCO2 of 25 mmHg

Question 2: Which finding indicates tension pneumothorax requiring immediate intervention?

A) Decreased breath sounds on one side with normal vital signs
B) Absent breath sounds, tracheal deviation, hypotension, and severe respiratory distress
C) Bilateral decreased breath sounds
D) Chest pain with shallow breathing

Question 3: A patient has blood at the urethral meatus after pelvic fracture. What should you do?

A) Insert Foley catheter immediately
B) Perform digital rectal exam first
C) Do not insert Foley until urethral injury ruled out
D) Insert smaller catheter gently

Question 4: Permissive hypotension in trauma resuscitation targets systolic blood pressure of:

A) 60-70 mmHg
B) 80-90 mmHg until hemorrhage control
C) 100-110 mmHg
D) Normal blood pressure always

Question 5: The most reliable early sign of compartment syndrome is:

A) Absent pulses
B) Paralysis
C) Pain out of proportion and pain with passive stretch
D) Pallor

Question 6: A patient with flail chest and severe respiratory distress needs:

A) Analgesics only
B) Positive pressure ventilation
C) Chest tube
D) External stabilization with sandbags

Question 7: Tranexamic acid (TXA) should be given within what timeframe for bleeding trauma patients?

A) 1 hour
B) 3 hours
C) 6 hours
D) 12 hours

Question 8: Which blood type is appropriate for emergency transfusion when patient type unknown?

A) AB positive
B) O positive
C) O negative
D) A negative

Question 9: A patient has seatbelt sign across the abdomen with free fluid on CT but no solid organ injury. This suggests:

A) Liver laceration
B) Splenic injury
C) Hollow viscus or mesenteric injury
D) Kidney contusion

Question 10: The primary survey follows which sequence?

A) SAMPLE
B) ABCDE
C) OPQRST
D) PEARRL

Question 11: Cushing's triad indicates increased intracranial pressure and includes:

A) Hypotension, tachycardia, tachypnea
B) Hypertension, bradycardia, irregular respirations
C) Hypotension, bradycardia, shallow breathing
D) Hypertension, tachycardia, deep breathing

Question 12: Each femur fracture can cause blood loss of approximately:

A) 250-500 mL
B) 500-750 mL
C) 1000-1500 mL
D) 2000-3000 mL

Question 13: A patient with knee dislocation and absent pulses needs:

A) X-ray before any intervention
B) Immediate reduction without waiting for imaging
C) CT angiography first
D) Observation for 30 minutes

Question 14: Beck's triad suggesting cardiac tamponade includes:

A) Hypotension, muffled heart sounds, JVD
B) Hypertension, clear heart sounds, flat neck veins
C) Hypotension, loud heart sounds, tachycardia
D) Normotension, irregular heartbeat, dyspnea

Question 15: The cricothyroid membrane is located:

A) Above the thyroid cartilage
B) Between the thyroid and cricoid cartilages
C) Below the cricoid cartilage
D) At the sternal notch

Question 16: A patient in Class III hemorrhagic shock has lost approximately:

A) Up to 15% blood volume
B) 15-30% blood volume
C) 30-40% blood volume
D) Over 40% blood volume

Question 17: Open pneumothorax should be initially managed with:

A) Immediate chest tube
B) Occlusive dressing taped on three sides
C) Occlusive dressing taped on all four sides
D) Packing the wound

Question 18: A pelvic binder should be placed:

A) Over the iliac crests
B) Around the greater trochanters
C) Around the waist
D) Around the thighs

Question 19: Which mechanism of injury requires trauma center transport per CDC guidelines?

A) Ground-level fall
B) Fall from 8 feet
C) Fall from 25 feet
D) Minor vehicle collision

Question 20: Rapid sequence intubation begins with:

A) Administering paralytic
B) Preoxygenation with 100% oxygen
C) Positioning the patient
D) Administering sedative

Question 21: A widened mediastinum on chest X-ray after high-speed deceleration suggests:

A) Pneumothorax
B) Traumatic aortic injury
C) Hemothorax
D) Pulmonary contusion

Question 22: Lactate level >2 mmol/L in trauma indicates:

A) Normal finding
B) Adequate tissue perfusion
C) Tissue hypoperfusion and anaerobic metabolism
D) Hyperglycemia

Question 23: A patient with posterior hip dislocation should be reduced within:

A) 2 hours
B) 6 hours to prevent avascular necrosis
C) 12 hours
D) 24 hours

Question 24: The jaw thrust maneuver is preferred in trauma because it:

A) Opens airway without extending the neck
B) Is easier to perform
C) Works better than head-tilt chin-lift
D) Requires no training

Question 25: Hemothorax on physical exam produces:

A) Hyperresonance to percussion
B) Dullness to percussion
C) Increased breath sounds
D) Tracheal deviation toward affected side

Question 26: Which patient requires massive transfusion protocol activation?

A) Stable patient with isolated extremity fracture
B) Patient in hemorrhagic shock transfusing >4 units in 1 hour
C) Any patient with trauma
D) Patient with minor bleeding

Question 27: Neurogenic shock presents with:

A) Tachycardia, hypotension, cool skin
B) Bradycardia, hypotension, warm skin below injury
C) Tachycardia, hypertension, warm skin
D) Bradycardia, hypertension, cool skin

Question 28: A patient has GCS 12 (E3, V4, M5). This indicates:

A) Severe brain injury
B) Moderate brain injury
C) Mild brain injury
D) Normal neurological function

Question 29: The preferred crystalloid for trauma resuscitation is:

A) D5W
B) 0.45% sodium chloride
C) Lactated Ringer's or normal saline
D) D5 normal saline

Question 30: Flail chest is defined as:

A) Single rib fracture
B) Multiple rib fractures on one side
C) Two or more ribs fractured in two or more places
D) Sternal fracture

Question 31: A patient post-splenectomy needs which vaccinations?

A) Influenza only
B) Pneumococcal, meningococcal, H. influenzae type B
C) Hepatitis only
D) No special vaccinations

Question 32: Compartment syndrome definitive treatment is:

A) Elevation and ice
B) Removing restrictive dressings
C) Fasciotomy
D) Pain medication

Question 33: Which finding suggests basilar skull fracture?

A) Scalp laceration
B) Battle's sign and raccoon eyes
C) Facial abrasions
D) Forehead contusion

Question 34: The FAST exam detects:

A) Specific organ injuries
B) Free fluid in abdomen and pericardium
C) All abdominal injuries
D) Hollow viscus perforations

Question 35: A chest tube drains 1600 mL immediately upon insertion. The appropriate action is:

A) Continue monitoring
B) Clamp the tube
C) Prepare for emergency thoracotomy
D) Remove and reinsert

Question 36: Which nerve is injured with midshaft humerus fracture?

A) Median
B) Ulnar
C) Radial
D) Axillary

Question 37: The leading preventable cause of death in trauma is:

A) Infection
B) Uncontrolled hemorrhage
C) Pulmonary embolism
D) Pneumonia

Question 38: Level I trauma centers require:

A) General surgery availability only
B) 24/7 in-house surgical teams and subspecialists
C) Transfer agreements only
D) Emergency physician coverage

Question 39: A patient with severe TBI should maintain cerebral perfusion pressure of:

A) 30-50 mmHg
B) 50-70 mmHg
C) 60-70 mmHg or higher
D) 80-100 mmHg

Question 40: Kehr's sign (left shoulder pain) in abdominal trauma suggests:

A) Clavicle fracture
B) Splenic injury with diaphragmatic irritation
C) Pneumothorax
D) Myocardial infarction

Question 41: The acceptable undertriage rate in trauma systems is:

A) <5%
B) <15%
C) 25-35%
D) <50%

Question 42: Which intervention should be avoided in increased ICP?

A) Elevating head of bed 30 degrees
B) Maintaining adequate blood pressure
C) Aggressive hyperventilation to PCO2 of 25 mmHg
D) Pain management

Question 43: A tourniquet should be placed:

A) Directly over the wound
B) 2-3 inches proximal to the wound
C) 2-3 inches distal to the wound
D) Over the nearest joint

Question 44: Intraperitoneal bladder rupture requires:

A) Foley catheter drainage only
B) Suprapubic catheter

C) Surgical repair
D) Observation

Question 45: The most common cause of airway obstruction in unconscious trauma patients is:

A) Blood or secretions
B) Tongue falling backward
C) Foreign body
D) Laryngeal edema

Question 46: A patient has epidural hematoma on CT. The classic presentation includes:

A) Immediate unconsciousness that persists
B) Brief loss of consciousness, lucid interval, then deterioration
C) Gradual onset of symptoms over days
D) No loss of consciousness

Question 47: Needle decompression for tension pneumothorax is performed at:

A) 4th intercostal space, anterior axillary line
B) 2nd intercostal space, midclavicular line
C) 5th intercostal space, midaxillary line
D) Suprasternal notch

Question 48: A balanced ratio for massive transfusion is:

A) PRBCs only
B) 2:1:1 (PRBCs:FFP:Platelets)
C) 1:1:1 (PRBCs:FFP:Platelets)
D) PRBCs and FFP only

Question 49: Which patient should be categorized as "Immediate" (Red) in START triage?

A) Walking with minor injuries
B) Not breathing after airway positioning
C) Respiratory rate 35 after airway positioned
D) Deceased

Question 50: The lethal triad in trauma includes:

A) Hemorrhage, infection, sepsis
B) Hypothermia, acidosis, coagulopathy
C) Hypoxia, hypotension, hypothermia
D) Pain, anxiety, fear

Question 51: A patient with open tibia fracture needs:

A) Immediate cast application
B) Antibiotics and tetanus prophylaxis
C) Observation only
D) Ice and elevation

Question 52: Traumatic brain injury is classified as severe when GCS is:

A) 13-15
B) 9-12
C) ≤8
D) <6

Question 53: The primary purpose of trauma registry is:

A) Billing
B) Performance improvement and outcomes tracking
C) Staff scheduling
D) Legal documentation

Question 54: Which represents secondary injury prevention?

A) Seatbelt laws
B) Airbags reducing injury severity
C) Rapid EMS response
D) Hospital care

Question 55: A subdural hematoma appears on CT as:

A) Lens-shaped (biconvex) hyperdensity
B) Crescent-shaped hyperdensity
C) Diffuse brain swelling
D) Midline shift only

Question 56: Pericardiocentesis is performed by inserting needle:

A) At cardiac apex
B) Below xiphoid toward left shoulder
C) Left 5th intercostal space
D) Right sternal border

Question 57: The purpose of damage control surgery is to:

A) Definitively repair all injuries
B) Control hemorrhage and contamination quickly
C) Avoid surgery completely
D) Perform diagnostic exploration only

Question 58: A patient develops fat embolism syndrome typically:

A) Immediately after fracture
B) 6-12 hours post-injury
C) 24-72 hours post-injury
D) 1-2 weeks later

Question 59: Which physiologic criterion in field triage mandates trauma center transport?

A) Heart rate 105 bpm
B) Systolic BP 85 mmHg
C) Respiratory rate 24/min
D) SpO2 93%

Question 60: Basilar skull fracture is associated with:

A) Scalp hematoma
B) CSF rhinorrhea or otorrhea
C) Facial lacerations
D) Neck pain

Question 61: The most common site of traumatic aortic injury is:

A) Ascending aorta
B) Aortic arch
C) Aortic isthmus (distal to left subclavian)
D) Abdominal aorta

Question 62: A patient with spinal cord injury at C5 level will have:

A) Quadriplegia
B) Paraplegia
C) No deficits
D) Arm weakness only

Question 63: Autotransfusion in hemothorax management allows:

A) Measuring blood loss only
B) Reinfusing patient's own drained blood
C) Testing for infection
D) Preventing clotting

Question 64: Which burn requires transfer to burn center?

A) Superficial burn of 8% TBSA in adult
B) Second-degree burn of 12% TBSA in adult
C) Second-degree burn involving hands, face, or genitals
D) Minor first-degree burn

Question 65: The Rule of Nines for burn assessment allocates what percentage to each entire leg in adults?

A) 9%
B) 18%
C) 14%
D) 36%

Question 66: Spinal shock is characterized by:

A) Immediate return of reflexes
B) Temporary loss of all neurologic function below injury level
C) Permanent paralysis
D) Hypertension and tachycardia

Question 67: Which finding indicates successful resuscitation from shock?

A) Normal temperature
B) Decreasing lactate level
C) Stable WBC count
D) Normal sodium

Question 68: A pulmonary contusion typically:

A) Improves immediately
B) Worsens over 24-48 hours
C) Has no clinical significance
D) Requires immediate surgery

Question 69: The appropriate tidal volume for bag-valve-mask ventilation in adults is:

A) 300-400 mL
B) 500-600 mL
C) 800-1000 mL
D) 1200-1500 mL

Question 70: Cervical spine clearance clinically requires:

A) Normal mental status, no midline tenderness, no neurological deficits, no distracting injuries
B) Normal X-ray only
C) CT scan only
D) Patient stating neck doesn't hurt

Question 71: A patient has decerebrate posturing. This indicates:

A) Cortical injury
B) Brainstem injury (more severe than decorticate)
C) Spinal cord injury
D) Peripheral nerve injury

Question 72: The primary complication of untreated hollow viscus perforation is:

A) Hemorrhage
B) Peritonitis and sepsis
C) Compartment syndrome
D) Renal failure

Question 73: Loop closure in performance improvement means:

A) Ending the program
B) Monitoring whether changes improved outcomes
C) Closing cases without review
D) Completing documentation

Question 74: Which patient needs immediate transfer from Level III to Level I trauma center?

A) Stable isolated extremity fracture
B) Ruptured abdominal aortic aneurysm
C) Minor head injury with normal CT
D) Simple rib fractures

Question 75: The primary goal of injury prevention programs is:

A) Generating revenue
B) Reducing injury incidence and severity
C) Meeting requirements only
D) Providing jobs

Question 76: Mean arterial pressure (MAP) is calculated as:

A) (Systolic + Diastolic) / 2
B) Systolic - Diastolic
C) [(2 × Diastolic) + Systolic] / 3
D) Systolic + Diastolic

Question 77: A patient with liver laceration managed non-operatively develops increasing pain and fever 3 days later. This suggests:

A) Normal healing
B) Bile leak or abscess
C) Pneumonia
D) Urinary tract infection

Question 78: Hard signs of vascular injury requiring immediate surgery include:

A) Proximity to major vessel
B) Pulsatile bleeding and absent pulse
C) Small hematoma
D) Mild pain

Question 79: The Haddon Matrix examines injury prevention across:

A) Time phases and factors
B) Only human factors
C) Post-injury only
D) Environmental factors only

Question 80: Increased ICP is indicated by:

A) ICP >5 mmHg
B) ICP >10 mmHg
C) ICP >15 mmHg
D) ICP >20 mmHg

Question 81: A concussion is best defined as:

A) Structural brain injury visible on CT
B) Alteration in mental status from trauma, may not involve LOC
C) Always involves loss of consciousness
D) Skull fracture with brain injury

Question 82: The Expectant category in disaster triage means:

A) Patient has died
B) Injuries incompatible with survival given resources
C) Will definitely survive
D) Treat first

Question 83: Which represents a process measure in trauma PI?

A) Mortality rate
B) Time from arrival to CT for severe TBI
C) Patient satisfaction
D) Hospital revenue

Question 84: Warm ischemia time for limb salvage is:

A) 1-2 hours
B) 4-6 hours
C) 8-10 hours
D) 12+ hours

Question 85: A patient with frontal lobe injury may exhibit:

A) Visual deficits
B) Personality changes and impaired judgment
C) Hearing loss
D) Paralysis only

Question 86: The sciatic nerve is most at risk with:

A) Anterior hip dislocation
B) Posterior hip dislocation
C) Knee dislocation
D) Ankle fracture

Question 87: Retroperitoneal air on CT suggests injury to:

A) Spleen
B) Duodenum or portions of colon
C) Liver
D) Kidney

Question 88: Brain herniation syndromes indicate:

A) Mild head injury
B) Critical increase in ICP with brain displacement
C) Scalp injury
D) Concussion

Question 89: The most common mechanism for duodenal injury is:

A) Gunshot wound
B) Motor vehicle crash
C) Handlebar injury compressing duodenum against spine
D) Fall from height

Question 90: Which medication reduces mortality in bleeding trauma patients?

A) Aspirin
B) Tranexamic acid (TXA)
C) Warfarin
D) Heparin

Question 91: A patient develops ARDS after trauma. This typically occurs:

A) Immediately
B) 24-72 hours post-injury
C) 1-2 weeks later
D) After discharge

Question 92: The primary purpose of cervical collar in trauma is:

A) Pain relief
B) Immobilizing cervical spine until injury ruled out
C) Supporting head
D) Preventing infection

Question 93: Which represents tertiary injury prevention?

A) Helmet laws
B) Airbags
C) DVT prophylaxis in hospitalized patients
D) Speed limits

Question 94: A patient with severe TBI should have head of bed elevated to:

A) Flat
B) 15 degrees
C) 30 degrees
D) 60 degrees

Question 95: Parkland formula for burn resuscitation calculates:

A) 2 mL × kg × % TBSA over 24 hours
B) 4 mL × kg × % TBSA over 24 hours
C) 6 mL × kg × % TBSA over 24 hours
D) 1 mL × kg × % TBSA over 24 hours

Question 96: A patient's pupils are unequal with one dilated and non-reactive. This suggests:

A) Normal variant
B) Uncal herniation with CN III compression
C) Medication effect only
D) Cataracts

Question 97: The Incident Command System (ICS) in disasters features:

A) Multiple supervisors per person
B) Unity of command with each person having one supervisor
C) No defined structure
D) Flat organization

Question 98: Which zone of the neck contains structures most accessible for surgical repair?

A) Zone I
B) Zone II
C) Zone III
D) All zones equal

Question 99: A patient with abdominal trauma and positive FAST who becomes unstable should:

A) Get CT scan
B) Proceed to OR immediately
C) Undergo angiography
D) Be observed

Question 100: The appropriate care for amputated body part includes:

A) Placing directly on ice
B) Wrapping in saline-moistened gauze, placing in plastic bag, then on ice
C) Leaving exposed to air
D) Wrapping in dry gauze only

Question 101: Autonomic dysreflexia in spinal cord injury above T6 presents with:

A) Hypotension and bradycardia
B) Severe hypertension and bradycardia
C) Hypotension and tachycardia
D) Normal vital signs

Question 102: Which test confirms endotracheal tube placement most reliably?

A) Chest rise
B) Breath sounds
C) Sustained end-tidal CO_2 waveform
D) Chest X-ray alone

Question 103: A patient with inhalation injury should be monitored for:

A) Immediate symptoms only
B) Delayed airway edema and respiratory failure over 24-48 hours
C) Skin burns only
D) No specific monitoring needed

Question 104: The preferred imaging for awake, alert patient with suspected cervical spine injury is:

A) Plain X-rays only
B) CT scan of cervical spine
C) MRI
D) Flexion-extension films

Question 105: Rhabdomyolysis after crush injury can cause:

A) Hyperglycemia
B) Renal failure from myoglobin
C) Bradycardia
D) Hypotension only

Question 106: A gunshot wound to the abdomen with evisceration requires:

A) Pushing organs back in
B) Covering with moist sterile dressing and immediate surgery
C) Dry dressing only
D) Observation

Question 107: The primary concern with first and second rib fractures is:

A) Severe pain
B) Underlying great vessel injury
C) Pneumothorax risk
D) Limited mobility

Question 108: Cerebral perfusion pressure (CPP) equals:

A) MAP + ICP
B) MAP - ICP
C) ICP - MAP
D) MAP × ICP

Question 109: Which patient should receive helicopter transport?

A) Stable patient 10 miles from hospital
B) Severe TBI 80 miles from Level I center
C) Minor injury any distance
D) Any fracture

Question 110: The purpose of permissive hypotension is to:

A) Save IV fluids
B) Prevent clot disruption before hemorrhage control
C) Avoid medication use
D) Reduce nursing workload

Question 111: A patient post-burn resuscitation develops decreased urine output and dark urine. This suggests:

A) Normal finding
B) Rhabdomyolysis from muscle injury
C) Dehydration only
D) Infection

Question 112: The Glasgow Coma Scale maximum score is:

A) 10
B) 12

C) 15
D) 20

Question 113: Neurogenic shock occurs with spinal injuries at or above:

A) L1
B) T12
C) T6
D) C7

Question 114: A patient with mandibular fracture is at risk for:

A) Visual deficits
B) Airway compromise from swelling or bleeding
C) Hearing loss
D) No specific risks

Question 115: The appropriate initial fluid for pediatric trauma resuscitation is:

A) 5 mL/kg
B) 10 mL/kg
C) 20 mL/kg
D) 40 mL/kg

Question 116: Cushing's reflex (response to increased ICP) includes:

A) Hypotension
B) Hypertension with widened pulse pressure
C) Tachycardia
D) Tachypnea

Question 117: A Le Fort fracture involves:

A) Mandible
B) Midface
C) Skull base
D) Cervical spine

Question 118: The primary role of Level III trauma centers is:

A) Definitive care for all injuries
B) Stabilization and appropriate transfer
C) Research
D) Only minor injury care

Question 119: Which finding indicates neurological deterioration requiring immediate intervention?

A) Stable GCS of 14
B) GCS drop from 14 to 10
C) Mild headache
D) Slight confusion that resolves

Question 120: Electrical burn injury requires assessment for:

A) Skin injury only
B) Cardiac dysrhythmias and deep tissue damage
C) Superficial burns only
D) No specific concerns

Question 121: The primary difference between concussion and contusion is:

A) Concussion has structural damage visible on CT
B) Contusion has structural damage (bruising) visible on CT
C) They are the same
D) Concussion is more severe

Question 122: Which patient requires neurosurgical consultation?

A) Mild concussion with normal CT
B) Epidural hematoma with midline shift
C) Scalp laceration only
D) Mild headache after trauma

Question 123: The goal of trauma system organization is:

A) Maximizing hospital revenue
B) Right patient, right resources, right time
C) Treating all patients at one facility
D) Avoiding transfers

Question 124: Blunt cardiac injury should be suspected with:

A) Any chest trauma
B) Sternal fracture or anterior chest impact
C) Rib fractures only
D) Back trauma

Question 125: A patient develops sudden severe headache and vomiting after minor head trauma 2 weeks ago. This suggests:

A) Migraine
B) Delayed intracranial hemorrhage (subdural)
C) Flu
D) Dehydration

Answer Key with Detailed Explanations

How to Use This Answer Key

Review your answers systematically. For questions you answered correctly, read the explanation to reinforce your understanding. For incorrect answers, understand why the correct answer is right and why you chose incorrectly. Identify patterns in your mistakes—are you missing questions in specific content areas? Are you misreading questions? This insight guides your continued study.

Remember: every mistake is a learning opportunity. The goal isn't perfection on this practice exam—it's identifying gaps and building confidence for the real test.

Question 1: B - Endotracheal intubation

Explanation: GCS ≤8 indicates severe traumatic brain injury with inability to protect the airway. Immediate intubation is the priority to secure the airway, prevent aspiration, and allow controlled ventilation (important for managing intracranial pressure). While CT scan, mannitol, and ventilation management will be needed, securing the airway comes first. Remember the primary survey: Airway is always the first priority.

Question 2: B - Absent breath sounds, tracheal deviation, hypotension, and severe respiratory distress

Explanation: This is the classic presentation of tension pneumothorax requiring immediate needle decompression. The combination of absent breath sounds, tracheal deviation away from affected side, hypotension (from decreased venous return), and severe respiratory distress indicates air under pressure compressing mediastinal structures. Don't wait for imaging—this is a clinical diagnosis requiring immediate intervention. Option A describes simple pneumothorax without tension physiology.

Question 3: C - Do not insert Foley until urethral injury ruled out

Explanation: Blood at the urethral meatus is a classic sign of urethral injury, particularly with pelvic fractures. Attempting catheter insertion can worsen the injury or create a false passage. The correct approach: perform retrograde urethrogram first to rule out injury. If urethral injury confirmed, place suprapubic catheter instead. Never blindly insert a Foley when urethral injury is suspected.

Question 4: B - 80-90 mmHg until hemorrhage control

Explanation: Permissive hypotension maintains systolic BP around 80-90 mmHg in hemorrhaging trauma patients until bleeding is surgically controlled. This prevents clot disruption from elevated blood pressure while maintaining adequate perfusion to vital organs. Exception: Don't use permissive hypotension in traumatic brain injury patients who need higher blood pressure for cerebral perfusion.

Question 5: C - Pain out of proportion and pain with passive stretch

Explanation: Early compartment syndrome presents with pain out of proportion to injury and severe pain with passive stretching of muscles in the affected compartment. These are the earliest and most reliable signs. Pulselessness, paralysis, and pallor are late signs indicating irreversible damage has occurred. By the time pulses disappear, you've missed the window for preventing permanent disability.

Question 6: B - Positive pressure ventilation

Explanation: Flail chest with severe respiratory distress requires positive pressure ventilation (BiPAP or mechanical ventilation after intubation) to provide internal pneumatic stabilization of the chest wall while supporting gas exchange through underlying pulmonary contusion. Analgesics alone are insufficient for severe distress. Chest tubes treat pneumothorax/hemothorax but don't stabilize flail segments. External stabilization methods are outdated and ineffective.

Question 7: B - 3 hours

Explanation: Tranexamic acid (TXA) reduces mortality in bleeding trauma patients when given within 3 hours of injury. The drug works by preventing clot breakdown (antifibrinolytic). Administration after 3 hours may actually increase mortality. Standard dose: 1 gram IV over 10 minutes, followed by 1 gram over 8 hours. TXA is now standard in massive transfusion protocols.

Question 8: C - O negative

Explanation: Type O negative is the universal donor blood type, lacking A, B, and Rh antigens, so it won't cause transfusion reactions in any blood type. It's used for emergency transfusion when patient type is unknown and no time exists for crossmatch. Type O positive can be used for males and post-menopausal females if O negative is unavailable, but O negative is universally safe.

Question 9: C - Hollow viscus or mesenteric injury

Explanation: Seatbelt sign with free fluid on CT but no solid organ injury strongly suggests hollow viscus (intestinal) or mesenteric injury. The compression force between seatbelt and spine can cause intestinal perforation or mesenteric tears. These injuries may show subtle or no CT findings initially but declare themselves over 12-24 hours as peritonitis develops. High clinical suspicion and serial exams are essential.

Question 10: B - ABCDE

Explanation: The primary survey follows ABCDE: Airway (with cervical spine protection), Breathing, Circulation, Disability (neurological status), Exposure (with environmental control). This sequence prioritizes immediate life threats. SAMPLE is used for patient history during secondary survey. The systematic ABCDE approach ensures no life-threatening condition is missed.

Question 11: B - Hypertension, bradycardia, irregular respirations

Explanation: Cushing's triad indicates severe increased intracranial pressure: hypertension with widened pulse pressure (compensatory response to maintain cerebral perfusion), bradycardia (vagal response), and irregular respirations (brainstem compression affecting respiratory centers). This is a late and ominous sign requiring immediate intervention to reduce ICP. The body is trying desperately to maintain brain perfusion despite critically elevated pressure.

Question 12: C - 1000-1500 mL

Explanation: Each femur fracture can cause 1000-1500 mL blood loss into the thigh compartment. This significant hemorrhage can lead to shock, especially with bilateral fractures (potential 2-3 liter loss). Understanding this blood loss potential guides resuscitation strategies and explains why patients with isolated long bone fractures can be in hemorrhagic shock.

Question 13: B - Immediate reduction without waiting for imaging

Explanation: Knee dislocation with absent pulses is a vascular emergency. The popliteal artery is likely injured or occluded. Immediate reduction should be performed without waiting for X-ray to restore blood flow and potentially save the limb. The "golden window" for limb salvage is 6-8 hours of ischemia. Time wasted on imaging costs precious minutes. After reduction, reassess pulses immediately.

Question 14: A - Hypotension, muffled heart sounds, JVD

Explanation: Beck's triad of cardiac tamponade: hypotension (decreased cardiac output from compression), muffled heart sounds (fluid in pericardium dampens sounds), and jugular venous distension (blood backs up because heart can't fill properly). While all three signs may not always be present, this classic triad indicates pericardial blood compressing the heart and requires immediate pericardiocentesis.

Question 15: B - Between the thyroid and cricoid cartilages

Explanation: The cricothyroid membrane is the soft space between the thyroid cartilage (Adam's apple) above and the cricoid cartilage below. This is the landmark for emergency cricothyroidotomy. The membrane is relatively avascular and superficial, making it the ideal site for surgical airway access when oral/nasal intubation fails or is contraindicated.

Question 16: C - 30-40% blood volume

Explanation: Class III hemorrhagic shock represents 30-40% blood loss (approximately 1500-2000 mL in adults). Signs include significant tachycardia (>120 bpm), hypotension, altered mental status, and decreased urine output. This requires aggressive resuscitation with blood products. Class I: <15%, Class II: 15-30%, Class IV: >40%.

Question 17: B - Occlusive dressing taped on three sides

Explanation: Open pneumothorax (sucking chest wound) requires occlusive dressing taped on three sides to create a flutter valve. This allows air to escape during exhalation but prevents air entry during inhalation. Taping all four sides risks creating tension pneumothorax. Chest tube placement follows but isn't the immediate first intervention.

Question 18: B - Around the greater trochanters

Explanation: Pelvic binders should be placed around the greater trochanters (hip level), not over the iliac crests. This position maximally reduces pelvic volume and provides optimal mechanical compression to tamponade bleeding from pelvic fractures. Correct placement is critical for effectiveness.

Question 19: C - Fall from 25 feet

Explanation: Falls >20 feet (one story = 10 feet) are high-energy mechanisms warranting trauma center transport per CDC field triage guidelines. This significant force transmission suggests potential for serious injuries that may not be immediately apparent. Mechanism alone (Step 3 criteria) indicates trauma center consideration even without obvious injuries.

Question 20: B - Preoxygenation with 100% oxygen

Explanation: Rapid sequence intubation begins with preoxygenation (3-5 minutes of 100% oxygen or 8 deep breaths). This provides an oxygen reservoir allowing several minutes of apnea during intubation without desaturation. After preoxygenation comes positioning, then medications (sedative and paralytic in rapid succession), then intubation with confirmation.

Question 21: B - Traumatic aortic injury

Explanation: Widened mediastinum (>8 cm) on chest X-ray after high-speed deceleration strongly suggests traumatic aortic injury. Other suggestive findings include obliterated aortic knob, tracheal deviation to the right, and depressed left mainstem bronchus. CT angiography confirms the diagnosis. The aortic isthmus (just distal to left subclavian artery) is the most common injury site from shearing forces.

Question 22: C - Tissue hypoperfusion and anaerobic metabolism

Explanation: Elevated lactate (>2 mmol/L) indicates tissue hypoperfusion leading to anaerobic metabolism. When cells don't receive adequate oxygen, they produce lactate. This confirms shock even when vital signs appear stable. Lactate is one of the best markers of tissue perfusion—rising lactate indicates worsening shock, decreasing lactate shows successful resuscitation.

Question 23: B - 6 hours to prevent avascular necrosis

Explanation: Hip dislocations should be reduced within 6 hours to minimize risk of avascular necrosis of the femoral head. Blood supply to the femoral head is compromised when the hip is dislocated. Prolonged ischemia leads to bone death. This time-sensitive nature makes hip dislocation an orthopedic emergency requiring urgent reduction.

Question 24: A - Opens airway without extending the neck

Explanation: The jaw thrust maneuver opens the airway by moving the mandible and tongue forward without extending the neck, making it safe for trauma patients with potential cervical spine injury. Head-tilt chin-lift extends the neck and is contraindicated in trauma. Place fingers at angle of mandible and lift anteriorly.

Question 25: B - Dullness to percussion

Explanation: Hemothorax (blood in pleural space) produces dullness to percussion because blood dampens the percussion sound. This distinguishes it from pneumothorax, which produces hyperresonance. Both cause decreased breath sounds, but percussion findings differentiate them. Hemothorax also causes decreased chest wall movement on the affected side.

Question 26: B - Patient in hemorrhagic shock transfusing >4 units in 1 hour

Explanation: Massive transfusion protocol is activated when patients require >4 units of blood in 1 hour with expectation of continued need, or when replacing one blood volume (approximately 10 units) in 24 hours. MTP ensures rapid delivery of balanced blood products (PRBCs, FFP, platelets in 1:1:1 ratio) without waiting for individual orders.

Question 27: B - Bradycardia, hypotension, warm skin below injury

Explanation: Neurogenic shock from spinal cord injury above T6 presents with the classic triad: bradycardia (can't mount compensatory tachycardia), hypotension (from vasodilation), and warm/dry skin below injury level (dilated vessels, not constricted). This presentation is opposite to hypovolemic shock (tachycardia, cool/clammy skin).

Question 28: B - Moderate brain injury

Explanation: GCS 9-12 indicates moderate traumatic brain injury. Score 13-15 is mild, ≤8 is severe (typically requires intubation). This patient (E3, V4, M5 = 12) needs close neurological monitoring, serial assessments, and likely CT imaging, but doesn't necessarily need immediate intubation unless other factors present.

Question 29: C - Lactated Ringer's or normal saline

Explanation: Lactated Ringer's or normal saline are the preferred crystalloid solutions for trauma resuscitation. Lactated Ringer's is slightly preferred as it more closely matches plasma electrolyte composition and doesn't cause hyperchloremic acidosis. D5W and hypotonic solutions are inappropriate for resuscitation.

Question 30: C - Two or more ribs fractured in two or more places

Explanation: Flail chest occurs when two or more adjacent ribs are fractured in two or more places each, creating a free-floating segment that moves paradoxically with respiration (inward during inspiration, outward during expiration). This requires significant blunt force and is usually associated with underlying pulmonary contusion.

Question 31: B - Pneumococcal, meningococcal, H. influenzae type B

Explanation: Post-splenectomy patients need vaccinations against encapsulated bacteria: pneumococcal (Pneumovax), meningococcal, and Haemophilus influenzae type B. The spleen normally filters these bacteria. Without it, patients have lifelong increased infection risk and should seek immediate care for fevers.

Question 32: C - Fasciotomy

Explanation: Fasciotomy (surgical release of fascia) is the only definitive treatment for compartment syndrome. While removing constrictive dressings and positioning at heart level may temporarily help, they don't replace surgical decompression when compartment syndrome is present. All compartments must be released (four in lower leg).

Question 33: B - Battle's sign and raccoon eyes

Explanation: Basilar skull fracture signs include Battle's sign (ecchymosis over mastoid process), raccoon eyes (periorbital ecchymosis), CSF rhinorrhea (clear fluid from nose), CSF otorrhea (clear fluid from ear), and hemotympanum (blood behind tympanic membrane). These indicate skull base fracture and potential dural tear.

Question 34: B - Free fluid in abdomen and pericardium

Explanation: FAST (Focused Assessment with Sonography for Trauma) rapidly detects free fluid (blood) in the peritoneal cavity and pericardium at bedside. It doesn't identify specific organ injuries or grade severity—that requires CT. FAST has limited sensitivity for hollow viscus injuries. It's a screening tool for free fluid requiring further evaluation.

Question 35: C - Prepare for emergency thoracotomy

Explanation: Immediate drainage >1500 mL from chest tube indicates massive hemothorax with ongoing hemorrhage requiring surgical control. This patient needs emergency thoracotomy for direct hemorrhage control. Simply monitoring allows continued blood loss. Never clamp chest tubes except briefly during tube changes—clamping can create tension hemothorax.

Question 36: C - Radial

Explanation: The radial nerve wraps around the humerus in a spiral groove, making it vulnerable to midshaft humerus fractures. Radial nerve injury causes wrist drop (inability to extend wrist), weak grip, and numbness over dorsum of hand. Always assess radial nerve function before and after manipulation of humerus fractures.

Question 37: B - Uncontrolled hemorrhage

Explanation: Uncontrolled hemorrhage is the leading preventable cause of trauma death. While infection, PE, and pneumonia cause morbidity and some mortality, immediate hemorrhage control saves more lives than any other intervention. This is why damage control resuscitation and rapid surgical hemorrhage control are fundamental to trauma care.

Question 38: B - 24/7 in-house surgical teams and subspecialists

Explanation: Level I trauma centers require 24/7 immediate availability of in-house surgical teams (general surgery, orthopedics, neurosurgery, anesthesia) and other subspecialists. They also have research programs, education/outreach, and serve as regional resources. This distinguishes them from Level II centers where some specialists may be on-call rather than in-house.

Question 39: C - 60-70 mmHg or higher

Explanation: Cerebral perfusion pressure (CPP = MAP - ICP) should be maintained at 60-70 mmHg or higher in severe TBI patients. This ensures adequate blood flow to the injured brain. CPP <60 mmHg indicates inadequate brain perfusion and requires intervention (increase blood pressure or decrease ICP).

Question 40: B - Splenic injury with diaphragmatic irritation

Explanation: Kehr's sign is referred pain to the left shoulder from diaphragmatic irritation by blood in the left upper quadrant, classically from splenic injury. The phrenic nerve (innervating diaphragm) shares nerve roots with shoulder nerves, causing referred pain. Similar right shoulder pain can occur with liver injury.

Question 41: A - <5%

Explanation: Acceptable undertriage rate (seriously injured patients not going to trauma centers) is <5% because it directly impacts survival. Systems accept 25-35% overtriage (minor injuries going to trauma centers) to keep undertriage low. The trade-off: bringing some minor injuries to trauma centers is acceptable to ensure severe injuries reliably reach appropriate care.

Question 42: C - Aggressive hyperventilation to PCO2 of 25 mmHg

Explanation: Aggressive hyperventilation to very low PCO2 (<30 mmHg) should be avoided in routine ICP management because it causes cerebral vasoconstriction and can worsen ischemia. Brief hyperventilation to PCO2 30-35 may be used for acute herniation, but prolonged aggressive hyperventilation is harmful. Elevating head of bed, maintaining adequate BP, and pain management are all appropriate.

Question 43: B - 2-3 inches proximal to the wound

Explanation: Tourniquets should be placed 2-3 inches proximal to the wound (toward the trunk). This placement occludes blood flow before it reaches the injury. Never place over joints or distal to wounds. Place directly on skin or over thin clothing, and tighten until bleeding stops. Document time of application.

Question 44: C - Surgical repair

Explanation: Intraperitoneal bladder rupture requires surgical repair because urine leaks into the peritoneal cavity, causing peritonitis. Extraperitoneal ruptures can often be managed with catheter drainage alone, but intraperitoneal ruptures need operative closure. Diagnosis is made with CT cystogram showing contrast in peritoneal cavity.

Question 45: B - Tongue falling backward

Explanation: The tongue falling backward is the most common cause of airway obstruction in unconscious trauma patients. Loss of muscle tone allows the tongue to block the posterior pharynx. This is why jaw thrust or chin lift are effective first interventions—they move the mandible and tongue forward, opening the airway.

Question 46: B - Brief loss of consciousness, lucid interval, then deterioration

Explanation: Epidural hematoma classically presents with brief loss of consciousness from impact, a lucid interval where patient seems fine, then rapid deterioration as the hematoma expands. This occurs because arterial bleeding (often middle meningeal artery) gradually accumulates. The lucid interval is the dangerous period where injury may be missed if not recognized. On CT, epidural hematomas appear lens-shaped (biconvex).

Question 47: B - 2nd intercostal space, midclavicular line

Explanation: Needle decompression for tension pneumothorax is performed at the 2nd intercostal space, midclavicular line on the affected side. Insert 14-gauge needle just above the rib (avoiding neurovascular bundle below). You should hear a rush of air. Chest tube placement in the safe triangle (4th-5th intercostal space) follows for definitive treatment.

Question 48: C - 1:1:1 (PRBCs:FFP:Platelets)

Explanation: Current evidence supports balanced 1:1:1 ratio of packed red blood cells, fresh frozen plasma, and platelets during massive transfusion. This approach replaces both oxygen-carrying capacity and clotting factors, preventing dilutional coagulopathy and improving survival compared to PRBC-heavy strategies.

Question 49: C - Respiratory rate 35 after airway positioned

Explanation: In START triage, respiratory rate >29 after positioning airway categorizes patients as Immediate (Red)—they need urgent intervention to survive. Walking patients are Minor (Green). Patients not breathing after airway positioning are Deceased/Expectant (Black)—in disasters, CPR isn't performed due to resource limitations.

Question 50: B - Hypothermia, acidosis, coagulopathy

Explanation: The "lethal triad" in trauma is hypothermia, acidosis, and coagulopathy. These three factors worsen each other in a vicious cycle and dramatically increase mortality. Hypothermia impairs clotting factors, acidosis from poor perfusion worsens with hypothermia, and coagulopathy from both causes more bleeding. Preventing and treating all three aggressively is critical.

Question 51: B - Antibiotics and tetanus prophylaxis

Explanation: Open fractures (bone exposed to environment) require immediate broad-spectrum IV antibiotics (within 1-3 hours) and tetanus prophylaxis to prevent infection. They also need surgical irrigation, debridement, and stabilization within 6-8 hours ideally. Cover wound with sterile saline-moistened dressing. Never apply cast to open fracture without surgical treatment first.

Question 52: C - ≤8

Explanation: Severe traumatic brain injury is defined as GCS ≤8. These patients typically cannot protect their airway and require intubation and mechanical ventilation. Mild TBI: GCS 13-15. Moderate TBI: GCS 9-12. The GCS score guides initial management and helps predict outcomes.

Question 53: B - Performance improvement and outcomes tracking

Explanation: The trauma registry's primary purpose is collecting data for performance improvement, benchmarking against national standards, research, and tracking outcomes. While data may support billing and documentation, the core purpose is improving trauma care quality through systematic data analysis and identifying improvement opportunities.

Question 54: B - Airbags reducing injury severity

Explanation: Secondary prevention reduces injury severity when incidents occur. Airbags are secondary prevention—they don't prevent crashes but reduce injury severity. Primary prevention stops injury before it happens (seatbelt laws, speed limits). Tertiary prevention reduces complications after injury (hospital care, DVT prophylaxis).

Question 55: B - Crescent-shaped hyperdensity

Explanation: Subdural hematoma appears on CT as crescent-shaped (concave) hyperdensity that follows brain contours. Epidural hematoma is lens-shaped (biconvex) and doesn't cross suture lines. Subdural bleeds from torn bridging veins, while epidural bleeds from arterial injury (often middle meningeal artery).

Question 56: B - Below xiphoid toward left shoulder

Explanation: Pericardiocentesis uses subxiphoid approach: insert needle just below and to the left of xiphoid, advancing at 45-degree angle toward left shoulder. This avoids coronary arteries and minimizes myocardial puncture risk. ECG monitoring during procedure helps detect ventricular contact. Even 20-30 mL removal can dramatically improve hemodynamics in tamponade.

Question 57: B - Control hemorrhage and contamination quickly

Explanation: Damage control surgery focuses on rapid hemorrhage control and contamination control in physiologically unstable patients (hypothermic, acidotic, coagulopathic). Definitive repairs are left for later when patient is warmer, better perfused, and coagulating. Goal is survival, not perfect repair initially. Patient returns to OR 24-72 hours later for definitive reconstruction.

Question 58: C - 24-72 hours post-injury

Explanation: Fat embolism syndrome typically develops 24-72 hours after long bone fractures (especially femur). Fat from bone marrow enters circulation and travels to lungs and brain, causing respiratory distress (hypoxemia), neurological symptoms (confusion), and petechial rash. Treatment is supportive—respiratory support, managing complications.

Question 59: B - Systolic BP 85 mmHg

Explanation: Systolic BP <90 mmHg is a Step 1 physiologic criterion requiring trauma center transport per CDC guidelines. This vital sign abnormality indicates shock requiring trauma center resources regardless of mechanism. RR threshold is <10 or >29, GCS ≤13. HR 105 and SpO2 93% don't meet specific triage criteria alone.

Question 60: B - CSF rhinorrhea or otorrhea

Explanation: Basilar skull fracture is associated with CSF rhinorrhea (clear fluid from nose) or otorrhea (clear fluid from ear), indicating dural tear. Other signs: Battle's sign (mastoid ecchymosis), raccoon eyes (periorbital ecchymosis), hemotympanum. These findings indicate skull base fracture and potential brain injury.

Question 61: C - Aortic isthmus (distal to left subclavian)

Explanation: The aortic isthmus (just distal to left subclavian artery) is the most common site of traumatic aortic disruption (80-90% of cases). This is where mobile aortic arch transitions to fixed descending aorta, creating shear forces during sudden deceleration. The aorta is tethered here by ligamentum arteriosum.

Question 62: A - Quadriplegia

Explanation: Spinal cord injury at C5 level (cervical spine) results in quadriplegia (paralysis of all four extremities). Cervical injuries above C4 also affect diaphragm function. Injuries below T1 cause paraplegia (lower extremity paralysis). The level of injury determines which muscles remain functional.

Question 63: B - Reinfusing patient's own drained blood

Explanation: Autotransfusion in hemothorax management collects blood drained from chest tube and reinfuses it to the patient. This provides immediate volume replacement with patient's own blood, avoiding transfusion reactions, conserving blood bank resources, and replacing volume quickly. Blood must be collected in sterile autotransfusion systems and reinfused within 4-6 hours.

Question 64: C - Second-degree burn involving hands, face, or genitals

Explanation: Burns involving hands, face, feet, genitals, perineum, or major joints require burn center care regardless of size due to functional and cosmetic importance. Other burn center criteria: partial-thickness >10% TBSA, full-thickness any size, electrical/chemical burns, inhalation injury, burns with major trauma, burns in very young/old/comorbid patients.

Question 65: B - 18%

Explanation: Rule of Nines for adults: Head 9%, each arm 9%, anterior trunk 18%, posterior trunk 18%, each entire leg 18%, perineum 1%. So each entire leg is 18% (anterior leg 9%, posterior leg 9%). Rule of Nines is modified for children (relatively larger head, smaller legs).

Question 66: B - Temporary loss of all neurologic function below injury level

Explanation: Spinal shock is temporary loss of all neurologic function (motor, sensory, reflex) below spinal cord injury level, typically lasting days to weeks. It's a physiologic response to spinal cord injury. When spinal shock resolves, reflexes return (often hyperactive) and the patient's permanent neurological status becomes clearer. This differs from neurogenic shock (hemodynamic changes).

Question 67: B - Decreasing lactate level

Explanation: Decreasing lactate level indicates improving tissue perfusion and resolution of anaerobic metabolism—one of the best markers of successful shock resuscitation. Lactate >2 mmol/L indicates tissue hypoperfusion. As resuscitation succeeds and perfusion improves, lactate decreases toward normal. Blood pressure and heart rate can be misleading; lactate directly reflects tissue-level perfusion.

Question 68: B - Worsens over 24-48 hours

Explanation: Pulmonary contusion (lung bruising) typically evolves and worsens over 24-48 hours after injury. Initial chest X-ray may be normal or show minimal changes. Progressive infiltrates and hypoxemia develop as inflammation and edema progress. This is why serial chest X-rays and close respiratory monitoring are essential after significant chest trauma.

Question 69: B - 500-600 mL

Explanation: Appropriate tidal volume for bag-valve-mask ventilation in adults is 500-600 mL (approximately 6-7 mL/kg), delivered over 1 second. This volume produces visible chest rise without excessive pressure. Smaller volumes don't provide adequate ventilation. Larger volumes increase risk of barotrauma, gastric inflation, and aspiration.

Question 70: A - Normal mental status, no midline tenderness, no neurological deficits, no distracting injuries

Explanation: Clinical cervical spine clearance (without imaging) requires all of these: alert/oriented, no midline cervical tenderness, no neurological deficits, no intoxication, and no distracting injuries that might mask pain. If all criteria met, the collar can be removed clinically. If any criterion fails, imaging is required (CT is now preferred over plain films).

Question 71: B - Brainstem injury (more severe than decorticate)

Explanation: Decerebrate posturing (extension of arms and legs) indicates brainstem injury and is more severe than decorticate posturing (flexion of arms, extension of legs indicating cortical injury). Both represent abnormal motor responses scored as 2 on GCS motor scale, but decerebrate suggests deeper, more severe injury with worse prognosis.

Question 72: B - Peritonitis and sepsis

Explanation: Hollow viscus perforation leaks intestinal contents into the peritoneum, causing peritonitis and eventually sepsis if untreated. While bleeding can occur, contamination and infection are the primary concerns requiring urgent surgical repair, washout, and antibiotics. Untreated perforation has high mortality from septic complications.

Question 73: B - Monitoring whether changes improved outcomes

Explanation: Loop closure in performance improvement means monitoring whether implemented changes actually produced the desired improvements. After identifying issues and making changes, you must verify the changes worked. This "closes the loop" by confirming interventions were effective or identifying need for further modification. Without this step, you don't know if improvements occurred.

Question 74: B - Ruptured abdominal aortic aneurysm

Explanation: Ruptured AAA requires vascular surgery expertise immediately available at Level I centers. Most Level III centers lack this capability. Stable extremity fractures can be managed at Level III before transfer. Minor head injury with normal CT and simple rib fractures don't require immediate transfer if the facility can provide appropriate monitoring and pain management.

Question 75: B - Reducing injury incidence and severity

Explanation: The fundamental purpose of injury prevention programs is reducing the burden of injury in the community—preventing injuries before they occur (primary prevention) and reducing severity when they do (secondary prevention). While programs may satisfy accreditation requirements, the core mission is actually preventing injuries and saving lives.

Question 76: C - [(2 × Diastolic) + Systolic] / 3

Explanation: Mean arterial pressure (MAP) = [(2 × Diastolic) + Systolic] / 3. This formula weights diastolic pressure more heavily because the heart spends more time in diastole. MAP represents average pressure in arteries during one cardiac cycle. MAP ≥65 mmHg is generally needed for adequate organ perfusion. CPP = MAP - ICP.

Question 77: B - Bile leak or abscess

Explanation: Increasing pain and fever 3 days after liver injury suggests bile leak (causing biloma or bile peritonitis) or abscess formation from infected hematoma. Liver injuries can develop these delayed complications even with successful non-operative management. Diagnosis with CT or HIDA scan. Treatment ranges from percutaneous drainage to ERCP with stent placement for bile leaks.

Question 78: B - Pulsatile bleeding and absent pulse

Explanation: Hard signs of vascular injury mandate immediate surgical exploration without delay for imaging: pulsatile bleeding, expanding/pulsatile hematoma, absent pulse distal to injury, bruit/thrill over injury site, and signs of acute ischemia. Soft signs (proximity, small stable hematoma, diminished pulse) warrant further investigation with imaging but may not require immediate surgery.

Question 79: A - Time phases and factors

Explanation: The Haddon Matrix analyzes injury prevention across three time phases (pre-event, event, post-event) and three factors (human, agent/vehicle, environment). This comprehensive framework identifies multiple intervention points for any injury type. For example, motor vehicle crash prevention addresses driver education (human/pre-event), airbags (agent/event), and rapid EMS (environment/post-event).

Question 80: D - ICP >20 mmHg

Explanation: Normal ICP is <10 mmHg. ICP >20 mmHg indicates increased intracranial pressure requiring intervention. Treatment aims to maintain ICP <20 mmHg and CPP (MAP - ICP) at 60-70 mmHg or higher. Elevated ICP can cause brain herniation if untreated. Interventions include elevating head of bed, osmotic therapy, sedation, and possibly surgery.

Question 81: B - Alteration in mental status from trauma, may not involve LOC

Explanation: Concussion is alteration in mental status from trauma that may or may not involve loss of consciousness. It's a functional (not structural) brain injury—CT scan is typically normal. Symptoms include confusion, amnesia, headache, dizziness, and cognitive difficulties. Most resolve within days to weeks. Structural injuries (contusions, hemorrhages) are visible on CT.

Question 82: B - Injuries incompatible with survival given resources

Explanation: Expectant (Black) category in disaster triage includes patients who are alive but have injuries so severe that survival is unlikely even with aggressive care given current resource limitations. Resources are directed to more salvageable patients. This isn't the same as deceased—these patients receive comfort care but not aggressive resuscitation. It's ethically appropriate when resources are genuinely insufficient.

Question 83: B - Time from arrival to CT for severe TBI

Explanation: Process measures track how care is delivered—times to interventions, protocol compliance, adherence to guidelines. Time from arrival to CT scan for severe TBI is a process measure indicating system efficiency. Outcome measures track results (mortality, complications). Patient satisfaction and revenue aren't clinical performance indicators.

Question 84: B - 4-6 hours

Explanation: Muscles tolerate 4-6 hours of warm ischemia before irreversible damage occurs. Beyond this "golden window," even with restoration of blood flow, muscle death and permanent disability or amputation may result. This creates urgency in managing vascular injuries, compartment syndrome, and limb-threatening trauma. Time from injury to revascularization is the most critical factor in limb salvage.

Question 85: B - Personality changes and impaired judgment

Explanation: The frontal lobe controls executive function, judgment, impulse control, and personality. Frontal lobe injury causes personality changes, impaired judgment, disinhibition, emotional lability, and difficulty with planning/organization. Patients may act inappropriately, make poor decisions, or exhibit changed personality. Occipital lobe injuries cause visual deficits, temporal lobe affects hearing/memory.

Question 86: B - Posterior hip dislocation

Explanation: The sciatic nerve courses behind the hip joint and is commonly injured with posterior hip dislocation (90% of hip dislocations). Injury causes foot drop, loss of ankle dorsiflexion/plantarflexion, and numbness in the foot. Always assess sciatic nerve function before and after hip reduction. Anterior dislocation risks femoral nerve/artery injury.

Question 87: B - Duodenum or portions of colon

Explanation: Retroperitoneal air on CT indicates perforation of a retroperitoneal structure, most commonly the duodenum (second through fourth portions) or portions of colon that are retroperitoneal (ascending and descending). This finding requires surgical exploration to identify and repair the perforation. Spleen and liver are intraperitoneal organs that would cause free intraperitoneal air.

Question 88: B - Critical increase in ICP with brain displacement

Explanation: Brain herniation syndromes occur when critically elevated ICP forces brain tissue through openings in the skull or between brain compartments. Types include uncal herniation (temporal lobe herniates through tentorium, compressing CN

III causing dilated pupil), central herniation (downward displacement), and tonsillar herniation (cerebellum through foramen magnum, affecting respirations). These are life-threatening emergencies.

Question 89: C - Handlebar injury compressing duodenum against spine

Explanation: Handlebar injuries (bicycle/motorcycle) classically cause duodenal trauma by compressing the duodenum against the spine. The duodenum is fixed retroperitoneally and vulnerable to this compression mechanism. These injuries can be difficult to diagnose, may present with delayed symptoms, and often involve pancreatic injury due to anatomical proximity.

Question 90: B - Tranexamic acid (TXA)

Explanation: Tranexamic acid reduces mortality in bleeding trauma patients when given within 3 hours of injury. TXA is an antifibrinolytic that prevents clot breakdown, giving the body time to control bleeding. Dose: 1 gram IV over 10 minutes, followed by 1 gram over 8 hours. Now standard in massive transfusion protocols. Aspirin, warfarin, and heparin worsen bleeding.

Question 91: B - 24-72 hours post-injury

Explanation: Acute Respiratory Distress Syndrome (ARDS) after trauma typically develops 24-72 hours post-injury as an inflammatory response to trauma, shock, or massive transfusion. Presents with bilateral infiltrates on chest X-ray, hypoxemia not explained by heart failure or fluid overload, and decreased lung compliance. Treatment is supportive with lung-protective ventilation.

Question 92: B - Immobilizing cervical spine until injury ruled out

Explanation: The cervical collar's primary purpose is immobilizing the cervical spine until injury is ruled out clinically or through imaging. Always assume cervical spine injury in trauma patients until proven otherwise. The collar alone doesn't provide complete immobilization—head blocks and backboard or appropriate padding are also needed. Collars don't treat pain or prevent infection.

Question 93: C - DVT prophylaxis in hospitalized patients

Explanation: Tertiary prevention reduces complications and disability after injury occurs. DVT prophylaxis in hospitalized trauma patients prevents thromboembolic complications. Primary prevention stops injury before it happens (helmet laws, speed limits). Secondary prevention reduces injury severity when incidents occur (airbags, crumple zones).

Question 94: C - 30 degrees

Explanation: Severe TBI patients should have head of bed elevated to 30 degrees to promote venous drainage from the head, reducing ICP. Keep head in midline position (no rotation). Flat positioning increases ICP. Extreme elevation (>45 degrees) can decrease cerebral perfusion pressure. The 30-degree position balances ICP reduction with maintaining adequate cerebral perfusion.

Question 95: B - 4 mL × kg × % TBSA over 24 hours

Explanation: Parkland formula for burn resuscitation: 4 mL × patient weight (kg) × % TBSA burned over 24 hours. Give half in first 8 hours, remaining half over next 16 hours. Uses lactated Ringer's. Example: 70 kg patient with 40% TBSA burn = 4 × 70 × 40 = 11,200 mL over 24 hours (5,600 mL in first 8 hours). Titrate to urine output 0.5-1 mL/kg/hr.

Question 96: B - Uncal herniation with CN III compression

Explanation: Unilateral dilated, non-reactive pupil in trauma patient indicates uncal herniation with compression of cranial nerve III (oculomotor nerve). This is a neurosurgical emergency requiring immediate intervention to reduce ICP. The temporal lobe herniates through the tentorium, compressing CN III and causing ipsilateral pupil dilation. Without treatment, herniation progresses to complete brain death.

Question 97: B - Unity of command with each person having one supervisor

Explanation: The Incident Command System (ICS) features unity of command—each person reports to one supervisor, preventing conflicting directions and maintaining clear accountability. Other ICS principles include span of control (supervisors manage 3-7 people), modular organization (structure expands/contracts based on needs), and common terminology. ICS provides standardized structure for all disaster responses.

Question 98: B - Zone II

Explanation: Zone II (mid-neck, from cricoid to angle of mandible) contains carotid arteries, jugular veins, trachea, and esophagus. It has the best surgical access and is most common injury location. Zone I (base of neck) and Zone III (upper neck to skull base) have difficult surgical access. Penetrating Zone II injuries with hard signs require immediate surgical exploration.

Question 99: B - Proceed to OR immediately

Explanation: Hemodynamically unstable patients with positive FAST exam (indicating intra-abdominal hemorrhage) need immediate surgical exploration. Don't delay for CT imaging—they're bleeding and need operative hemorrhage control now. CT is appropriate for stable patients to define specific injuries and guide management decisions. Unstable patients with positive FAST go directly to OR.

Question 100: B - Wrapping in saline-moistened gauze, placing in plastic bag, then on ice

Explanation: Proper care of amputated parts: wrap in saline-moistened gauze, place in sealed plastic bag, then place bag on ice (not directly on ice, which causes frostbite damage). This preserves tissue for possible replantation while preventing freezing injury. Transport with patient even if part doesn't seem viable—surgeons will decide replantation feasibility.

Question 101: B - Severe hypertension and bradycardia

Explanation: Autonomic dysreflexia in spinal cord injury above T6 is a life-threatening emergency: severe hypertension (can cause stroke), bradycardia, pounding headache, flushing above injury level, and pallor below. Triggered by noxious stimuli below injury level (distended bladder, fecal impaction, pressure ulcer). Treatment: elevate head, identify and remove trigger, antihypertensives if needed. Prevent by avoiding triggers.

Question 102: C - Sustained end-tidal CO_2 waveform

Explanation: End-tidal CO_2 detection showing sustained waveform is the most reliable objective confirmation of tracheal (not esophageal) placement. While visualizing tube passing through cords is excellent, it's not always possible. Breath sounds can be misleading (esophageal sounds transmit). Chest X-ray confirms position but shouldn't delay other immediate confirmation methods. Use multiple methods together.

Question 103: B - Delayed airway edema and respiratory failure over 24-48 hours

Explanation: Inhalation injury often shows delayed effects. Initial assessment may seem reassuring, but airway edema, bronchospasm, and respiratory failure develop over 24-48 hours as inflammation progresses. Monitor closely for worsening respiratory status, stridor, increased work of breathing. Have low threshold for early intubation before edema makes it impossible. Inhalation injury significantly increases mortality in burn patients.

Question 104: B - CT scan of cervical spine

Explanation: CT scan of the cervical spine is now the preferred imaging for suspected cervical spine injury in trauma patients, especially in those who can't be clinically cleared (altered mental status, intoxication, distracting injuries, or positive clinical findings). CT is more sensitive than plain X-rays for bony injury. MRI is used for ligamentous injury or neurological deficits with negative CT.

Question 105: B - Renal failure from myoglobin

Explanation: Rhabdomyolysis (muscle breakdown) from crush injury releases myoglobin, which damages kidneys and can cause acute renal failure. Signs: dark tea-colored urine, elevated creatine kinase (CK), elevated potassium, metabolic acidosis. Treatment: aggressive IV hydration to maintain high urine output (flush myoglobin through kidneys), alkalinize urine, monitor electrolytes (watch for hyperkalemia), possibly dialysis if renal failure develops.

Question 106: B - Covering with moist sterile dressing and immediate surgery

Explanation: Evisceration (abdominal contents protruding through wound) requires covering with moist sterile dressing and immediate surgical exploration. Never push organs back in—this introduces contamination deep into abdomen. Keep organs moist with sterile saline-soaked dressings while preparing for OR. These injuries require surgical repair without delay. Penetrating abdominal trauma with evisceration is absolute surgical indication.

Question 107: B - Underlying great vessel injury

Explanation: First and second rib fractures require tremendous force because these ribs are protected by shoulder girdle and clavicle. The force needed to fracture them suggests possible injury to underlying great vessels (subclavian artery/vein, aorta). These patients need vascular imaging (CT angiography) to rule out life-threatening vascular injuries. Ribs 9-12 fractures suggest liver/spleen injury risk.

Question 108: B - MAP - ICP

Explanation: Cerebral perfusion pressure (CPP) = Mean Arterial Pressure (MAP) - Intracranial Pressure (ICP). CPP represents the pressure gradient driving blood flow to the brain. Target CPP 60-70 mmHg or higher in TBI. If ICP increases or MAP decreases, CPP drops, potentially causing brain ischemia. Treatment focuses on maintaining adequate MAP and reducing ICP to optimize CPP.

Question 109: B - Severe TBI 80 miles from Level I center

Explanation: Helicopter transport is indicated for time-critical patients (like severe TBI) when distance is 50-150 miles from appropriate facility and time savings would significantly impact outcome. Short distances (<50 miles) typically use ground. Very long distances (>150 miles) may use fixed-wing aircraft. Minor injuries don't justify helicopter cost/risk. Weather and patient condition must also be considered.

Question 110: B - Prevent clot disruption before hemorrhage control

Explanation: Permissive hypotension (maintaining systolic BP 80-90 mmHg until surgical hemorrhage control) prevents clot disruption from elevated blood pressure while maintaining adequate vital organ perfusion. Raising BP before controlling bleeding increases hemorrhage. This strategy is used in penetrating trauma with uncontrolled bleeding. Not appropriate for traumatic brain injury patients who need higher BP for cerebral perfusion.

Question 111: B - Rhabdomyolysis from muscle injury

Explanation: Decreased urine output with dark, tea-colored urine after burn injury (especially electrical or deep burns) suggests rhabdomyolysis from muscle damage. Myoglobin released from damaged muscle causes dark urine and kidney damage. Treatment: increase IV fluid rate to maintain high urine output (200 mL/hr for adults until urine clears), alkalinize urine, monitor for acute kidney injury and electrolyte abnormalities.

Question 112: C - 15

Explanation: Glasgow Coma Scale (GCS) maximum score is 15, indicating normal consciousness: Eye opening 4 (spontaneous), Verbal 5 (oriented), Motor 6 (obeys commands). Minimum score is 3 (completely unresponsive). GCS helps classify injury severity: 13-15 mild, 9-12 moderate, ≤8 severe. Score guides initial management and helps predict outcomes.

Question 113: C - T6

Explanation: Neurogenic shock occurs with spinal cord injuries at or above T6 because sympathetic nervous system control is disrupted. Loss of sympathetic tone causes vasodilation (hypotension) and prevents compensatory tachycardia (bradycardia instead). Classic triad: hypotension, bradycardia, warm/dry skin below injury level. Lower injuries don't affect enough sympathetic system to cause neurogenic shock.

Question 114: B - Airway compromise from swelling or bleeding

Explanation: Mandibular fractures risk airway compromise from soft tissue swelling, hematoma, or loss of tongue support (tongue attaches to mandible—bilateral fractures can cause posterior tongue displacement). Monitor closely for airway obstruction. Secure airway early if concerns develop. Other risks: malocclusion, infection (if open fracture into oral cavity), nerve injury.

Question 115: C - 20 mL/kg

Explanation: Pediatric trauma resuscitation begins with 20 mL/kg bolus of isotonic crystalloid (lactated Ringer's or normal saline). Reassess after each bolus. If ongoing signs of shock after 2-3 boluses (40-60 mL/kg total), begin blood transfusion (10 mL/kg PRBCs). Children compensate well initially but decompensate suddenly, so close monitoring is essential.

Question 116: B - Hypertension with widened pulse pressure

Explanation: Cushing's reflex (response to critically elevated ICP) includes hypertension with widened pulse pressure (body trying to maintain cerebral perfusion despite high ICP), bradycardia (vagal response), and irregular respirations (brainstem compression). This triad indicates impending herniation requiring immediate intervention. Don't confuse with Cushing's triad, which is the same clinical presentation.

Question 117: B - Midface

Explanation: Le Fort fractures involve the midface and are classified as Le Fort I (horizontal maxillary fracture), Le Fort II (pyramidal fracture through maxilla and nasal bones), or Le Fort III (complete craniofacial separation). These high-energy injuries often involve airway compromise from swelling, bleeding, or unstable facial structures. May need advanced airway management. Associated with significant facial deformity and CSF leak risk.

Question 118: B - Stabilization and appropriate transfer

Explanation: Level III trauma centers provide prompt assessment, resuscitation, emergency operations if needed, and stabilization before transfer to higher-level centers for definitive care. They're critical in rural areas where travel to Level I/II centers takes hours. They have general surgery availability (may be on-call) and transfer agreements with higher-level centers.

Question 119: B - GCS drop from 14 to 10

Explanation: Declining GCS indicates neurological deterioration requiring immediate intervention. A drop of 2 or more points is significant. This patient dropped 4 points, suggesting evolving intracranial hemorrhage, increased ICP, or herniation. Requires immediate CT scan, neurosurgical consultation, and interventions to reduce ICP. Don't wait for further deterioration—act immediately on declining neurological status.

Question 120: B - Cardiac dysrhythmias and deep tissue damage

Explanation: Electrical burns cause injury along electrical current path through body. Entrance and exit wounds may seem small, but deep tissue destruction occurs (muscle, nerves, blood vessels, organs). Cardiac monitoring required—dysrhythmias can occur immediately or delayed. Also assess for compartment syndrome (deep muscle injury), rhabdomyolysis, neurological deficits, and vascular injury. Surface appearance underestimates injury severity.

Question 121: B - Contusion has structural damage (bruising) visible on CT

Explanation: Concussion is functional brain injury without structural damage—CT is typically normal. Contusion is brain bruising with structural damage visible on CT as areas of hemorrhage and edema. Both result from trauma, but contusion is more severe with visible tissue injury. Concussions are more common and usually resolve fully. Contusions have higher risk of complications and delayed hemorrhage.

Question 122: B - Epidural hematoma with midline shift

Explanation: Epidural hematoma with midline shift indicates significant mass effect requiring neurosurgical evaluation for possible evacuation. Midline shift (displacement of brain structures from normal position) suggests the hematoma is large enough to compress brain tissue. Not all epidural hematomas need surgery—small ones without shift may be observed—but shift indicates need for surgical consultation immediately.

Question 123: B - Right patient, right resources, right time

Explanation: The goal of trauma system organization is ensuring the right patient gets to the right resources at the right time. This means appropriate field triage, efficient transfer protocols, and facility capabilities matching patient needs. Not all patients need Level I centers, and concentrating all care at one facility reduces access. The system balances capability with geographic coverage.

Question 124: B - Sternal fracture or anterior chest impact

Explanation: Blunt cardiac injury should be suspected with sternal fractures, anterior chest impact, or significant chest trauma. The sternum protects the heart—fracturing it requires significant force transmitted to underlying heart. Patients need cardiac monitoring (watch for dysrhythmias), ECG, and possibly troponin levels or echocardiogram. Most injuries are contusions managed supportively; rarely, serious structural damage occurs.

Question 125: B - Delayed intracranial hemorrhage (subdural)

Explanation: Sudden severe headache and vomiting weeks after minor head trauma suggests delayed intracranial hemorrhage, most commonly chronic subdural hematoma. Initial trauma tears bridging veins, but bleeding is slow. Hematoma gradually expands over days to weeks, eventually causing symptoms. More common in elderly (brain atrophy allows more space before symptoms) and patients on anticoagulants. Requires CT scan and possible surgical evacuation.

Interpreting Your Score

Now that you've reviewed all the answers, let's talk about what your score means and how to move forward.

Scoring Ranges:

106-125 correct (85-100%): Outstanding! You're demonstrating strong mastery of trauma nursing concepts. Your understanding of assessment priorities, injury patterns, and interventions is solid. Continue reviewing areas where you missed questions, but you're on track for TCRN success. Focus your remaining study time on:

Areas where you missed questions

Integrating knowledge across content areas

Test-taking strategies to maximize your score

Building confidence through additional practice

94-105 correct (75-84%): Very good! You have a solid foundation with some areas needing strengthening. This is a passing score on most practice exams, but aim higher for comfort on test day. Your study plan should:

Identify patterns in missed questions (specific content areas? Question types?)

Deep dive into weak areas with focused review

Practice more questions in challenging topics

Review test-taking strategies, especially for priority questions

81-93 correct (65-74%): Good progress, but targeted study is needed. You understand many concepts but need to strengthen several areas before feeling confident on exam day. Don't be discouraged—you're building knowledge that will get you there. Next steps:

Thoroughly review all missed questions—understand why you got them wrong

Identify your 2-3 weakest content areas and study them intensively

Go back to relevant chapters and re-read with focus on application

Practice more questions to reinforce learning

Consider additional practice exams after targeted review

Below 81 (Below 65%): You're building foundational knowledge but need significant additional preparation. This is feedback, not failure—it tells you what to focus on. Create a comprehensive study plan:

Review each content chapter systematically

Don't just read—actively engage (make notes, explain concepts aloud, teach someone else)

Focus on understanding "why" behind answers, not just memorizing facts

Build on strengths while addressing weaknesses

Consider study group or mentor support

Take more time before exam if possible—preparation is key to success

Pattern Analysis:

Look beyond your overall score. Identify patterns:

Content area patterns: Did you miss most questions on a specific topic (neurological trauma, compartment syndrome, etc.)? This tells you where to focus study time.

Question type patterns:

Missing priority questions? Review ABCDE approach and primary survey principles

Missing "why" questions? Focus on pathophysiology understanding

Missing mechanism questions? Study injury patterns and mechanisms

Common mistakes:

Misreading questions (read completely before answering)

Choosing "possible" answer over "most correct" answer

Not recognizing time-sensitive emergencies

Forgetting exceptions to rules (like permissive hypotension doesn't apply to TBI)

Next Steps for Success

If you scored well (85%+):

Review missed questions thoroughly—even small gaps matter

Take Practice Exam 2 to confirm consistency

Focus final study on high-yield topics and test-taking strategies

Build confidence through positive self-talk and visualization

Schedule your exam with confidence

If you need additional preparation:

- Don't rush—give yourself adequate preparation time
- Create focused study plan targeting weak areas
- Use multiple study methods (reading, practice questions, teaching others)
- Take Practice Exam 2 after targeted review
- Track improvement to stay motivated
- Consider delaying exam if needed—better to be ready than rush

Remember:

- This practice exam is a learning tool, not a prediction of failure
- Every nurse preparing for TCRN has strengths and weaknesses
- Improvement comes from identifying gaps and addressing them systematically
- Consistent, focused study pays off on exam day
- You've already invested significant time in preparation—see it through

Moving Forward:

Take a short break, then review your performance objectively. Make a plan for your continued preparation based on what this exam revealed. Whether you're fine-tuning knowledge or building foundational understanding, you're making progress toward your goal.

The TCRN certification demonstrates your commitment to excellence in trauma nursing. This practice exam is one step on that journey. Use it wisely, learn from it, and let it guide your preparation strategy.

You're capable of achieving this certification. Keep working, stay focused, and believe in your ability to master this material. Every trauma nurse who's earned TCRN certification started where you are now—preparing, practicing, and persevering.

Your dedication to this preparation process shows you're already thinking like a trauma nurse. Now continue building the knowledge and confidence you need to prove it on exam day.

Remember: Review isn't just about checking answers—it's about understanding concepts. Use this answer key as a learning tool, not just a scoring guide. Each explanation reinforces trauma nursing principles that will serve you on exam day and throughout your career.

Practice Exam 2

Instructions

Welcome to your second full-length practice exam. This exam provides another opportunity to assess your knowledge, build test-taking stamina, and identify any remaining areas needing review.

Exam Format:

125 questions covering all TCRN content areas

150 minutes (2.5 hours) to complete

Simulates actual TCRN exam experience

Before You Begin:

Choose a quiet, distraction-free environment

Have scratch paper available for calculations

Set timer for 150 minutes

Commit to completing the exam in one sitting if possible

Answer every question—there's no penalty for guessing

How to Use This Exam:

If this is your first practice exam, use it to identify your baseline and areas needing focus. If you've taken Practice Exam 1, compare your performance to track improvement and ensure consistent understanding across different question sets.

Mindset for Success:

Approach this exam with confidence. You've prepared systematically. Trust your knowledge and clinical judgment. Remember: you're not just memorizing facts—you're demonstrating the expertise that defines excellent trauma nursing.

Take a deep breath. You're ready. Let's begin.

Practice Exam 2 - Questions

Question 1: What is the first priority when a trauma patient arrives with active arterial bleeding from an extremity wound?

A) Establish IV access
B) Apply direct pressure to control hemorrhage
C) Obtain vital signs
D) Administer pain medication

Question 2: A patient has a GCS of 6 after motor vehicle crash. What intervention is most critical?

A) CT scan
B) Immediate endotracheal intubation
C) Neurosurgery consultation
D) Mannitol administration

Question 3: Which burn depth involves destruction of epidermis and dermis with white, leathery appearance?

A) Superficial (first-degree)
B) Superficial partial-thickness (second-degree)
C) Deep partial-thickness
D) Full-thickness (third-degree)

Question 4: A patient with pelvic fracture develops hypotension despite fluid resuscitation and pelvic binder. What is the next intervention?

A) More crystalloid fluids
B) CT scan
C) Angiography with embolization or preperitoneal packing
D) Observation

Question 5: The primary survey is interrupted when:

A) Family arrives
B) Life-threatening condition is identified requiring immediate intervention
C) Physician orders tests
D) Patient needs to be moved

Question 6: Which finding suggests increased intracranial pressure?

A) Hypotension, tachycardia, rapid breathing
B) Hypertension, bradycardia, irregular respirations
C) Normal vital signs with headache
D) Fever and confusion

Question 7: A hemodynamically stable patient with Grade II splenic laceration should be managed with:

A) Immediate splenectomy
B) Non-operative management with close monitoring
C) Angiography and embolization
D) Exploratory laparotomy

Question 8: What is the most sensitive indicator of adequate resuscitation?

A) Blood pressure normalization
B) Heart rate <100 bpm
C) Urine output 0.5-1 mL/kg/hr
D) Normal temperature

Question 9: A patient with suspected cervical spine injury is alert, has no midline tenderness, no neurological deficits, and no distracting injuries. The appropriate action is:

A) Keep collar on indefinitely
B) Clinical clearance without imaging
C) CT scan required
D) MRI required

Question 10: Massive hemothorax is defined as:

A) Any blood in chest
B) ≥500 mL in chest
C) ≥1500 mL or one-third blood volume
D) ≥3000 mL in chest

Question 11: Which nerve injury causes foot drop?

A) Femoral nerve
B) Sciatic or common peroneal nerve
C) Tibial nerve
D) Saphenous nerve

Question 12: A patient arrives with impaled knife in abdomen. The correct management is:

A) Remove knife and pack wound
B) Leave knife in place and transport to OR
C) Remove knife and apply pressure
D) Push knife deeper to stop bleeding

Question 13: The secondary survey begins:

A) Immediately upon patient arrival
B) After the primary survey is complete
C) When family requests information
D) After all lab results return

Question 14: Which patient meets criteria for trauma center transport per CDC guidelines?

A) Isolated wrist fracture
B) GCS 12 after head trauma
C) Minor vehicle damage with no injuries
D) Abrasion on knee

Question 15: Recommended depth for chest compressions in adults is:

A) 1-2 inches
B) At least 2 inches (5 cm)
C) 3-4 inches
D) As deep as possible

Question 16: A patient with abdominal trauma has a positive FAST exam but stable vital signs. The next step is:

A) Immediate surgery
B) CT scan to characterize injuries
C) Observation only
D) Repeat FAST in 1 hour

Question 17: Which medication is given for severe traumatic brain injury to reduce intracranial pressure?

A) Furosemide
B) Mannitol or hypertonic saline
C) Dopamine
D) Morphine

Question 18: A tourniquet should be loosened periodically to check if still needed.

A) True
B) False - leave in place until surgical evaluation

Question 19: The most common cause of shock in trauma patients is:

A) Cardiogenic
B) Neurogenic
C) Hypovolemic from hemorrhage
D) Septic

Question 20: Which position is appropriate for a patient with suspected spinal injury during log roll?

A) Keep spine aligned in neutral position
B) Hyperextend neck
C) Flex hips completely
D) Twist at waist

Question 21: A patient develops stridor 6 hours after neck trauma. This indicates:

A) Normal finding
B) Developing airway edema requiring urgent evaluation

C) Vocal cord paralysis that will resolve
D) Anxiety

Question 22: Class II hemorrhagic shock involves loss of:

A) Up to 15% blood volume
B) 15-30% blood volume
C) 30-40% blood volume
D) Over 40% blood volume

Question 23: The best position for a pregnant trauma patient in third trimester is:

A) Supine flat
B) Left lateral tilt or manual uterine displacement
C) Trendelenburg
D) Right lateral

Question 24: A patient with open femur fracture needs antibiotics within what timeframe?

A) 24 hours
B) 12 hours
C) 6 hours
D) 1-3 hours

Question 25: Which lab value indicates rhabdomyolysis?

A) Elevated glucose
B) Elevated creatine kinase (CK)
C) Decreased sodium
D) Elevated white blood cells

Question 26: Normal cerebral perfusion pressure should be maintained at:

A) 30-40 mmHg
B) 40-50 mmHg
C) 60-70 mmHg or higher
D) 80-100 mmHg

Question 27: A patient with rib fractures should avoid:

A) Deep breathing and coughing
B) Adequate pain control
C) Incentive spirometry
D) Early mobilization

Question 28: Which represents appropriate prehospital spinal immobilization?

A) Cervical collar only
B) Cervical collar, backboard, and head blocks
C) Head blocks only
D) Patient preference

Question 29: A child in compensated shock will have:

A) Hypotension
B) Normal blood pressure with tachycardia and poor perfusion
C) Bradycardia
D) Hypertension

Question 30: The appropriate response to a patient pulling at their endotracheal tube is:

A) Immediately extubate
B) Apply restraints without assessment
C) Assess for hypoxia, pain, or agitation and address causes
D) Ignore the behavior

Question 31: Which finding indicates successful cricothyroidotomy?

A) Subcutaneous emphysema
B) Easy ventilation with chest rise and CO2 return
C) Bleeding from site
D) Difficulty advancing tube

Question 32: A patient's blood pressure is 88/62, heart rate 118, with cool extremities. The primary concern is:

A) Pain
B) Anxiety
C) Hemorrhagic shock
D) Neurogenic shock

Question 33: Pediatric trauma differs from adult trauma in that children:

A) Never develop shock
B) Compensate longer but decompensate suddenly
C) Always need surgery
D) Don't need fluid resuscitation

Question 34: The "golden hour" in trauma refers to:

A) Exact 60 minutes from injury
B) Critical early period when intervention most impacts survival
C) Time from 911 call to hospital
D) First hour in the emergency department

Question 35: A patient with suspected cardiac tamponade should be positioned:

A) Flat or slightly elevated to optimize venous return
B) Trendelenburg
C) High Fowler's
D) Prone

Question 36: Which assessment finding requires immediate chest tube placement?

A) Minor rib fracture pain
B) Tension pneumothorax after needle decompression
C) Mild hemoptysis
D) Chest wall contusion

Question 37: The AVPU scale assesses:

A) Pupil size
B) Level of consciousness
C) Pain intensity
D) Blood pressure

Question 38: A patient with severe facial trauma and airway compromise may require:

A) Nasotracheal intubation
B) Surgical airway (cricothyroidotomy)
C) Bag-valve-mask only
D) Nasal cannula oxygen

Question 39: Which medication should be avoided in hypovolemic shock?

A) Vasopressors before adequate volume resuscitation
B) Crystalloids
C) Blood products
D) Antibiotics

Question 40: A patient develops sudden hypotension after central line placement. This suggests:

A) Sepsis
B) Tension pneumothorax from procedure
C) Normal response
D) Anxiety

Question 41: The appropriate needle size for needle decompression is:

A) 18-20 gauge
B) 14-16 gauge
C) 22 gauge
D) Any size

Question 42: Which patient requires emergent dialysis?

A) Creatinine 1.5 mg/dL
B) Potassium 7.2 mEq/L with peaked T waves
C) Sodium 132 mEq/L
D) Glucose 150 mg/dL

Question 43: A trauma patient suddenly becomes agitated and confused. The first assessment should be:

A) Psychiatric evaluation
B) Oxygen saturation and perfusion status
C) Blood alcohol level
D) Social work consultation

Question 44: The purpose of log rolling a trauma patient is to:

A) Make them comfortable
B) Examine posterior while maintaining spinal alignment
C) Change sheets
D) Prevent pressure ulcers only

Question 45: Which intervention is appropriate for patient with severe epistaxis after facial trauma?

A) Have patient tilt head back
B) Apply pressure to bridge of nose, lean forward, ice
C) Insert nasopharyngeal airway
D) Lie patient flat

Question 46: A patient with suspected pneumothorax should have chest tube inserted:

A) In the 2nd intercostal space, midclavicular line
B) In the 4th-5th intercostal space, "safe triangle"
C) At the site of rib fracture
D) Wherever is easiest

Question 47: The primary complication of hypothermia in trauma is:

A) Shivering
B) Discomfort
C) Coagulopathy impairing clotting
D) Fever

Question 48: A patient's pupils are bilaterally dilated and non-reactive after head trauma. This indicates:

A) Normal response to light
B) Severe brainstem injury or herniation
C) Opiate administration
D) Cataracts

Question 49: Which injury pattern suggests child abuse?

A) Single bruise on shin
B) Fractures at different healing stages with inconsistent history
C) Skinned knee
D) Minor abrasion

Question 50: The most appropriate initial fluid bolus for adult trauma patient in shock is:

A) 500 mL crystalloid
B) 1-2 liters crystalloid rapidly
C) 100 mL crystalloid
D) Blood products only

Question 51: A patient with inhalation injury should be intubated:

A) Never
B) Prophylactically before airway edema makes it impossible
C) Only after respiratory failure
D) Only if burns >50% TBSA

Question 52: Which statement about organ donation is correct?

A) Trauma patients cannot be organ donors
B) Family must bring up donation
C) Designated requestor should discuss donation after death determination
D) Organ donation always delays care

Question 53: The appropriate management for mild traumatic brain injury (concussion) includes:

A) Immediate return to normal activities
B) Graduated return to activity with symptom monitoring
C) Bed rest for 6 months
D) No follow-up needed

Question 54: A patient receiving massive transfusion should be monitored for:

A) Hypernatremia
B) Hypocalcemia from citrate in blood products

C) Hyperglycemia only
D) Hypokalemia

Question 55: The appropriate assessment for potential spinal cord injury includes:

A) Asking about pain only
B) Complete motor and sensory exam of all extremities
C) Reflex testing only
D) MRI immediately

Question 56: Which medication reverses opioid-induced respiratory depression?

A) Flumazenil
B) Naloxone
C) Atropine
D) Epinephrine

Question 57: A patient with severe burns requires:

A) Oral fluids only
B) IV fluid resuscitation based on burn size and weight
C) No fluids for first 24 hours
D) Minimal fluids to avoid overload

Question 58: The most common long bone fracture in adults is:

A) Humerus
B) Femur
C) Radius
D) Tibia

Question 59: A patient develops paradoxical chest wall movement after trauma. This indicates:

A) Normal breathing
B) Flail chest from multiple rib fractures
C) Pneumothorax
D) Anxiety

Question 60: Which patient should be transported to a burn center?

A) Superficial burn 5% TBSA
B) Partial-thickness burn 15% TBSA in adult
C) Minor first-degree sunburn
D) Small blister on finger

Question 61: The appropriate position for shock patient (without spinal injury) is:

A) Sitting upright
B) Supine or legs elevated if tolerated
C) Prone
D) Trendelenburg (head down)

Question 62: A patient's Glasgow Coma Scale decreases from 15 to 10 over 2 hours. This requires:

A) Routine monitoring
B) Immediate evaluation for expanding intracranial hemorrhage
C) Observation for 24 hours
D) No intervention

Question 63: The most common organism causing infection in trauma patients is:

A) Virus
B) Fungus
C) Bacteria (Staphylococcus and gram-negatives)
D) Parasite

Question 64: A patient with gunshot wound to chest has absent breath sounds on right. The immediate intervention is:

A) Wait for chest X-ray
B) Chest tube placement
C) CT scan
D) Antibiotics only

Question 65: Which finding indicates adequate pain management?

A) Patient reports 0/10 pain
B) Patient comfortable with acceptable pain level and can participate in care
C) Patient sleeping continuously
D) Patient not asking for medication

Question 66: The appropriate method to clear cervical spine in obtunded patient is:

A) Clinical exam only
B) CT scan of cervical spine
C) Patient report
D) No imaging needed

Question 67: A patient with electrical injury should be monitored for:

A) Superficial burns only
B) Cardiac dysrhythmias and deep tissue injury
C) Nothing specific
D) Infection only

Question 68: The primary purpose of rehabilitation after trauma is:

A) Preventing hospital readmission
B) Maximizing functional recovery and independence
C) Reducing hospital costs
D) Satisfying insurance requirements

Question 69: A patient develops sudden dyspnea and chest pain 3 days post-trauma. This suggests:

A) Anxiety
B) Pulmonary embolism
C) Rib fracture pain
D) Pneumonia

Question 70: Which laboratory value indicates acute kidney injury?

A) Glucose 110 mg/dL
B) Rising creatinine and decreased urine output
C) Sodium 140 mEq/L
D) Normal potassium

Question 71: The appropriate initial management of open fracture includes:

A) Immediate casting
B) Covering with sterile dressing, antibiotics, tetanus prophylaxis
C) Letting wound air dry
D) Immediate ambulation

Question 72: A patient with head injury should avoid:

A) Adequate oxygenation
B) Hypotension and hypoxia
C) Pain management
D) Monitoring

Question 73: Which finding suggests basilar skull fracture?

A) Forehead laceration
B) CSF otorrhea and Battle's sign
C) Scalp hematoma
D) Facial abrasion

Question 74: The most appropriate pain assessment tool for nonverbal trauma patient is:

A) Numeric rating scale
B) Behavioral pain scale or observation
C) No assessment needed
D) Verbal descriptor scale

Question 75: A patient with spinal cord injury at T4 level will have:

A) Quadriplegia
B) Paraplegia
C) No deficits
D) Only arm weakness

Question 76: Which intervention prevents pressure injuries in trauma patients?

A) Keeping patient completely still
B) Regular turning and pressure redistribution
C) Applying extra padding only
D) Waiting until injuries heal

Question 77: A patient develops decreased urine output despite fluid resuscitation. The next step is:

A) Give more fluids
B) Assess for urethral injury, bladder dysfunction, or acute kidney injury
C) Wait 24 hours
D) Ignore finding

Question 78: The appropriate management for traumatic amputation includes:

A) Attempting replantation for all amputations
B) Controlling hemorrhage, preserving part properly, evaluating for replantation
C) Discarding amputated part
D) Immediate closure without evaluation

Question 79: Which patient requires immediate surgical intervention?

A) Stable patient with minor laceration
B) Unstable patient with ruptured spleen and ongoing hemorrhage
C) Patient with healed fracture
D) Patient with resolved pneumothorax

Question 80: The primary goal in disaster triage is:

A) Optimal individual care
B) Doing the most good for the most people
C) Treating immediate category only
D) Ignoring minor injuries

Question 81: A patient's ICP reading is 28 mmHg. This indicates:

A) Normal pressure
B) Elevated ICP requiring intervention
C) Low pressure
D) Measurement error

Question 82: Which medication is appropriate for procedural sedation during fracture reduction?

A) Insulin
B) Fentanyl and midazolam
C) Antibiotics only
D) Aspirin

Question 83: The appropriate initial management of suspected spinal cord injury includes:

A) Immediate surgery
B) Spinal immobilization and preventing secondary injury
C) Hyperextension of spine
D) No specific interventions

Question 84: A patient with severe bleeding should receive:

A) Crystalloids only
B) Blood products with balanced ratios
C) No fluids
D) Dextrose solutions

Question 85: Which assessment indicates effective bag-valve-mask ventilation?

A) No chest rise
B) Chest rise, oxygen saturation improving, CO2 detected
C) Gurgling sounds
D) Cyanosis worsening

Question 86: The most common cause of preventable in-hospital trauma death is:

A) Missed injuries
B) Infection
C) Equipment failure
D) Medication errors

Question 87: A patient with abdominal trauma develops sudden hypotension and rigid abdomen. This suggests:

A) Constipation
B) Intra-abdominal hemorrhage or perforation
C) Urinary retention
D) Normal finding

Question 88: The appropriate needle insertion site for pericardiocentesis is:

A) Left 5th intercostal space
B) Subxiphoid approach directed toward left shoulder
C) Right sternal border
D) Suprasternal notch

Question 89: Which intervention reduces ventilator-associated pneumonia risk?

A) Keeping head of bed flat
B) Elevating head of bed 30-45 degrees
C) Never suctioning
D) Discontinuing all nutrition

Question 90: A trauma patient's family is distressed. The appropriate nursing action is:

A) Ignore family
B) Provide information, support, and facilitate presence when appropriate
C) Ask family to leave
D) Focus only on patient

Question 91: Which finding suggests compartment syndrome in lower leg?

A) Mild soreness
B) Severe pain with passive dorsiflexion of foot
C) No symptoms
D) Palpable pulses only

Question 92: The appropriate management of suspected elder abuse includes:

A) Ignoring concerns
B) Reporting to appropriate authorities and ensuring safety
C) Confronting family only
D) Sending patient home

Question 93: A patient with chest tube develops sudden respiratory distress and subcutaneous emphysema. This suggests:

A) Normal finding
B) Tube dislodgement or air leak
C) Infection
D) Pain only

Question 94: Which laboratory value indicates transfusion reaction?

A) Normal temperature
B) Hemoglobinuria and fever
C) Stable vital signs
D) Normal potassium

Question 95: The appropriate management of avulsed tooth includes:

A) Discarding tooth
B) Preserving in milk or saline and seeking dental care
C) Attempting immediate reimplantation without evaluation
D) Cleaning with alcohol

Question 96: A patient develops acute onset of severe back pain after fall. This suggests:

A) Muscle strain only
B) Possible spinal fracture requiring imaging
C) Normal soreness
D) No intervention needed

Question 97: Which intervention prevents deep vein thrombosis in trauma patients?

A) Complete bed rest
B) Sequential compression devices and/or pharmacologic prophylaxis
C) Avoiding all movement
D) No prophylaxis needed

Question 98: The most appropriate initial imaging for suspected hollow viscus injury is:

A) Ultrasound
B) CT scan with oral and IV contrast
C) Plain X-rays only
D) MRI

Question 99: A patient with traumatic brain injury develops diabetes insipidus. This indicates:

A) Pancreatic injury
B) Pituitary dysfunction from brain injury
C) Kidney stones
D) Normal response

Question 100: Which medication is appropriate for agitation in intubated trauma patient?

A) Nothing - ignore agitation
B) Sedation after ruling out hypoxia and pain
C) Restraints only
D) Extubation

Question 101: The appropriate management of penetrating neck injury with hard signs includes:

A) Observation only
B) Immediate surgical exploration
C) CT scan and delay
D) Discharge home

Question 102: A patient's end-tidal CO2 suddenly drops to zero. This indicates:

A) Normal finding
B) Tube dislodgement, obstruction, or cardiac arrest
C) Hyperventilation
D) Adequate ventilation

Question 103: Which finding indicates transfusion-related acute lung injury (TRALI)?

A) Normal oxygenation
B) Acute hypoxemia and bilateral infiltrates during transfusion
C) Stable vital signs
D) No respiratory symptoms

Question 104: The appropriate position for patient with maxillofacial trauma and bleeding is:

A) Supine flat to prevent aspiration
B) Sitting upright or lateral to prevent aspiration
C) Prone
D) Trendelenburg

Question 105: A patient develops oliguria (<0.5 mL/kg/hr) despite resuscitation. This suggests:

A) Normal kidney function
B) Inadequate perfusion or acute kidney injury
C) Overhydration
D) No concern

Question 106: The most common cause of hypoxia in trauma patients is:

A) Pneumonia
B) Airway obstruction or inadequate ventilation
C) Cardiac arrest
D) Anemia only

Question 107: Which intervention is appropriate for hypothermic trauma patient?

A) Cold fluids
B) Warming interventions (warm fluids, warming devices, warm room)
C) Ice packs
D) Keeping patient wet

Question 108: A patient with pelvic fracture has blood at urethral meatus. The appropriate diagnostic test is:

A) Attempting Foley placement
B) Retrograde urethrogram
C) Cystoscopy immediately
D) No testing needed

Question 109: The appropriate management of snake bite includes:

A) Tourniquet and ice
B) Immobilization, supportive care, antivenom if indicated

C) Cutting and sucking venom
D) Applying heat

Question 110: Which patient requires helicopter transport?

A) Stable patient 10 miles away
B) Severe multi-system trauma 75 miles from Level I center
C) Minor laceration
D) Resolved symptoms

Question 111: A patient develops sudden vision loss after facial trauma. This suggests:

A) Normal response
B) Retrobulbar hemorrhage or globe injury requiring urgent evaluation
C) Fatigue
D) No intervention needed

Question 112: The appropriate management of impaled object in eye includes:

A) Removing object
B) Stabilizing object, protecting eye, immediate ophthalmology consultation
C) Applying pressure to eye
D) Flushing vigorously

Question 113: Which finding indicates successful tube thoracostomy?

A) Continued respiratory distress
B) Chest re-expansion, drainage, improved oxygenation
C) No drainage
D) Worsening hypotension

Question 114: A patient develops stridor immediately after extubation. The appropriate intervention is:

A) Observation only
B) Racemic epinephrine and preparation for reintubation
C) Discharge home
D) Antibiotics only

Question 115: The most common site for pressure injury in immobilized trauma patient is:

A) Elbow
B) Sacrum and heels
C) Forehead
D) Hands

Question 116: Which intervention prevents catheter-associated urinary tract infection?

A) Leaving catheter in indefinitely
B) Removing catheter as soon as not needed
C) Never emptying drainage bag
D) Breaking sterile technique

Question 117: A patient with chemical burn should receive:

A) No treatment
B) Copious water irrigation after removing contaminated clothing
C) Application of neutralizing agent
D) Covering without irrigation

Question 118: The appropriate management of tension pneumothorax in pregnant patient is:

A) No intervention
B) Needle decompression in higher intercostal space due to elevated diaphragm
C) Observation only
D) Immediate delivery

Question 119: Which assessment indicates adequate perfusion?

A) Weak pulses, confusion
B) Strong pulses, alert mental status, adequate urine output
C) Hypotension
D) Cool extremities

Question 120: A patient with abdominal trauma refuses surgery despite life-threatening injuries. The appropriate response is:

A) Forcing treatment
B) Assessing decision-making capacity and respecting informed refusal if patient competent
C) Ignoring patient wishes
D) Discharging immediately without discussion

Question 121: The primary purpose of damage control resuscitation is:

A) Definitive treatment
B) Temporary hemorrhage control and correction of lethal triad
C) Complete repair of all injuries
D) Avoiding surgery

Question 122: Which finding suggests meningitis in trauma patient?

A) Headache only
B) Fever, nuchal rigidity, altered mental status
C) Normal neurological exam
D) No symptoms

Question 123: The appropriate management of ruptured globe includes:

A) Applying pressure to eye
B) Eye shield without pressure, NPO, immediate ophthalmology consultation
C) Flushing eye vigorously
D) Discharging home

Question 124: A patient develops acute onset facial droop and slurred speech after head trauma. This suggests:

A) Normal response
B) Stroke or intracranial hemorrhage requiring immediate imaging
C) Anxiety
D) No concern

Question 125: The most important factor in trauma patient outcomes is:

A) Hospital size
B) Time to appropriate definitive care
C) Patient's insurance
D) Day of week

End of Practice Exam 2 Questions

Next Steps:

Score your exam

Review the answer key on the following pages

Identify patterns in missed questions

Compare performance to Practice Exam 1 if taken

Focus continued study on areas needing improvement

Practice Exam 2 - Complete Answer Key with Explanations

How to Use This Answer Key

Welcome to the complete answer explanations for Practice Exam 2. This isn't just an answer key—it's a learning tool designed to deepen your understanding of trauma nursing concepts.

For each question:

Review the correct answer and understand why it's right

Identify why incorrect options are wrong

Connect the concept to clinical practice

Note any patterns in questions you missed

Compare your performance: If you took Practice Exam 1, compare scores to track improvement. Consistent performance indicates solid understanding. Improvement shows your study is working. Persistent weak areas need focused review.

Remember: Missing questions isn't failure—it's identifying exactly what you need to review. Every question, right or wrong, teaches you something valuable for exam day.

Let's review your answers and strengthen your knowledge.

Answer Key with Detailed Explanations

Question 1: B - Apply direct pressure to control hemorrhage

Explanation: In the primary survey, Circulation assessment includes immediate hemorrhage control. Active arterial bleeding is immediately life-threatening and takes priority. Direct pressure is the fastest, most effective initial intervention. While IV access, vital signs, and pain management are important, they come after controlling life-threatening bleeding. Remember: You can't resuscitate a patient who's actively hemorrhaging—stop the bleeding first.

Question 2: B - Immediate endotracheal intubation

Explanation: GCS ≤8 indicates severe traumatic brain injury with inability to protect the airway, requiring immediate intubation. This secures the airway, prevents aspiration, and allows controlled ventilation for ICP management. While CT scan, neurosurgery consultation, and mannitol will be needed, securing the airway is the first priority. A patient who can't protect their airway will die before you can treat their brain injury.

Question 3: D - Full-thickness (third-degree)

Explanation: Full-thickness burns destroy both epidermis and dermis, appearing white, brown, or black with a leathery texture. They're insensate (no pain) because nerve endings are destroyed. Superficial burns are red and painful. Superficial partial-thickness are blistered and very painful. Deep partial-thickness are white/red with decreased sensation. Full-thickness burns require grafting for healing.

Question 4: C - Angiography with embolization or preperitoneal packing

Explanation: Pelvic fracture patients with persistent hypotension despite binder and resuscitation need definitive hemorrhage control. Options include angiography with embolization (for arterial bleeding) or preperitoneal packing in OR (for venous bleeding). More crystalloid won't stop ongoing bleeding. CT delays definitive treatment in unstable patients. This patient needs hemorrhage control now.

Question 5: B - Life-threatening condition is identified requiring immediate intervention

Explanation: The primary survey is interrupted only when a life-threatening condition requiring immediate intervention is identified. For example, if you discover tension pneumothorax during breathing assessment, you stop to perform needle decompression before continuing. You don't interrupt for tests, family arrivals, or routine movement. The systematic approach prevents missing life threats, but identified problems are treated immediately.

Question 6: B - Hypertension, bradycardia, irregular respirations

Explanation: Cushing's triad indicates critically elevated ICP: hypertension with widened pulse pressure (body trying to perfuse brain), bradycardia (vagal response), and irregular respirations (brainstem compression). This late sign indicates impending herniation requiring immediate intervention. Normal vital signs with headache might be benign. Hypotension and tachycardia suggest shock, not increased ICP.

Question 7: B - Non-operative management with close monitoring

Explanation: Hemodynamically stable patients with Grade I-II splenic lacerations are typically managed non-operatively with ICU monitoring, serial exams, and serial hemoglobin checks. Most low-grade splenic injuries stop bleeding spontaneously. Preserving the spleen maintains immune function. Surgery is reserved for unstable patients or those who fail conservative management. Success rate for non-operative management of Grade II injuries is >90%.

Question 8: C - Urine output 0.5-1 mL/kg/hr

Explanation: Urine output is one of the best indicators of adequate tissue perfusion. Normal output (0.5-1 mL/kg/hr, approximately 30-50 mL/hr for average adult) indicates kidneys are adequately perfused, reflecting whole-body perfusion. Blood pressure and heart rate can be misleading—compensatory mechanisms maintain them despite inadequate perfusion. Temperature doesn't directly measure perfusion. Urine output reflects end-organ perfusion.

Question 9: B - Clinical clearance without imaging

Explanation: Alert, oriented patients with no midline cervical tenderness, no neurological deficits, no intoxication, and no distracting injuries can have cervical spine cleared clinically without imaging. All criteria must be met. If any criterion fails, imaging (CT scan preferred) is required. This evidence-based approach reduces unnecessary imaging while maintaining safety.

Question 10: C - ≥1500 mL or one-third blood volume

Explanation: Massive hemothorax is defined as ≥1500 mL blood in chest cavity or one-third of patient's blood volume. This amount compromises both breathing (lung compression) and circulation (hemorrhagic shock). Treatment requires large-bore chest tube for drainage, fluid resuscitation, and often surgical intervention if bleeding continues. Smaller amounts are significant but don't meet "massive" criteria.

Question 11: B - Sciatic or common peroneal nerve

Explanation: Foot drop (inability to dorsiflex foot) results from sciatic nerve injury or common peroneal nerve injury (branch of sciatic). Sciatic nerve is injured with posterior hip dislocation or proximal femur fracture. Common peroneal nerve wraps around fibular head and is injured with knee trauma or proximal fibula fracture. Patients can't lift foot and drag toes when walking.

Question 12: B - Leave knife in place and transport to OR

Explanation: Impaled objects should never be removed in the field or ED—they may be tamponading bleeding vessels. Leave object in place, stabilize it to prevent movement, and transport to OR where it can be removed under controlled conditions with immediate ability to control hemorrhage if needed. Removing impaled objects outside the OR has caused fatal exsanguination.

Question 13: B - After the primary survey is complete

Explanation: The secondary survey (head-to-toe examination) begins only after the primary survey is complete and immediate life threats are addressed. The primary survey identifies and treats conditions that will kill the patient in minutes. Once those are managed, the detailed secondary survey identifies all other injuries. Never skip the primary survey or start the secondary survey during resuscitation of unstable patients.

Question 14: B - GCS 12 after head trauma

Explanation: GCS ≤13 is a Step 1 physiologic criterion requiring trauma center transport per CDC field triage guidelines. This altered mental status indicates potential serious brain injury requiring trauma center resources. Isolated extremity fractures, minor vehicle damage without injuries, and minor abrasions don't meet trauma center criteria.

Question 15: B - At least 2 inches (5 cm)

Explanation: Current CPR guidelines recommend chest compression depth of at least 2 inches (5 cm) in adults, with rate of 100-120 compressions per minute. Adequate depth is critical for generating forward blood flow. Too shallow compressions are ineffective. Allow complete chest recoil between compressions. Minimize interruptions—continuous quality compressions save lives.

Question 16: B - CT scan to characterize injuries

Explanation: Stable patients with positive FAST (free fluid indicating bleeding) should undergo CT scan to identify specific organ injuries, grade severity, and guide management decisions. Immediate surgery is for unstable patients. Observation alone misses the opportunity to define injuries. CT determines whether non-operative management is appropriate or surgery is needed. Stable patients have time for detailed evaluation.

Question 17: B - Mannitol or hypertonic saline

Explanation: Mannitol (osmotic diuretic) or hypertonic saline reduce ICP by creating osmotic gradient that pulls fluid from brain tissue into blood vessels. Mannitol: 0.25-1 g/kg IV bolus. Hypertonic saline: 3% or 23.4% solutions. Monitor serum osmolality—keep <320 mOsm/L. These are first-line medical treatments for elevated ICP. Furosemide alone isn't appropriate. Dopamine is a vasopressor. Morphine can worsen ICP.

Question 18: B - False - leave in place until surgical evaluation

Explanation: Never loosen tourniquets to "check if still needed"—this restarts bleeding and defeats the purpose. Once applied, tourniquets stay in place until surgical evaluation. Document time of application. Modern evidence shows properly applied tourniquets are safe for several hours. Loosening risks uncontrolled bleeding and tourniquet failure. Remove only in controlled OR setting.

Question 19: C - Hypovolemic from hemorrhage

Explanation: Hypovolemic shock from hemorrhage is by far the most common cause of shock in trauma patients. In trauma, assume shock is from bleeding until proven otherwise. Cardiogenic, neurogenic, and septic shock occur but are much less common in acute trauma. The most common mistake is attributing shock to other causes when the patient is simply bleeding.

Question 20: A - Keep spine aligned in neutral position

Explanation: During log roll, maintain spine in neutral alignment—no flexion, extension, or rotation. One person controls the head, maintaining alignment with body. Others roll patient as a unit. This prevents secondary spinal cord injury. Hyperextension, hip flexion, or twisting at waist can worsen spinal injuries. The entire spine moves as one piece.

Question 21: B - Developing airway edema requiring urgent evaluation

Explanation: Stridor (high-pitched breath sound) developing hours after neck trauma indicates progressive airway edema and impending obstruction. This is an airway emergency. The patient needs immediate evaluation, preparation for intubation, and possibly fiberoptic intubation or surgical airway. Delaying intervention risks complete airway obstruction requiring emergent cricothyroidotomy. Airway edema worsens over time—act before it's too late.

Question 22: B - 15-30% blood volume

Explanation: Class II hemorrhagic shock: 15-30% blood loss (750-1500 mL in adults). Signs include tachycardia (100-120 bpm), narrowed pulse pressure, mild anxiety, cool extremities. Blood pressure usually remains normal due to compensatory mechanisms. Treatment: crystalloid fluids usually sufficient. Class I: <15%, Class III: 30-40%, Class IV: >40%.

Question 23: B - Left lateral tilt or manual uterine displacement

Explanation: After 20 weeks gestation, the gravid uterus compresses the inferior vena cava when supine, decreasing venous return and cardiac output. Position pregnant trauma patients in left lateral tilt (15-30 degrees) or manually displace uterus to the left. This relieves IVC compression while allowing spinal precautions if needed. Supine positioning can cause supine hypotensive syndrome.

Question 24: D - 1-3 hours

Explanation: Open fractures require immediate IV antibiotics (within 1-3 hours ideally) to prevent infection. Bacterial contamination occurs at time of injury. Early antibiotics significantly reduce infection rates. First-generation cephalosporin for Type I-II, add aminoglycoside for Type III. Also give tetanus prophylaxis and plan surgical debridement within 6-8 hours. Delayed antibiotics increase osteomyelitis risk.

Question 25: B - Elevated creatine kinase (CK)

Explanation: Rhabdomyolysis (muscle breakdown) from crush injury, electrical burns, or prolonged immobilization causes markedly elevated creatine kinase (CK), often >5,000-10,000 U/L. Other findings: myoglobinuria (dark tea-colored urine), hyperkalemia, hypocalcemia, metabolic acidosis. Myoglobin damages kidneys causing acute renal failure. Treatment: aggressive IV hydration, maintain high urine output, monitor electrolytes.

Question 26: C - 60-70 mmHg or higher

Explanation: Cerebral perfusion pressure (CPP = MAP - ICP) should be maintained at 60-70 mmHg or higher in severe TBI to ensure adequate brain blood flow. CPP <60 mmHg indicates inadequate cerebral perfusion causing secondary brain injury. Treatment focuses on maintaining adequate MAP (through blood pressure support) and reducing ICP (through positioning, osmotic therapy, sedation, sometimes surgery).

Question 27: A - Deep breathing and coughing

Explanation: Rib fracture patients should NOT avoid deep breathing and coughing—they need adequate pain control TO ALLOW deep breathing and coughing. Splinting (shallow breathing to avoid pain) leads to atelectasis and pneumonia. The goal is aggressive pain management (opioids, nerve blocks, epidural) that enables effective pulmonary toilet. Incentive spirometry, deep breathing, and early mobilization all prevent complications.

Question 28: B - Cervical collar, backboard, and head blocks

Explanation: Complete spinal immobilization requires all three: rigid cervical collar, backboard (or vacuum splint/scoop stretcher), and head blocks with straps. Collar alone provides inadequate immobilization. Use minimal movement to place on backboard, then secure with straps across forehead and collar. Remove from backboard as soon as safely possible to prevent pressure injuries.

Question 29: B - Normal blood pressure with tachycardia and poor perfusion

Explanation: Children compensate remarkably well for blood loss, maintaining blood pressure through vasoconstriction and tachycardia much longer than adults. Compensated shock in children shows tachycardia, delayed capillary refill, cool extremities, but normal BP. When BP finally drops (decompensated shock), they crash suddenly. Don't wait for hypotension to recognize shock in children—tachycardia and poor perfusion signs indicate shock requiring aggressive intervention.

Question 30: C - Assess for hypoxia, pain, or agitation and address causes

Explanation: Patients pulling at ET tubes ("self-extubation attempts") are usually hypoxic, in pain, or inadequately sedated—they're not being difficult. First assess: Is patient hypoxic (check sat, ventilator)? In pain (treat pain)? Inadequately sedated (adjust sedation)? Appropriately responding (may be ready to extubate)? Never immediately extubate or apply restraints without assessment. Address underlying cause.

Question 31: B - Easy ventilation with chest rise and CO_2 return

Explanation: Successful cricothyroidotomy is confirmed by easy ventilation with bag-valve device, visible chest rise, breath sounds bilaterally, and end-tidal CO_2 detection. Subcutaneous emphysema suggests placement outside trachea. Bleeding is concerning. Difficulty advancing tube may indicate incorrect placement. If ventilation is difficult or CO2 absent, reassess position—may need to remove and re-attempt.

Question 32: C - Hemorrhagic shock

Explanation: Hypotension, tachycardia, and cool extremities are classic signs of hypovolemic (hemorrhagic) shock. Peripheral vasoconstriction causes cool skin. This patient is in Class III shock requiring immediate intervention: hemorrhage control, IV access, blood products. Pain and anxiety don't cause sustained hypotension with cool skin. Neurogenic shock shows warm skin, not cool.

Question 33: B - Compensate longer but decompensate suddenly

Explanation: Children's physiology allows them to compensate for blood loss longer than adults through robust vasoconstriction and tachycardia, maintaining blood pressure despite significant volume loss. However, when compensation fails, they decompensate suddenly and dramatically. This makes early recognition crucial—don't wait for hypotension. Tachycardia, poor perfusion, and altered mental status indicate shock requiring immediate aggressive resuscitation.

Question 34: B - Critical early period when intervention most impacts survival

Explanation: The "golden hour" is a concept (not a literal 60 minutes) representing the critical early period after injury when rapid assessment and appropriate intervention most significantly impact survival. It emphasizes importance of minimizing time from injury to definitive care. Some injuries (exsanguinating hemorrhage) have shorter windows; others allow more time. The principle is rapid recognition and treatment of life threats.

Question 35: A - Flat or slightly elevated to optimize venous return

Explanation: Cardiac tamponade patients need adequate venous return to maximize cardiac filling despite pericardial compression. Position flat or slightly elevated (15-30 degrees). Trendelenburg may worsen respiratory compromise. High Fowler's decreases venous return. Supine positioning optimizes preload while preparing for pericardiocentesis. Aggressive fluid resuscitation before decompression helps temporarily but definitive treatment is removing pericardial blood.

Question 36: B - Tension pneumothorax after needle decompression

Explanation: After needle decompression of tension pneumothorax, chest tube placement is immediate next step for definitive treatment. Needle decompression is temporizing—it converts tension to simple pneumothorax but doesn't provide ongoing drainage. Chest tube in "safe triangle" (4th-5th intercostal space) allows complete lung re-expansion and continuous drainage. Minor rib fracture pain doesn't need chest tube.

Question 37: B - Level of consciousness

Explanation: AVPU scale rapidly assesses level of consciousness: Alert, responds to Verbal stimuli, responds to Painful stimuli, Unresponsive. It's quicker than Glasgow Coma Scale for initial assessment. Alert patients are awake and oriented. Verbal response patients respond to voice. Pain response patients respond only to painful stimuli. Unresponsive patients don't respond to any stimuli. AVPU helps quickly identify decreased consciousness requiring intervention.

Question 38: B - Surgical airway (cricothyroidotomy)

Explanation: Severe facial trauma with airway compromise often precludes oral or nasal intubation due to distorted anatomy, bleeding, or edema. Surgical airway (cricothyroidotomy) may be necessary. Nasotracheal intubation is contraindicated in facial fractures (risk of intracranial placement if skull base fracture). BVM is temporary. Nasal cannula insufficient for airway compromise. Have low threshold for surgical airway in severe maxillofacial trauma.

Question 39: A - Vasopressors before adequate volume resuscitation

Explanation: Giving vasopressors to hypovolemic patients without adequate volume resuscitation is harmful—"clamping down empty vessels" worsens tissue perfusion and can cause end-organ damage. Hypovolemic shock requires volume replacement (crystalloids initially, then blood products). Vasopressors are for distributive shock (neurogenic, septic) after adequate volume. Give volume first, then consider vasopressors if still hypotensive after adequate resuscitation.

Question 40: B - Tension pneumothorax from procedure

Explanation: Sudden hypotension after central line placement suggests tension pneumothorax from inadvertent lung puncture during subclavian or internal jugular line insertion. Immediate assessment: breath sounds (decreased on affected side), respiratory distress, possibly tracheal deviation. Treat with needle decompression then chest tube. Chest X-ray confirms but don't delay treatment for imaging if high clinical suspicion. This is a known complication requiring immediate recognition and treatment.

Question 41: B - 14-16 gauge

Explanation: Needle decompression for tension pneumothorax requires 14-16 gauge catheter to ensure adequate air flow. Smaller needles may be too short (especially in obese/muscular patients) or may kink. Insert at 2nd intercostal space, midclavicular line, just above rib (avoiding neurovascular bundle below). Some guidelines now recommend longer needles (6-8 cm) or anterior axillary line placement for better success.

Question 42: B - Potassium 7.2 mEq/L with peaked T waves

Explanation: Severe hyperkalemia (K >6.5 mEq/L, especially >7 mEq/L) with ECG changes (peaked T waves, widened QRS, sine wave) is life-threatening cardiac emergency requiring emergent dialysis. Can cause fatal arrhythmias. Immediate treatment before dialysis: calcium gluconate (cardiac membrane stabilization), insulin with glucose (shift K intracellularly), possibly albuterol. Other values don't require emergent dialysis.

Question 43: B - Oxygen saturation and perfusion status

Explanation: Sudden agitation/confusion in trauma patients is hypoxia or hypoperfusion until proven otherwise. Immediately assess: Is patient adequately oxygenated? Perfusion adequate? These cause altered mental status more commonly than psychiatric issues or intoxication. Check airway patency, oxygen saturation, blood pressure, perfusion signs. Correct physiologic derangements before attributing behavior to other causes. Brain needs oxygen and blood flow.

Question 44: B - Examine posterior while maintaining spinal alignment

Explanation: Log rolling allows examination of entire posterior body surface (back, buttocks, posterior legs) while maintaining spinal alignment in patients with suspected spinal injury. One person controls head, others roll patient as unit. This prevents missed posterior injuries (penetrating wounds, pressure areas, fractures). Always log roll trauma patients during secondary survey—you can't assess what you can't see.

Question 45: B - Apply pressure to bridge of nose, lean forward, ice

Explanation: Severe epistaxis management: Have patient lean forward (prevents blood swallowing/aspiration), pinch soft part of nose firmly for 10-15 minutes without releasing, apply ice to bridge. Tilting head back causes blood to run down throat. NPAs can worsen bleeding. If bleeding continues, may need packing or ENT consultation. Severe facial trauma epistaxis may indicate skull base fracture requiring imaging.

Question 46: B - In the 4th-5th intercostal space, "safe triangle"

Explanation: Chest tubes are placed in "safe triangle" (4th-5th intercostal space, between anterior and posterior axillary lines) for pneumothorax or hemothorax. This location avoids major muscles, breast tissue, and provides good drainage. 2nd intercostal space is for needle decompression only. Never insert at rib fracture site (may extend injury). Safe triangle placement is standard technique.

Question 47: C - Coagulopathy impairing clotting

Explanation: Hypothermia's most dangerous effect in trauma is coagulopathy—clotting factors and platelets function poorly when cold, worsening bleeding. Hypothermia is part of "lethal triad" (hypothermia, acidosis, coagulopathy) dramatically increasing mortality. Also causes arrhythmias, decreased immune function, impaired drug metabolism. Prevent hypothermia: warm room, warm fluids, warming devices. Treat aggressively—maintaining temperature >35°C (95°F) is critical.

Question 48: B - Severe brainstem injury or herniation

Explanation: Bilateral dilated, non-reactive pupils after head trauma indicate severe brainstem injury or complete herniation—ominous sign with very poor prognosis. Both parasympathetic pathways (CN III) are affected. This differs from unilateral dilated pupil (uncal herniation with ipsilateral CN III compression). Bilateral suggests global brainstem dysfunction. Immediate neurosurgery consultation and aggressive ICP management, though prognosis is grave.

Question 49: B - Fractures at different healing stages with inconsistent history

Explanation: Multiple fractures at different healing stages (shown on X-ray) with history inconsistent with injuries strongly suggests non-accidental trauma (child abuse). Other red flags: injuries in non-mobile infants, delay seeking care, implausible mechanisms, spiral fractures in non-ambulatory children, pattern injuries (belt marks, grab marks), retinal hemorrhages. Healthcare providers are mandated reporters—report suspicions to child protective services.

Question 50: B - 1-2 liters crystalloid rapidly

Explanation: Initial resuscitation for adult trauma patients in shock: 1-2 liters crystalloid (Lactated Ringer's or normal saline) given rapidly (wide open). Reassess after each liter. If shock persists after 2 liters, begin blood products. Current evidence supports limiting crystalloid to prevent dilutional coagulopathy. 500 mL or 100 mL boluses are inadequate. Blood products are started if shock persists, but crystalloid is initial fluid.

Question 51: B - Prophylactically before airway edema makes it impossible

Explanation: Inhalation injury patients should be intubated prophylactically before progressive airway edema makes intubation impossible. Signs of inhalation injury: facial burns, singed nasal hair, carbonaceous sputum, hoarseness, stridor. Airway edema worsens over 24-48 hours. Early intubation (when still possible) is safer than waiting for respiratory failure when edema makes intubation extremely difficult or impossible, necessitating emergency cricothyroidotomy.

Question 52: C - Designated requestor should discuss donation after death determination

Explanation: Organ donation discussions should be conducted by trained designated requestors (organ procurement organization staff) after death has been determined and family has been informed. Separating roles (healthcare team determines death, OPO discusses donation) is more effective and ethical. Healthcare team focuses on saving life; OPO focuses on donation after death. Trauma patients can be organ donors. Donation doesn't delay necessary care for living patients.

Question 53: B - Graduated return to activity with symptom monitoring

Explanation: Mild TBI (concussion) management: Initial rest (24-48 hours), then graduated return to physical and cognitive activities guided by symptom tolerance. Return to play/work follows stepwise progression—if symptoms return at any level, drop back and advance more slowly. Most concussions resolve within days to weeks. Prolonged bed rest isn't beneficial. Patients need symptom monitoring, education about warning signs, and follow-up.

Question 54: B - Hypocalcemia from citrate in blood products

Explanation: Massive transfusion patients risk hypocalcemia because citrate (preservative in blood products) binds calcium. Signs: prolonged QT interval, hypotension, decreased cardiac contractility, tetany. Treatment: calcium chloride or calcium gluconate IV. Also monitor for hypothermia (cold blood products), hyperkalemia (K+ leaks from stored RBCs), acid-base disturbances, and dilutional coagulopathy. Give blood through fluid warmer when possible.

Question 55: B - Complete motor and sensory exam of all extremities

Explanation: Spinal cord injury assessment requires systematic evaluation of all extremities: motor function (strength testing in major muscle groups), sensory function (light touch, pain in dermatome distribution), reflexes (initially absent in spinal shock, later hyperactive). Also assess rectal tone, perianal sensation (sacral sparing indicates incomplete injury with better prognosis). Document exam carefully—baseline assessment guides detection of neurological changes.

Question 56: B - Naloxone

Explanation: Naloxone (Narcan) is opioid antagonist that rapidly reverses opioid-induced respiratory depression. Dose: 0.4-2 mg IV, titrated to effect. Can be repeated. Duration shorter than most opioids, so patient needs monitoring for recurrent depression. Flumazenil reverses benzodiazepines. Atropine treats bradycardia. Epinephrine treats anaphylaxis/cardiac arrest. For respiratory depression from opioids, naloxone is specific reversal agent.

Question 57: B - IV fluid resuscitation based on burn size and weight

Explanation: Severe burns require massive IV fluid resuscitation to replace fluid losses from damaged capillaries and evaporation. Parkland formula: 4 mL × kg × % TBSA burned over 24 hours (half in first 8 hours). Use Lactated Ringer's. Titrate to urine output 0.5-1 mL/kg/hr. Oral fluids inadequate. Withholding fluids causes hypovolemic shock and acute renal failure. Proper resuscitation is critical for survival.

Question 58: D - Tibia

Explanation: The tibia (shinbone) is the most commonly fractured long bone in adults because it's subcutaneous (minimal soft tissue protection) and vulnerable to direct trauma. Tibia fractures have high compartment syndrome risk due to tight fascial compartments. Open fractures are common because bone is just beneath skin. Management includes splinting, neurovascular monitoring, and often surgical fixation.

Question 59: B - Flail chest from multiple rib fractures

Explanation: Paradoxical chest wall movement (segment moves inward during inspiration, outward during expiration—opposite of normal) indicates flail chest: two or more adjacent ribs fractured in two or more places each, creating free-floating segment. Usually accompanied by underlying pulmonary contusion. Treatment: pain control, positive pressure ventilation if severe respiratory distress. Paradoxical motion impairs ventilation.

Question 60: B - Partial-thickness burn 15% TBSA in adult

Explanation: Burn center criteria include: partial-thickness burns >10% TBSA, full-thickness burns any size, burns to face/hands/feet/genitals/perineum/major joints, electrical/chemical burns, inhalation injury, burns with trauma, circumferential burns, burns in very young/old, burns in patients with comorbidities. 15% partial-thickness meets criteria for burn center transfer. Superficial burns <10% don't require burn center.

Question 61: B - Supine or legs elevated if tolerated

Explanation: Shock patients (without spinal injury) should be positioned supine or with legs elevated (if tolerated) to improve venous return and cardiac output. Sitting upright decreases venous return, worsening hypotension. Trendelenburg (head down) not recommended—doesn't improve outcomes and may worsen respiratory function. Prone is inappropriate. Simple supine positioning optimizes hemodynamics while allowing access for interventions.

Question 62: B - Immediate evaluation for expanding intracranial hemorrhage

Explanation: Declining GCS (drop of 2+ points) indicates neurological deterioration suggesting expanding intracranial hemorrhage, increased ICP, or herniation. This patient dropped 5 points (15 to 10)—significant decline requiring immediate CT scan, neurosurgery consultation, and interventions to reduce ICP. Never assume "wait and see" with declining neuro status—deterioration indicates evolving injury requiring urgent intervention.

Question 63: C - Bacteria (Staphylococcus and gram-negatives)

Explanation: Bacterial infections are most common in trauma patients, particularly Staphylococcus aureus (including MRSA) from skin flora and gram-negative bacteria (E. coli, Pseudomonas, Klebsiella) from environmental contamination or instrumentation. Open wounds, invasive lines, urinary catheters, and ventilators all create infection risk. Prevention: proper sterile technique, appropriate antibiotic prophylaxis, timely removal of devices, wound care.

Question 64: B - Chest tube placement

Explanation: Gunshot wound to chest with absent breath sounds indicates pneumothorax or hemothorax (or both) requiring immediate chest tube placement. Don't wait for chest X-ray if patient unstable or in respiratory distress—clinical diagnosis based on mechanism and exam is sufficient for intervention. CT scan would delay treatment. Antibiotics needed but chest tube is priority. Penetrating chest trauma with respiratory compromise needs immediate thoracic decompression.

Question 65: B - Patient comfortable with acceptable pain level and can participate in care

Explanation: Adequate pain management means patient reports acceptable pain level (not necessarily 0—that may require excessive sedation), can take deep breaths, cooperate with care, and maintain reasonable comfort. Goal isn't complete pain elimination but comfortable functionality. Continuous sleeping may indicate oversedation. Not asking for medication doesn't mean comfortable—some patients don't request help. Assess pain regularly using appropriate scales.

Question 66: B - CT scan of cervical spine

Explanation: Obtunded (altered mental status) trauma patients cannot reliably report pain or cooperate with clinical exam, so cervical spine clearance requires imaging. CT of cervical spine is standard—more sensitive than plain X-rays for bony injury. MRI may be needed if neurological deficits present with negative CT (to assess ligamentous injury). Clinical exam alone is insufficient when patient can't participate in assessment.

Question 67: B - Cardiac dysrhythmias and deep tissue injury

Explanation: Electrical injuries cause current flow through body along nerves, vessels, and muscles, creating deep tissue destruction far beyond surface appearance. Cardiac monitoring is mandatory—dysrhythmias can occur immediately or delayed. Also assess for compartment syndrome (deep muscle injury causes swelling), rhabdomyolysis, neurological deficits, and vascular injury. Small entry/exit wounds don't reflect internal damage extent.

Question 68: B - Maximizing functional recovery and independence

Explanation: Rehabilitation's primary goal is maximizing functional recovery and patient independence after trauma. This includes physical therapy (strength, mobility), occupational therapy (activities of daily living), speech therapy if needed, psychological support, and preparing for return to work/home. Early rehabilitation improves outcomes. While reducing readmissions and costs matter, the core purpose is restoring maximum function and quality of life.

Question 69: B - Pulmonary embolism

Explanation: Sudden dyspnea and chest pain days after trauma suggests pulmonary embolism (PE) from deep vein thrombosis. Trauma patients have high VTE risk from immobilization, vascular injury, and hypercoagulability. PE presents with sudden-onset dyspnea, chest pain, tachycardia, and hypoxemia. Diagnosis: CT pulmonary angiography. Treatment: anticoagulation. This is why VTE prophylaxis (compression devices, pharmacologic agents when safe) is critical in trauma patients.

Question 70: B - Rising creatinine and decreased urine output

Explanation: Acute kidney injury (AKI) is indicated by rising creatinine (>0.3 mg/dL increase from baseline) and decreased urine output (<0.5 mL/kg/hr for >6 hours). Causes in trauma: hypovolemia, rhabdomyolysis (myoglobin damages kidneys), nephrotoxic medications, direct renal injury. Treatment addresses underlying cause: fluid resuscitation for hypovolemia, aggressive hydration for rhabdomyolysis, possible dialysis for severe AKI.

Question 71: B - Covering with sterile dressing, antibiotics, tetanus prophylaxis

Explanation: Open fracture management: Cover wound with sterile saline-moistened dressing (protects from further contamination), start IV antibiotics immediately (within 1-3 hours), give tetanus prophylaxis, splint fracture, plan surgical irrigation/debridement within 6-8 hours. Never apply cast to open fracture without surgical treatment first. Never push protruding bone back in or let wound dry out.

Question 72: B - Hypotension and hypoxia

Explanation: Head injury patients must avoid hypotension (SBP <90 mmHg) and hypoxia (SpO2 <90%) as these worsen secondary brain injury by reducing cerebral oxygen delivery. Even brief episodes significantly increase mortality and morbidity. Maintain adequate blood pressure, oxygenation, and ventilation. Pain management and monitoring are important, but preventing hypotension/hypoxia is critical for neuroprotection.

Question 73: B - CSF otorrhea and Battle's sign

Explanation: Basilar skull fracture signs include CSF otorrhea (clear fluid from ear), CSF rhinorrhea (clear fluid from nose), Battle's sign (ecchymosis over mastoid), raccoon eyes (periorbital ecchymosis), and hemotympanum. These indicate skull base fracture with potential dural tear. Risk of meningitis if CSF leak present. Most CSF leaks resolve spontaneously, but some require surgical repair.

Question 74: B - Behavioral pain scale or observation

Explanation: Nonverbal patients (intubated, altered mental status, pediatric, cognitively impaired) need behavioral pain assessment tools like Behavioral Pain Scale (BPS), Critical-Care Pain Observation Tool (CPOT), or FLACC for children. These assess facial expression, body movements, muscle tension, ventilator compliance, and vocalizations. Numeric/verbal scales require patient communication. All patients deserve pain assessment and management.

Question 75: B - Paraplegia

Explanation: Spinal cord injury at T4 (thoracic level) causes paraplegia—paralysis of lower extremities and trunk below injury level. Upper extremities remain functional. Quadriplegia results from cervical injuries affecting all four extremities. Injury level determines which muscles function: higher injuries affect more body areas. T4 injury also affects trunk muscles and sympathetic nervous system control.

Question 76: B - Regular turning and pressure redistribution

Explanation: Preventing pressure injuries requires regular turning (every 2 hours minimum), pressure redistribution surfaces (specialized mattresses), keeping skin clean and dry, optimizing nutrition, and mobilizing as soon as safely possible. Keeping patients completely still causes pressure injuries. Extra padding alone insufficient. Pressure injury prevention starts immediately—don't wait for injuries to heal before implementing prevention strategies.

Question 77: B - Assess for urethral injury, bladder dysfunction, or acute kidney injury

Explanation: Decreased urine output despite adequate resuscitation requires systematic assessment: Is catheter functioning? (Check for kinks, blockage). Urethral injury? (Blood at meatus suggests don't force catheter). Bladder injury? (Unable to pass catheter, hematuria). Acute kidney injury? (Rising creatinine, other causes). Neurogenic bladder from spinal injury? Don't just give more fluids without determining cause of oliguria.

Question 78: B - Controlling hemorrhage, preserving part properly, evaluating for replantation

Explanation: Traumatic amputation priorities: Control hemorrhage (direct pressure, pressure dressing, tourniquet if needed), care for amputated part properly (wrap in saline-moistened gauze, place in sealed bag on ice—not directly on ice), transport patient and part to facility with replantation capability. Not all amputations are replantable (crush vs. clean mechanism, ischemia time, patient factors), but preserve part for surgical evaluation.

Question 79: B - Unstable patient with ruptured spleen and ongoing hemorrhage

Explanation: Hemodynamically unstable patients with ongoing hemorrhage from solid organ injury require immediate surgical intervention for hemorrhage control. This patient is actively dying from bleeding—surgery can't wait. Stable patients with minor injuries, healed fractures, or resolved conditions don't need emergency surgery. Emergency surgery indications: uncontrolled hemorrhage, peritonitis, expanding hematomas, vascular injuries.

Question 80: B - Doing the most good for the most people

Explanation: Disaster triage shifts from individual optimal care (routine nursing) to maximizing population benefit—doing the most good for the most people with limited resources. This requires difficult decisions: directing resources to salvageable patients rather than those unlikely to survive. It's ethically appropriate when resources are genuinely insufficient. Goal is saving maximum lives given resource constraints.

Question 81: B - Elevated ICP requiring intervention

Explanation: ICP 28 mmHg is significantly elevated (normal <10 mmHg, treat when >20 mmHg). This requires immediate intervention: elevate head of bed 30 degrees, ensure adequate sedation/analgesia, osmotic therapy (mannitol or hypertonic saline), maintain adequate MAP for cerebral perfusion, consider EVD placement if not already present, neurosurgery consultation. Sustained ICP >20 mmHg causes secondary brain injury.

Question 82: B - Fentanyl and midazolam

Explanation: Procedural sedation for fracture reduction typically uses combination of opioid (fentanyl for analgesia) and benzodiazepine (midazolam for anxiolysis and amnesia). Provides pain relief and sedation while maintaining spontaneous breathing. Requires monitoring (continuous pulse oximetry, capnography, blood pressure), reversal agents available (naloxone for fentanyl, flumazenil for midazolam), appropriate personnel, and equipment for airway management.

Question 83: B - Spinal immobilization and preventing secondary injury

Explanation: Initial spinal cord injury management focuses on immobilization (prevent further damage) and preventing secondary injury (maintain adequate blood pressure for spinal cord perfusion, avoid hypoxia, careful handling). High-dose steroids previously used but now controversial. Some injuries need surgical decompression/stabilization, but timing is individualized. Never hyperextend spine. Goal is preventing worsening of initial injury.

Question 84: B - Blood products with balanced ratios

Explanation: Severe bleeding requires blood products in balanced ratios (1:1:1 PRBCs:FFP:Platelets) to replace both oxygen-carrying capacity and clotting factors. Limit crystalloid to 1-2 liters to avoid dilutional coagulopathy. Give tranexamic acid within 3 hours. Dextrose solutions are inappropriate for hemorrhage. Crystalloid alone worsens outcomes in major hemorrhage. Massive transfusion protocol ensures rapid balanced product delivery.

Question 85: B - Chest rise, oxygen saturation improving, CO2 detected

Explanation: Effective bag-valve-mask ventilation is confirmed by visible chest rise with each breath, improving oxygen saturation, and end-tidal CO2 detection (confirms air reaching lungs). Adequate seal between mask and face essential. Rate should be 10-12 breaths/min for adults. No chest rise suggests inadequate seal, airway obstruction, or esophageal ventilation. Gurgling or worsening cyanosis indicate ineffective ventilation requiring troubleshooting.

Question 86: A - Missed injuries

Explanation: Missed injuries are the most common cause of preventable in-hospital trauma deaths. These occur when injuries aren't identified during initial evaluation, causing delayed diagnosis and treatment. Common missed injuries: hollow viscus perforations, diaphragm injuries, some fractures, vascular injuries. Prevention: systematic primary and secondary surveys, appropriate imaging, maintaining high suspicion, serial exams, and having structured tertiary survey process.

Question 87: B - Intra-abdominal hemorrhage or perforation

Explanation: Sudden hypotension with rigid abdomen in trauma patient indicates intra-abdominal catastrophe: hemorrhage from solid organ injury or peritonitis from hollow viscus perforation. Rigid abdomen (involuntary muscle spasm) indicates peritoneal irritation. This patient needs immediate surgical exploration. Don't delay for imaging if unstable. Peritonitis plus shock is absolute indication for emergency laparotomy.

Question 88: B - Subxiphoid approach directed toward left shoulder

Explanation: Pericardiocentesis uses subxiphoid approach: insert needle just below and left of xiphoid process, advance at 45-degree angle toward left shoulder while aspirating. ECG monitoring during procedure helps detect ventricular contact (ST elevation). Ultrasound guidance when available. Even small volume removal (20-30 mL) can dramatically improve hemodynamics in tamponade. Definitive treatment is surgical repair of cardiac injury.

Question 89: B - Elevating head of bed 30-45 degrees

Explanation: Ventilator-associated pneumonia (VAP) prevention bundle includes: head of bed elevation 30-45 degrees (reduces aspiration), daily sedation vacation and assessment of extubation readiness, peptic ulcer prophylaxis, DVT prophylaxis, oral care with chlorhexidine, maintaining endotracheal cuff pressure 20-30 cm H_2O. These evidence-based interventions significantly reduce VAP incidence.

Question 90: B - Provide information, support, and facilitate presence when appropriate

Explanation: Family-centered care in trauma includes keeping family informed (within HIPAA limits), providing emotional support, answering questions honestly, and facilitating family presence during resuscitation when appropriate (with dedicated support person). Research shows family presence during resuscitation doesn't interfere with care and helps families process the event. Balance family needs with patient care priorities.

Question 91: B - Severe pain with passive dorsiflexion of foot

Explanation: Compartment syndrome's most reliable early sign is severe pain with passive stretch of muscles in affected compartment. For lower leg anterior compartment syndrome, passive plantarflexion (stretching dorsiflexors) causes excruciating pain. Pain out of proportion to injury is cardinal sign. Palpable pulses don't rule out compartment syndrome—capillary pressure is exceeded long before arterial pressure. Early recognition prevents permanent disability.

Question 92: B - Reporting to appropriate authorities and ensuring safety

Explanation: Suspected elder abuse requires reporting to Adult Protective Services (or equivalent), documenting findings objectively, ensuring patient safety, and social work consultation. Healthcare providers are mandated reporters. Signs: unexplained injuries, poor hygiene, malnutrition, medications mismanaged, patient fearful of caregiver, injuries inconsistent with history. Never confront suspected abusers alone—this can endanger patient. Follow institutional protocols.

Question 93: B - Tube dislodgement or air leak

Explanation: Sudden respiratory distress and subcutaneous emphysema after chest tube placement suggests tube dislodgement (tube outside pleural space, allowing air into subcutaneous tissue) or significant air leak. Assess tube position, connections, and patient respiratory status. May need tube repositioning or replacement. Subcutaneous emphysema can be extensive but is concerning because it indicates air going where it shouldn't.

Question 94: B - Hemoglobinuria and fever

Explanation: Transfusion reactions present with fever, chills, hemoglobinuria (dark urine from hemolyzed red blood cells), back/flank pain, hypotension, and possibly DIC. Acute hemolytic reactions are most serious. If suspected: Stop transfusion immediately, maintain IV access with saline, notify blood bank and physician, send samples for testing, monitor urine output and kidney function, supportive care. Prevention requires meticulous attention to blood type matching.

Question 95: B - Preserving in milk or saline and seeking dental care

Explanation: Avulsed (completely knocked out) teeth can potentially be reimplanted if handled properly: Don't touch root surface, rinse gently with saline if dirty, place in milk (best) or saline, seek dental care immediately (within 30 minutes optimal). Some sources suggest attempting immediate reimplantation by holder, but professional evaluation is essential. Don't clean with alcohol or let tooth dry out.

Question 96: B - Possible spinal fracture requiring imaging

Explanation: Severe back pain after fall suggests possible spinal fracture. Mechanism (fall) and pain warrant imaging even without neurological deficits. Compression fractures are common, especially in elderly or osteoporotic patients. Some are stable and managed conservatively, but unstable fractures need surgical stabilization. Never assume "just muscle strain" after trauma—evaluate appropriately. Maintain spinal precautions until fracture ruled out.

Question 97: B - Sequential compression devices and/or pharmacologic prophylaxis

Explanation: VTE prophylaxis in trauma patients includes mechanical methods (sequential compression devices on legs) and/or pharmacologic prophylaxis (low-molecular-weight heparin or unfractionated heparin) when not contraindicated by bleeding risk. Start as soon as safe. Early mobilization also helps. Trauma patients have multiple VTE risk factors: immobility, vascular injury, hypercoagulability. Prophylaxis significantly reduces VTE incidence and associated mortality.

Question 98: B - CT scan with oral and IV contrast

Explanation: Hollow viscus injury suspicion warrants CT scan with IV contrast (shows enhancement patterns) and oral contrast when time/patient condition allows (helps identify bowel perforation). CT may show free air (perforation), free fluid without solid organ injury, bowel wall thickening, or mesenteric hematoma. However, many hollow viscus injuries show subtle findings initially—high clinical suspicion and serial exams remain crucial.

Question 99: B - Pituitary dysfunction from brain injury

Explanation: Diabetes insipidus (DI) after traumatic brain injury indicates posterior pituitary dysfunction (located in brain). DI causes massive dilute urine output (>200-300 mL/hr), hypernatremia, and increased serum osmolality. Treatment: desmopressin (DDAVP), fluid replacement matching output. DI can indicate severe brain injury and is common after significant head trauma. Monitor fluid/electrolyte balance closely.

Question 100: B - Sedation after ruling out hypoxia and pain

Explanation: Agitation in intubated patients requires assessment before sedation: Is patient hypoxic? (Check ventilator, suction if needed). In pain? (Treat pain first). Adequately sedated? (May need sedation adjustment). Fighting ventilator appropriately? (Ventilator settings may need adjustment). Never sedate without assessment—hypoxia and pain cause agitation and must be addressed. After ruling out physiologic causes, appropriate sedation improves comfort and ventilator synchrony.

Question 101: B - Immediate surgical exploration

Explanation: Penetrating neck injuries (especially Zone II) with hard signs (expanding hematoma, active bleeding, airway compromise, shock, bruit/thrill) require immediate surgical exploration without delay for imaging. These indicate vascular injury, aerodigestive injury, or both—life-threatening conditions needing operative control. Soft signs warrant imaging (CT angiography) but hard signs mandate emergency surgery.

Question 102: B - Tube dislodgement, obstruction, or cardiac arrest

Explanation: End-tidal CO_2 suddenly dropping to zero indicates: endotracheal tube dislodged (no longer in trachea), tube obstructed (mucus plug, biting), or cardiac arrest (no pulmonary blood flow to carry CO_2). Immediately assess: Is patient being ventilated? (Check chest rise, breath sounds). Is tube in correct position? Patient's pulse/perfusion status? This is an emergency requiring immediate intervention—check tube position, assess patient, be prepared for airway re-establishment.

Question 103: B - Acute hypoxemia and bilateral infiltrates during transfusion

Explanation: Transfusion-related acute lung injury (TRALI) presents with acute respiratory distress, hypoxemia, and bilateral pulmonary infiltrates during or within 6 hours of transfusion, without evidence of volume overload. Caused by antibodies in donor plasma reacting with recipient white cells. Treatment: stop transfusion, supportive care with oxygen/ventilation, diuretics generally not helpful (not volume overload). Most cases resolve with supportive care.

Question 104: B - Sitting upright or lateral to prevent aspiration

Explanation: Maxillofacial trauma patients with bleeding should sit upright or be positioned laterally to prevent aspiration of blood into airway. Never position supine—blood runs down throat causing airway obstruction and aspiration. Allow blood to drain forward. Suction carefully to prevent triggering gag/vomiting. Monitor airway closely—facial trauma can cause airway compromise from swelling, bleeding, or structural damage.

Question 105: B - Inadequate perfusion or acute kidney injury

Explanation: Oliguria (<0.5 mL/kg/hr) despite adequate resuscitation suggests either continued inadequate perfusion (need more resuscitation) or acute kidney injury developing. Assess: Fluid status adequate? Blood pressure adequate for renal perfusion? Catheter functioning? Urethral/bladder injury? Monitor creatinine, electrolytes. Treatment depends on cause: more fluids if underperfused, address AKI if developing, manage complications.

Question 106: B - Airway obstruction or inadequate ventilation

Explanation: Hypoxia in trauma patients most commonly results from airway obstruction (tongue, blood, foreign body, swelling) or inadequate ventilation (rib fractures causing splinting, hemopneumothorax, flail chest, decreased consciousness). Address airway first (jaw thrust, suction, airway adjuncts, intubation if needed), then breathing (supplemental oxygen, assisted ventilation, chest decompression if needed). Circulation problems cause hypoperfusion but airway/breathing issues cause hypoxia.

Question 107: B - Warming interventions (warm fluids, warming devices, warm room)

Explanation: Hypothermic trauma patients need active rewarming: Warm IV fluids (fluid warmers), forced-air warming devices (Bair Hugger), warm room temperature, warm blood products, possibly warmed humidified oxygen. Remove wet clothing. Core rewarming for severe hypothermia. Never give cold fluids or apply ice—worsens hypothermia. Maintaining temperature >35°C (95°F) is critical for clotting function and overall outcomes.

Question 108: B - Retrograde urethrogram

Explanation: Blood at urethral meatus with pelvic fracture indicates urethral injury. Never attempt Foley catheter—could worsen injury or create false passage. Retrograde urethrogram is diagnostic test: inject contrast through urethra under fluoroscopy, looking for extravasation. If urethral injury confirmed, place suprapubic catheter for bladder drainage. Cystoscopy can be done after diagnosis but urethrogram is initial diagnostic test.

Question 109: B - Immobilization, supportive care, antivenom if indicated

Explanation: Snake bite management: Immobilize affected extremity below heart level, remove jewelry (swelling will occur), transport to hospital, supportive care (IV access, monitoring), antivenom for significant envenomations (pit vipers, coral snakes). Don't: apply tourniquet (worsens ischemia), apply ice (worsens tissue damage), cut and suck (ineffective, causes more tissue damage), use heat. Mark swelling extent with time-stamped marks to track progression.

Question 110: B - Severe multi-system trauma 75 miles from Level I center

Explanation: Helicopter transport appropriate for: Time-critical patients (severe trauma, TBI, burns) when distance is 50-150 miles from appropriate facility and time savings would significantly impact outcome, difficult ground access, or when ground transport time exceeds air transport time significantly. Short distances use ground. Very long distances may use fixed-wing. Minor injuries don't justify helicopter cost/risk.

Question 111: B - Retrobulbar hemorrhage or globe injury requiring urgent evaluation

Explanation: Sudden vision loss after facial trauma indicates serious orbital/ocular injury: retrobulbar hemorrhage (bleeding behind eye compressing optic nerve—requires lateral canthotomy for decompression), globe rupture, retinal detachment, or optic nerve injury. This is an ophthalmologic emergency. Assess: visual acuity, pupil reactivity, eye movements, globe integrity. Immediate ophthalmology consultation. Protect eye with shield (no pressure).

Question 112: B - Stabilizing object, protecting eye, immediate ophthalmology consultation

Explanation: Impaled objects in eye: NEVER remove (may be tamponading bleeding or preventing further vitreous loss), stabilize object to prevent movement, protect with rigid shield (cup, cone) without applying pressure to globe, cover uninjured eye (reduces consensual eye movement), keep patient NPO, give analgesia, immediate ophthalmology consultation. Object removed only in OR under controlled conditions.

Question 113: B - Chest re-expansion, drainage, improved oxygenation

Explanation: Successful chest tube placement is indicated by: lung re-expansion on chest X-ray, drainage of blood/air, improved oxygenation and respiratory status, resolution of respiratory distress, and tidaling (fluid level fluctuation with breathing) in water seal chamber. No drainage doesn't mean unsuccessful—may not be blood/air present. Continued distress or worsening suggests either tube malposition or additional problem.

Question 114: B - Racemic epinephrine and preparation for reintubation

Explanation: Stridor immediately post-extubation indicates laryngeal edema causing upper airway obstruction—serious complication. Immediate treatment: Racemic epinephrine nebulizer (reduces airway edema), elevate head of bed, supplemental oxygen, monitor closely, have reintubation equipment ready. If stridor worsens or respiratory distress develops, reintubate. Never discharge patient with post-extubation stridor—this can progress to complete obstruction.

Question 115: B - Sacrum and heels

Explanation: Most common pressure injury sites in immobilized trauma patients: sacrum (if supine), heels (constant pressure), occiput (back of head in some patients), and shoulder blades. These bony prominences bear weight when patient lies still. Prevention: turn every 2 hours minimum, pressure redistribution surfaces, heel protectors, keep skin clean/dry, optimize nutrition, mobilize early when possible.

Question 116: B - Removing catheter as soon as not needed

Explanation: CAUTI (catheter-associated urinary tract infection) prevention: Remove catheter as soon as clinically unnecessary (daily assessment of need), use aseptic insertion technique, maintain closed drainage system, keep bag below bladder level, secure catheter to prevent urethral trauma, perform hand hygiene before/after manipulation, catheter care per protocol. Leaving catheters in longer than needed dramatically increases infection risk.

Question 117: B - Copious water irrigation after removing contaminated clothing

Explanation: Chemical burn management: Remove patient from source, remove all contaminated clothing (chemicals continue burning), copious water irrigation (20+ minutes) for most chemicals, protect staff with appropriate PPE. Don't apply neutralizing agents (exothermic reactions can worsen injury). Exceptions: Dry chemicals should be brushed off before water (some react with water). Specific chemicals (hydrofluoric acid, white phosphorus) need specialized treatment.

Question 118: B - Needle decompression in higher intercostal space due to elevated diaphragm

Explanation: Pregnancy after 20 weeks elevates diaphragm, raising position of abdominal contents and lungs. Tension pneumothorax in pregnant patients may need needle decompression in higher intercostal space (3rd-4th rather than 2nd) to reach pleural space above elevated diaphragm. Otherwise treat same as non-pregnant patients. Consider fetal monitoring if viable gestational age. Delivery isn't required for pneumothorax treatment.

Question 119: B - Strong pulses, alert mental status, adequate urine output

Explanation: Adequate perfusion indicators: Strong pulses, normal capillary refill (<2 seconds), alert and oriented mental status, urine output 0.5-1 mL/kg/hr, warm extremities, normal skin color, lactate <2 mmol/L. These signs indicate blood is reaching tissues and organs effectively. Weak pulses, confusion, hypotension, and cool extremities all indicate inadequate perfusion requiring intervention.

Question 120: B - Assessing decision-making capacity and respecting informed refusal if patient competent

Explanation: Competent adult patients have right to refuse treatment even if life-threatening. Assess decision-making capacity: Does patient understand condition, treatment options, and consequences of refusal? Not influenced by temporary factors (intoxication, medications)? If competent, document thorough discussion, ensure informed refusal, offer alternatives, involve family if patient consents. Don't force treatment on competent adults. If capacity questionable, involve ethics committee.

Question 121: B - Temporary hemorrhage control and correction of lethal triad

Explanation: Damage control resuscitation focuses on rapidly controlling hemorrhage, contamination control, and correcting lethal triad (hypothermia, acidosis, coagulopathy) in physiologically unstable patients. Definitive repairs are delayed until patient warmed, resuscitated, and coagulopathy corrected. Patient returns to OR 24-72 hours later for definitive reconstruction. Goal: survival, not perfect repair initially. This staged approach improves outcomes in severely injured patients.

Question 122: B - Fever, nuchal rigidity, altered mental status

Explanation: Meningitis in trauma patients (especially with basilar skull fracture or penetrating head trauma) presents with classic triad: fever, nuchal rigidity (stiff neck), and altered mental status. May also have headache, photophobia, positive Kernig/Brudzinski signs. Diagnosis: lumbar puncture (if no contraindications). Treatment: immediate empiric antibiotics, then adjust based on cultures. High mortality if untreated. Preventive antibiotics controversial for basilar skull fractures.

Question 123: B - Eye shield without pressure, NPO, immediate ophthalmology consultation

Explanation: Ruptured globe (full-thickness eye wall injury) management: Apply rigid eye shield without applying pressure (no patch—pressure worsens injury), cover both eyes (reduces consensual movement), keep NPO (will need surgery), give analgesia, antiemetics (prevent vomiting which increases intraocular pressure), immediate ophthalmology consultation, IV antibiotics, tetanus prophylaxis. Never apply pressure, instill medications, or manipulate the eye.

Question 124: B - Stroke or intracranial hemorrhage requiring immediate imaging

Explanation: Acute onset focal neurological deficits (facial droop, slurred speech, weakness) after head trauma indicate stroke from traumatic vascular injury or expanding intracranial hemorrhage. This requires immediate CT scan, neurosurgery consultation, and possible intervention (evacuation of hematoma, vascular repair). Time is critical—rapid diagnosis and treatment improve outcomes. Never assume "just confused" when focal neuro deficits present.

Question 125: B - Time to appropriate definitive care

Explanation: The single most important factor in trauma outcomes is minimizing time from injury to appropriate definitive care. This means: Rapid field triage to appropriate facility, efficient prehospital transport, immediate assessment and resuscitation, timely operative intervention when needed, and early intensive care. Organized trauma systems reduce mortality by ensuring patients reach right resources quickly. Hospital size, insurance, and day of week matter far less than timely appropriate care.

Interpreting Your Results - Practice Exam 2

Comparing Exam 1 and Exam 2:

If you took both practice exams, comparing your scores reveals important insights about your preparation:

Improved Score: Excellent! Your study efforts are working. You're retaining information and applying it more effectively. Continue your current study approach while addressing remaining weak areas.

Similar Score: Consistency is good—you're maintaining your knowledge level. If both scores are strong (85%+), you're ready. If both need improvement, intensify your study in weak areas identified by both exams.

Decreased Score: Don't panic. Different question emphasis or test-day factors may have affected performance. Review both exams' missed questions to identify patterns. Fatigue, rushing, or specific content gaps may explain the difference. Adjust your study approach based on what you learn.

Content Area Analysis:

Look for patterns across both exams:

- Consistently strong areas: Your strengths—maintain with light review
- Consistently weak areas: Priority for intensive study
- Strong on one exam, weak on other: Review those concepts more deeply

Question Type Patterns:

Are you missing:

- Priority questions? Review primary survey and ABCDE
- Application questions? Focus on understanding "why," not just memorizing facts
- Specific content (neuro, ortho, systems)? Deep dive into those chapters

Next Steps Based on Your Total Score:

106-125 (85-100%): You're demonstrating exam readiness. Fine-tune weak areas, review test-taking strategies, schedule your exam with confidence. Focus remaining study on highest-yield topics and maintaining knowledge.

94-105 (75-84%): Solid foundation with room for improvement. Target your weak areas intensively, practice more questions, review missed concepts thoroughly. You're close to consistent passing performance—focused effort will get you there.

81-93 (65-74%): Meaningful progress but needs more preparation. Review core chapters for weak areas, practice questions extensively, ensure you understand concepts not just memorize. Don't rush to schedule exam—invest time in thorough preparation.

Below 81 (<65%): Comprehensive review needed. Systematically work through content chapters, actively engage with material (teach concepts aloud, make connections), practice questions daily, consider additional resources or study support. Success requires dedicated preparation time.

General Recommendations:

Within 2 weeks of exam:

- Complete any remaining content review
- Practice test-taking strategies
- Review high-yield topics daily
- Maintain confidence—you're prepared

2-4 weeks from exam:

- Intensive review of weak areas
- Daily practice questions
- Review all missed questions from both exams
- Create summary notes for quick review

More than 4 weeks from exam:

- Systematic content review
- Build understanding progressively
- Regular practice questions
- Track improvement over time

Remember:

- These practice exams predict readiness but aren't perfect predictors
- Exam day performance includes knowledge, strategies, and composure
- Every nurse who's earned TCRN certification studied, practiced, and persevered
- Your dedication to preparation positions you for success

Final Encouragement

You've completed two full-length practice exams—a significant accomplishment that demonstrates your commitment to TCRN certification. Whether your scores show readiness or areas needing work, you've gained valuable insights about your preparation.

Key Insights from Your Practice:

These exams revealed your strengths and identified specific areas needing attention. This information is invaluable—it tells you exactly where to focus your remaining study time. Rather than studying everything equally, you can now target your efforts where they'll make the most difference.

Understanding Your Journey:

Every certified trauma nurse once stood where you are now—preparing, practicing, sometimes frustrated, but committed to excellence. The difference between those who succeed and those who don't isn't innate ability—it's persistence, strategic preparation, and refusing to give up when challenged.

What Success Looks Like:

Success isn't scoring perfectly on every practice question. Success is:

Understanding why you missed questions and learning from them

Seeing improvement between practice exams

Building confidence in your trauma nursing knowledge

Developing test-taking strategies that work for you

Maintaining persistence even when preparation feels difficult

Your Path Forward:

Based on your performance across both practice exams, you now have a clear roadmap:

Review all missed questions from both exams—these are your most valuable learning tools

Identify patterns in what you're missing—content areas, question types, reasoning errors

Create a focused study plan targeting your specific weak areas

Practice consistently rather than cramming—daily engagement beats marathon sessions

Believe in your preparation—you're investing significant effort in this goal

The Reality of Exam Preparation:

Preparing for TCRN certification is challenging. That's by design—the certification means something because it requires demonstrable expertise. Feeling challenged during preparation doesn't mean you're failing. It means you're pushing yourself to grow, which is exactly what this process requires.

Some days, studying will feel productive and concepts will click. Other days, you'll struggle with material that seemed clear before. This is normal. Learning isn't linear—it includes advances, plateaus, and occasional setbacks. What matters is consistent forward movement over time.

Building Confidence:

Confidence comes from preparation. Each practice question you answer, each concept you master, each clinical scenario you reason through builds the foundation for exam-day confidence. You're not hoping to remember information on exam day—you're building understanding that allows you to reason through any question.

When exam day arrives, you'll draw on hundreds of hours of study, thousands of practice questions, and all the clinical experience you bring as a trauma nurse. That preparation is your foundation. Trust it.

Practical Final Steps:

As you approach your exam date:

2-3 weeks before:

- Complete final content review of weak areas
- Practice questions daily (50-100 questions)
- Review both practice exams' explanations
- Simulate test conditions with timed practice

1 week before:

- Light review only—no new content
- Focus on high-yield topics and test-taking strategies
- Maintain normal sleep schedule
- Exercise and manage stress
- Trust your preparation

Day before:

- Minimal studying (review one page of key concepts at most)
- Prepare everything for test day (ID, confirmation, directions)
- Do something relaxing
- Get adequate sleep

Exam day:

- Eat a good breakfast
- Arrive early
- Trust your preparation
- Read each question completely
- Remember: You're prepared for this

A Final Word:

The TCRN certification validates your expertise in trauma nursing. It demonstrates to employers, colleagues, and patients that you've met rigorous standards in this specialized field. More importantly, it represents your commitment to providing the highest quality trauma care.

This certification journey—the studying, the practice exams, the moments of frustration and triumph—is developing you into a more knowledgeable, confident trauma nurse. The learning doesn't end with the exam, but the certification opens doors and validates the expertise you've worked hard to build.

You've invested significant time and effort in this preparation. You've completed comprehensive content review, answered hundreds of practice questions, and worked through complex clinical scenarios. That investment positions you for success.

Believe in your preparation. Trust your clinical judgment. Approach the exam with confidence. You're ready to demonstrate your trauma nursing expertise.

The journey to TCRN certification is challenging, but you've done the work. Now it's time to show what you know.

You've got this. Go earn your certification.

Best wishes for your success,

The Nedrial TestPrep Team

Made in the USA
Monee, IL
05 November 2026

67985673R10306